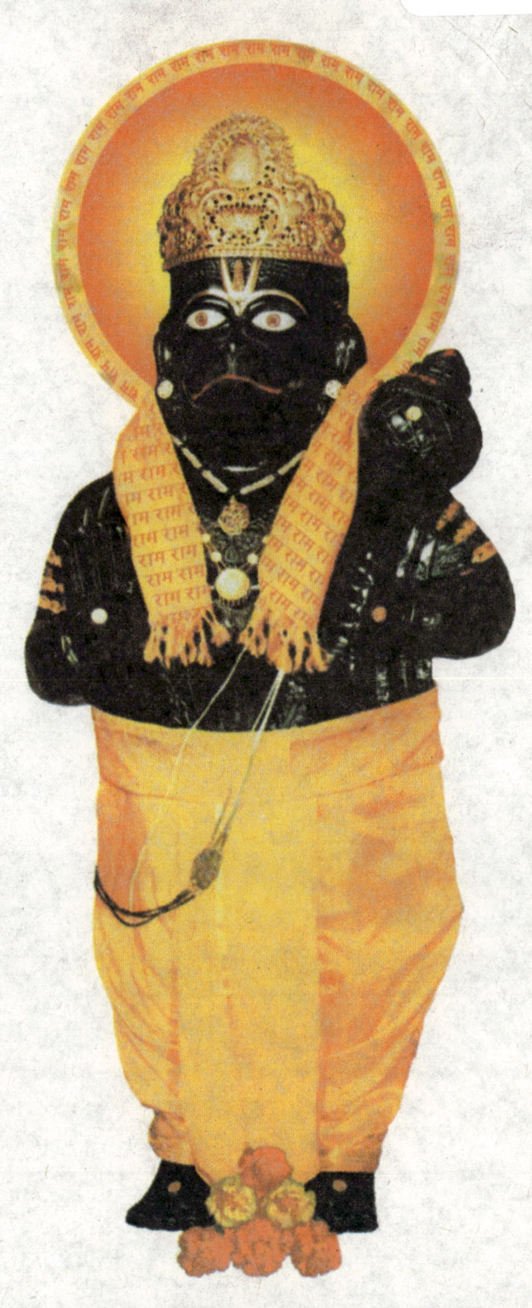

तेरा तुझको अर्पण

PREFACE

The second edition of *"A Question Bank in Life Sciences"* is based on the new examination scheme of CSIR initiated in June 2011. This new edition of the book is divided into 12 chapters according to the syllabus of CSIR. Each of the chapters contains two parts: Part B and Part C. Questions of part B are concept and fact based. These questions test the conceptual and factual knowledge of students and provide them with recent information regarding the topics. The questions of part C are of analytical type which requires in-depth knowledge and scientific approach to solve them. Since there is no standard question bank available in the market that fulfills the requirements of the students and judges their approach to study, I am most certain that my endeavors would achieve the results intended in terms of assessment and evaluation.

As the saying goes the more you sweat in training the less you bleed in War. Most students believe that the more questions they solve for practice before the examination the better. However this school of thought can backfire if precious time is wasted on substandard questions. Students in the practice phase of their preparation should emphasis on solving standard questions. Keeping this in mind, the below standard questions have been done away with in the final manuscript.

Many people have helped me in the regeneration of the book. I would like to reach out in upmost gratitude to Mr. Ram Chandra Suthar from Rampura urf Ramsara,Hanuman Garh, Rajasthan, who provided me with many standard questions on animal systems, Mr. Shatrujeet Pandey who kept reminding me to write the contents according to new examination pattern of CSIR, Dr. Shailesh Shrivastava of Shia PG College, Mr. P. K. Singh, Ankur Srivastav, my niece Sonali and Gaurav Singh for their support.

Rajveer Singh Chauhan

16 February 2012

CONTRIBUTORS

Ravi Shanker Yadav, a postgraduate in Biotechnology who has qualified CSIR-UGC NET with JRF. He is currently pursuing research in IITR, Lucknow on Colon cancer. The topics of his interest are Cancer Biology and Functional Genomics. His contributions in the chapters Cell Biology, Molecular Biology, Animal Physiology and Genetics are worth mentioning.

Abhishek Jauhari has a post graduate degree in Biotechnology. He joined the IITR, Lucknow after qualifying CSIR-UGC NET with JRF. He is working on the role of microRNA in neurodifferentiation and neurodegeneration. The topics of his interest are Instrumentation Biology, Immunology and Gene regulation. He has contributed in the chapters Developmental Biology, Immunology, Life forms and Applied Biology and Biological Techniques in the book.

Ruby Singh earned her M. Sc. in Zoology from CSJM University, Kanpur. The topic of her interest is Cell Physiology. She has contributed in chapters Cell Biology, Animal Physiology and Evolution & Behaviour in the book.

CONTENTS

Host parasite interaction Recognition and entry processes of different pathogens like bacteria, viruses into animal and plant host cells, alteration of host cell behavior by pathogens, virus-induced cell transformation, pathogen-induced diseases in animals and plants, cell-cell fusion in both normal and abnormal cells.

Cell signaling Hormones and their receptors, cell surface receptor, signaling through G-protein coupled receptors, signal transduction pathways, second messengers, regulation of signaling pathways, bacterial and plant two- component systems, light signaling in plants, bacterial chemotaxis and quorum sensing.

Cellular communication Regulation of hematopoiesis, general principles of cell communication, cell adhesion and roles of different adhesion molecules, gap junctions, extracellular matrix, integrins, neurotransmission and its regulation.

Cancer Genetic rearrangements in progenitor cells, oncogenes, tumor suppressor genes, cancer and the cell cycle, virus-induced cancer, metastasis, interaction of cancer cells with normal cells, apoptosis, therapeutic interventions of uncontrolled cell growth. Programmed cell death, aging and senescence

3. MOLECULAR BIOLOGY 99

DNA replication, repair and recombination (Unit of replication, enzymes involved, replication origin and replication fork, fidelity of replication, extrachromosomal replicons, DNA damage and repair mechanisms, homologous and site-specific recombination). Conformation of nucleic acids (helix (A, B, Z), t-RNA, micro-RNA). Stability of proteins and nucleic acids.

RNA synthesis and processing (transcription factors and machinery, formation of initiation complex, transcription activator and repressor, RNA polymerases, capping, elongation, and termination, RNA processing, RNA editing, splicing, and polyadenylation, structure and function of different types of RNA, RNA transport).

Protein synthesis and processing (Ribosome, formation of initiation complex, initiation factors and their regulation, elongation and elongation factors, termination, genetic code, aminoacylation of tRNA, tRNA-identity, aminoacyl tRNA synthetase, and translational proof-reading, translational inhibitors, Post-translational modification of proteins).

Respiratory system - Comparison of respiration in different species, anatomical considerations, transport of gases, exchange of gases, waste elimination, neural and chemical regulation of respiration.

Nervous system - Neurons, action potential, gross neuroanatomy of the brain and spinal cord, central and peripheral nervous system, neural control of muscle tone and posture.

Sense organs - Vision, hearing and tactile response.

Excretory system - Comparative physiology of excretion, kidney, urine formation, urine concentration, waste elimination, micturition, regulation of water balance, blood volume, blood pressure, electrolyte balance, acid-base balance.

Thermoregulation - Comfort zone, body temperature – physical, chemical, neural regulation, acclimatization.

Stress and adaptation

Digestive system - Digestion, absorption, energy balance, BMR.

Endocrinology and reproduction - Endocrine glands, basic mechanism of hormone action, hormones and diseases; reproductive processes, gametogenesis, ovulation, neuroendocrine regulation

Mendelian principles : Dominance, segregation, independent assortment.

Concept of gene : Allele, multiple alleles, pseudoallele, complementation tests

Extensions of Mendelian principles : Codominance, incomplete dominance, gene interactions, pleiotropy, genomic imprinting, penetrance and expressivity, phenocopy, linkage and crossing over, sex linkage, sex limited and sex influenced characters.

Gene mapping methods : Linkage maps, tetrad analysis, mapping with molecular markers, mapping by using somatic cell hybrids, development of mapping population in plants.

Extra chromosomal inheritance : Inheritance of Mitochondrial and chloroplast genes, maternal inheritance.

Microbial genetics : Methods of genetic transfers – transformation, conjugation, transduction and sex-duction, mapping genes by interrupted mating, fine structure analysis of genes.

Human genetics : Pedigree analysis, lod score for linkage testing, karyotypes, genetic disorders.

Quantitative genetics : Polygenic inheritance, heritability and its measurements, QTL mapping.

Mutation : Types, causes and detection, mutant types – lethal, conditional, biochemical, loss of function, gain of function, germinal verses somatic mutants, insertional mutagenesis.

Structural and numerical alterations of chromosomes : Deletion, duplication, inversion, translocation, ploidy and their genetic implications.

Recombination : Homologous and non-homologous recombination including transposition.

9. ECOLOGICAL PRINCIPLES 303

The Environment: Physical environment; biotic environment; biotic and abiotic interactions.

Habitat and Niche: Concept of habitat and niche; niche width and overlap; fundamental and realized niche; resource partitioning; character displacement.

Population Ecology: Characteristics of a population; population growth curves; population regulation; life history strategies (*r* and *K* selection); concept of metapopulation – demes and dispersal, interdemic extinctions, age structured populations.

Species Interactions: Types of interactions, interspecific competition, herbivory, carnivory, pollination, symbiosis.

Community Ecology: Nature of communities; community structure and attributes; levels of species diversity and its measurement; edges and ecotones.

Ecological Succession: Types; mechanisms; changes involved in succession; concept of climax.

Ecosystem Ecology: Ecosystem structure; ecosystem function; energy flow and mineral cycling (C,N,P); primary production and decomposition; structure and function of some Indian ecosystems: terrestrial (forest, grassland) and aquatic (fresh water, marine, eustarine).

Biogeography: Major terrestrial biomes; theory of island biogeography; biogeographical zones of India.

Applied Ecology: Environmental pollution; global environmental change; biodiversity: status, monitoring and documentation; major drivers of biodiversity change; biodiversity management approaches.

Conservation Biology: Principles of conservation, major approaches to management, Indian case studies on conservation/management strategy (Project Tiger, Biosphere reserves).

Emergence of evolutionary thoughts: Lamarck; Darwin–concepts of variation, adaptation, struggle, fitness and natural selection; Mendelism; Spontaneity of mutations; The evolutionary synthesis.

Origin of cells and unicellular evolution: Origin of basic biological molecules; Abiotic synthesis of organic monomers and polymers; Concept of Oparin and Haldane; Experiement of Miller (1953); The first cell; Evolution of prokaryotes; Origin of eukaryotic cells; Evolution of unicellular eukaryotes; Anaerobic metabolism, photosynthesis and aerobic metabolism.

Paleontology and Evolutionary History: The evolutionary time scale; Eras, periods and epoch; Major events in the evolutionary time scale; Origins of unicellular and multi cellular organisms; Major groups of plants and animals; Stages in primate evolution including Homo.

Molecular Evolution: Concepts of neutral evolution, molecular divergence and molecular clocks; Molecular tools in phylogeny, classification and identification; Protein and nucleotide sequence analysis; origin of new genes and proteins; Gene duplication and divergence.

The Mechanisms: Population genetics – Populations, Gene pool, Gene frequency; Hardy-Weinberg Law; concepts and rate of change in gene frequency through natural selection, migration and random genetic drift; Adaptive radiation; Isolating mechanisms; Speciation; Allopatricity and Sympatricity; Convergent evolution; Sexual selection; Co-evolution.

Brain, Behavior and Evolution: Approaches and methods in study of behavior; Proximate and ultimate causation; Altruism and evolution-Group selection, Kin selection, Reciprocal altruism; Neural basis of learning, memory, cognition, sleep and arousal; Biological clocks; Development of behavior; Social communication; Social dominance; Use of space and territoriality; Mating systems,

Parental investment and Reproductive success; Parental care; Aggressive behavior; Habitat selection and optimality in foraging; Migration, orientation and navigation; Domestication and behavioral changes.

11. LIFE FORMS & APPLIED BIOLOGY 403

Principles & methods of taxonomy: Concepts of species and hierarchical taxa, biological nomenclature, classical & quantititative methods of taxonomy of plants, animals and microorganisms.

Levels of structural organization: Unicellular, colonial and multicellular forms. Levels of organization of tissues, organs & systems. Comparative anatomy, adaptive radiation, adaptive modifications.

Outline classification of plants, animals & microorganisms: Important criteria used for classification in each taxon. Classification of plants, animals and microorganisms. Evolutionary relationships among taxa.

Natural history of Indian subcontinent: Major habitat types of the subcontinent, geographic origins and migrations of species. Comman Indian mammals, birds. Seasonality and phenology of the subcontinent.

Organisms of health & agricultural importance: Common parasites and pathogens of humans, domestic animals and crops.

Organisms of conservation concern: Rare, endangered species. Conservation strategies.

Microbial fermentation and production of small and macro molecules.

Application of immunological principles, vaccines, diagnostics. Tissue and cell culture methods for plants and animals.

Transgenic animals and plants, molecular approaches to diagnosis and strain identification.

Genomics and its application to health and agriculture, including gene therapy.

Bioresource and uses of biodiversity.

Breeding in plants and animals, including marker – assisted selection

Bioremediation and phytoremediation

Biosensors

12. BIOLOGICAL TECHNIQUES 425

Molecular Biology and Recombinant DNA methods: Isolation and purification of RNA , DNA (genomic and plasmid) and proteins, different separation methods.

Analysis of RNA, DNA and proteins by one and two dimensional gel electrophoresis, Isoelectric focusing gels.

Molecular cloning of DNA or RNA fragments in bacterial and eukaryotic systems.

Expression of recombinant proteins using bacterial, animal and plant vectors.

Isolation of specific nucleic acid sequences

Generation of genomic and cDNA libraries in plasmid, phage, cosmid, BAC and YAC vectors.

In vitro mutagenesis and deletion techniques, gene knock out in bacterial and eukaryotic organisms.

Protein sequencing methods, detection of post translation modification of proteins.

DNA sequencing methods, strategies for genome sequencing.

Methods for analysis of gene expression at RNA and protein level, large scale expression, such as micro array based techniques

Isolation, separation and analysis of carbohydrate and lipid molecules RFLP, RAPD and AFLP techniques

Histochemical and Immunotechniques: Antibody generation, Detection of molecules using ELISA, RIA, western blot, immunoprecipitation, fluocytometry and immunofluorescence microscopy, detection of molecules in living cells, in situ localization by techniques such as FISH and GISH.

Biophysical Method: Molecular analysis using UV/visible, fluorescence, circular dichroism, NMR and ESR spectroscopy Molecular structure determination using X-ray diffraction and NMR, Molecular analysis using light scattering, different types of mass spectrometry and surface plasma resonance methods.

Statisitcal Methods: Measures of central tendency and dispersal; probability distributions (Binomial, Poisson and normal); Sampling distribution; Difference between parametric and non-parametric statistics; Confidence Interval; Errors; Levels of significance;

Regression and Correlation; t-test; Analysis of variance; X^2 test;; Basic introduction to Muetrovariate statistics, etc.

Radiolabeling techniques: Detection and measurement of different types of radioisotopes normally used in biology, incorporation of radioisotopes in biological tissues and cells, molecular imaging of radioactive material, safety guidelines.

Microscopic techniques: Visulization of cells and subcellular components by light microscopy, resolving

powers of different microscopes, microscopy of living cells, scanning and transmission microscopes, different fixation and staining techniques for EM, freeze-etch and freeze-fracture methods for EM, image processing methods in microscopy.

Electrophysiological methods: Single neuron recording, patch-clamp recording, ECG, Brain activity recording, lesion and stimulation of brain, pharmacological testing, PET, MRI, fMRI, CAT.

Methods in field biology: Methods of estimating population density of animals and plants, ranging patternsthrough direct, indirect and remote observations, sampling methods in the study of behavior, habitat characterization: ground and remote sensing methods.

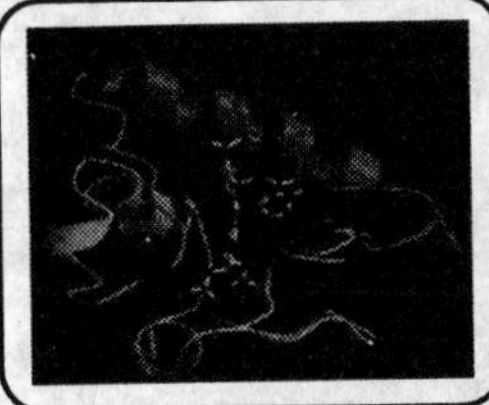

Chapter 1 Biochemistry

Part B

1. A polypeptide having 15 amino acid residues can form any of the
   a) 15 amino acid sequences b) 15^{20} amino acid sequences
   c) 20^{15} amino acid sequences d) 20x15 amino acid sequences

2. Agar - agar is the polymer of
   a) Glucose b) Fructose
   c) Xylose d) Galactose

3. Alcohol is used as disinfectant because it can destroy the surrounding bacteria by breaking
   a) Ionic bonds of bacterial proteins
   b) Hydrogen bonds of bacterial proteins
   c) Vander Waals forces of bacterial proteins
   d) Hydrophobic and disulphide bonds of bacterial proteins

4. Anomeric carbon is not found in
   a) Glucose b) Fructose
   c) Lactose d) Dihydroxyacetone

5. Arachidonic acid may be formed from dietary
   a) Oleic acid b) Linoleic acid
   c) Linolenic acid d) Palmitoleic acid

6. Blood group deciding antigens are :
   a) Glycoproteins b) Glycolipids
   c) Phospholipids d) Peripheral proteins

7. β-1, 4 glycosidic linkage is not found in
   a) Chitin b) Lactose
   c) Cellulose d) Sucrose

8. α-helix is stabilized through
   a) Hydrophobic interactions b) Ionic bonds
   c) Hydrogen bonds d) All of the above

9. Chitin is found in the exoskeleton of
   a) Annelids b) Insects
   c) Echinoderms d) Bryozoans

10. Chitin occurs in cell wall of fungus. It is polymer of
   a) Glucose b) Sucrose
   c) Amino sugars d) Galactose

11. Cooperativity effect in proteins is the result of
   a) Super secondary structure of proteins
   b) Secondary structure of proteins
   c) Tertiary structure of proteins
   d) Quaternary structure of proteins

12. Disulfide bond formation in proteins takes place in
   a) Cytosol b) Smooth ER
   c) Rough ER d) Golgi complex

13. Disulphide bond can not be formed within cytosol becuase
   a) It lacks PDI
   b) It's environment is highly reducing due to presence of free radicals
   c) It's environment is highly reducing due to presence of glutathione
   d) Cytosolic proteins are more prone to destruction in the presence of disulphide bond

14. Hydrogen bonds are especially important for living organisms because
   a) They occur only inside of organisms
   b) They are very strong and maintain the physical stability of molecules
   c) They allow biological molecules to dissolve in water, which is the universal medium for living processes
   d) They are responsible for liquid phase of water

15. Hydrophobic interactions
   a) are stronger than covalent bonds.
   b) are stronger than hydrogen bonds.
   c) can hold two ions.
   d) can hold two non-polar molecules together.

16. Which statement about thermodynamics is true?
   a) Free energy is used up in an exergonic reaction.
   b) Free energy can not be used to do work, such as chemical transformations.
   c) Free energy can be kinetic but not potential energy.
   d) Entropy tends always to a maximum.

17. Intrachain hydrogen bonding in α-helix occurs between
a) 1 and 4 amino acid
b) 1 and 5 amino acid
c) 2 and 4 amino acid
d) 1 and 6 amino acid

18. Maltose is disaccharide of
a) Glucose + Galactose
b) Glucose + Sucrose
c) Glucose + Fructose
d) Glucose + Glucose

19. What is the most important factor in determining the native, 3-D structure of proteins?
a) The number of disulphide bonds
b) The sequence of amino acids in proteins
c) Interaction of the protein molecules with solvent
d) The origin of the protein

20. Secondary structures of proteins are stabilized by
a) Disulphide bonds
b) Hydrogen bonds between back bone atoms
c) Hydrogen bonds between R groups
d) Ionic Bonds and hydrogen bonds between R groups.

21. Which one of the following is the weakest bond found in proteins?
a) Hydrophobic bond
b) Ionic bond
c) Hydrogen bond
d) Disulphide bond

22. The imidazole groups are parts of the active sites of many enzymes. This group is found in
a) Proline
b) Glutamine
c) Histidine
d) Asparagine

23. The main force in membrane resealing of ruptured biomembrane in aqueous environment is
a) Ionic interactions between membrane lipids
b) Force between proteins and lipids
c) Covalent forces between membrane lipids
d) Hydrophobic forces between membrane lipids

24. Trehalose is found in the exoskeleton of insects, it is
a) Disaccharide
b) Trisaccharide
c) Polysaccharide
d) Oligosaccaride

25. Under what thermodynamic conditions will a reaction proceed spontaneously?
a) $\Delta H<0$
b) $\Delta G=0$
c) $\Delta S<0$
d) $\Delta S=0$

26. What is the maximum number of hydrogen bonds that can be formed by each molecule of water?
    a) 1 b) 2
    c) 4 d) 3
27. When the forces arise from the electrostatic attraction between the positively charged nucleus of one atom and the negatively charged electrons of the other it is called
    a) Ionic bonding b) Stacking force
    c) Hydrogen bonding d) Van der Waals force
28. Which of the following amino acid can easily be ionized at cellular pH?
    a) Arginine b) Lysine
    c) Histidine d) Tryptophan
29. Which of the following can not be obtained from plants
    a) Vitamin-D b) Vitamin-B12
    c) Folic acid d) Vitamin C

[CSIR (NET/JRF) Exam. June. 2002]

30. Which of the following interactions is responsible for curly hair?
    a) Hydrogen boding b) Hydrophobic interaction
    c) Disulphide bond d) Ionic bond
31. Which of the following is a non- reducing sugar
    a) Lactose b) Fructose
    c) Maltose d) Sucrose
32. Which of the following is not a group of amphipathic molecules in biological membranes?
    a) Phosphoglycerides b) Glycolipids
    c) Cholesterol d) None of the above
33. Which of the following is not found in myoglobin?
    a) Primary structure b) Secondary structure
    c) Tertiary structure d) Quaternary structure
34. Which of the following is not optically active biomolecule
    a) Glucose b) Proline
    c) Dihydroxy acetone d) None of the above
35. Which of the following is the constituent of fungal cell wall
    a) Cutin b) Chitin
    c) Cellulose d) Pectin
36. Which of the following is the energy-storage molecule in fruits and honey ?
    a) Glucose b) Sucrose
    c) Glycogen d) Fructose

37. Which of the following non-covalent interaction plays a pivotal role in protein folding?
a) Ionic interactions b) Hydrogen bonds
c) Vander waal forces d) Hydrophobic interactions

38. Which one of the following amino acid is never found in α-helix
a) Alanine b) Serine
c) Phenylalanine d) Proline

39. Which of the following protein is involved in the correct folding of proteins?
a) Ubiquitin b) Chaperon
c) SUMO d) Clathrin

40. Which of the following reagent can be used to detect tyrosine residue in the active site of an enzyme
a) Iodoacetamide b) Phenylglyoxal
c) Tetranitromethane d) Pyridoxal phosphate

41. Which of the following statement is correct?
a) Formation of disulphide bond is must to stabilize the native conformation of a protein
b) Detergents can be used to break ionic bonds
c) Reducing environment of the cytosol promotes formation of disulphide bonds in proteins.
d) Three dimensional structure of a protein is determined by its primary structure

42. Which of the following statements is correct for α-helix?
a) It is stabilized by hydrogen bonding between peptide bonds and side chain groups
b) Proline promotes formation of α-helix
c) Spider web contain α-helix
d) It is a secondary structure of proteins

43. Which of the following statement is correct?
a) Fatty acids found in glycerophospholipids of plasma membrane have trans-double bonds
b) Cholesterol is a storage lipid
c) Sphingoglycolopids are equally distributed in the inner and outer leaflets of plasma membrane
d) Length and saturation level of fatty acids play a pivotal role in determining the fluidity of biological membranes

44. Which of the following statements is not correct?
   a) We can not digest cellulose because of the absence of enzyme that hydrolyses β-1, 4-glycosidic bonds.
   b) Plants transport sugar in the form of sucrose.
   c) Animals store glucose in the form of glycogen because it can change osmolarity of cells according to need.
   d) Starch includes amylose and amylopectin.

45. Which of the following statements is not true for enzymes?
   a) They have no effect on thermodynamics of reaction
   b) They are not used in reaction
   c) They can change equilibrium of the reaction
   d) They decrease activation energy of the substrate

46. What biochemical is the immediate source of cytoplasmic acetyl-Co-A used in fatty acid biosynthesis?
   a) Malate
   b) Glucose
   c) Citrate
   d) Oxaloacetate

47. A bond may be 'high energy' for any of the following reasons except
   a) Products of its cleavage are more resonance stabilized than the original compound.
   b) The bond is usually stable, requiring a large energy input to cleave it.
   c) Electrostatic repulsion is relieved when the bond is cleaved.
   d) A cleavage product may be unstable, tautomerizing to a more stable form.

48. Abzymes are
   a) Enzymes that are highly specific like antibodies
   b) Antibodies that have catalytic activities
   c) Also referred to as zymogens
   d) Enzymes that hydrolyze antibodies

49. Although enzymic catalysis is reversible, a given reaction may appear irreversible
   a) If the products are thermodynamically far more stable than the reactants
   b) Under equilibrium conditions
   c) At high enzyme concentrations
   d) At high temperatures

50. Among the following which amino acid can act as buffer against addition of acid
   a) Glycine
   b) Histidine
   c) Arginine
   d) Phenylalanine

[CSIR (NET/JRF) Exam. Dec 2004]

51. An allosteric modulator influences enzyme's activity by
   a) Competing for the catalytic site with the substrate
   b) Binding to a site on the enzymes molecule distinct from the catalytic site
   c) Changing nature of the product formed
   d) Covalently modifying the enzyme
52. An enzyme inhibitor which decreases both Vmax and Km comes under
   a) Competitive inhibitor b) Mixed inhibitor
   c) Uncompetitive inhibitor d) Irreversible inhibitor
53. ATP is used as "energy currency" in cells because it
   a) Is high energy-compound
   b) Is kinetically stable and thermodynamically unstable
   c) Has "intermediate energy"
   d) All of the above
54. Which statement is true regarding the action of an enzyme?
   a) An enzyme usually binds the substrate more tightly than the transition state.
   b) An enzyme usually binds the product more tightly than the transition state.
   c) An enzyme stabilizes the transition state for the reaction more than the ES complex.
   d) An enzyme usually binds S and P with equal affinity.
55. Binding mode of enzymatic catalysis employ
   a) Acid-base catalysis
   b) Covalent catalysis
   c) Induced fit
   d) Proximity effect
56. Biological activity of X molecule was inactivated by heating at 65°C. The X molecule is
   a) Protein b) DNA
   c) Carbohydrate d) Lipid

[CSIR (NET/JRF) Exam. June- 2005]

57. Biotin is a cofactor of the enzyme
   a) Pyruvate carboxylase b) Superoxide dismutase
   c) Nitrate reductase d) Pyruvate dehydrogenase

58. Buttermilk is produced by inoculating milk with *Streptococcus lactis*, which causes curdling and coagulation of protein. This is due to
   a) Breakage of disulfide bond.
   b) Breakage of peptide bond.
   c) Disruption of hydrophobic interaction.
   d) Formation of lactic acid

59. Which statement is not true for allosteric enzymes?
   a) They often do not exhibit typical Michaelis-Menton kinetics
   b) They are often larger than other enzymes
   c) They can be regulated by allosteric regulators which irreversibly and covalently bind to these enzymes.
   d) They show cooperativity effect

60. Chaperon proteins help in
   a) Protein folding and assembly
   b) Protein stability
   c) Both of the above
   d) None of the above

61. Crocodiles can remain underwater without breathing for periods of over one hour. It is possible because
   a) They can survive anaerobically for a long time
   b) They have relatively changed primary structure of haemoglobin
   c) They can use dissolved oxygen of water
   d) Oxygen demand is very low in these organisms

62. Detergents can denature the proteins by disrupting
   a) Ionic bonds b) Hydrogen bonds
   c) Hydrophobic bonds d) Disulphide bond

63. During inhibition of enzyme action Vmax remains unchanged while Km is altered. The inhibition is
   a) Competitive b) Non-compettive
   c) Uncompetitive d) Allosteric

[CSIR (NET/JRF) Exam. June 2005]

64. EIS complex is formed in
   a) Non-competitive inhibition
   b) Uncompetitive inhibition
   c) Competitive inhibition
   d) Both (a) and (b)

65. Enzymes are called biocatalyst as it increases the rate of a reaction by
   a) Increasing the free energy of activation
   b) Increasing the free energy change of the reaction

c) Decreasing the energy of activation
d) Changing the equilibrium constant of the reaction

[CSIR (NET/JRF) Exam. Dec 2002]

66. False statement of competitive inhibition is
a) Structure same as substrate
b) Inhibits substrate binding
c) Binds to active site
d) Reaction can not be favorably biased by increasing substrate concentration

67. Fats are the most concentrated form of dietary energy because
a) In fats carbon atoms of fatty acids are more reduced than those of sugars
b) They are insoluble in water
c) They contain high energy bonds
d) They have high molecular weight

68. Fats give more energy than glucose because
a) They are highly reduced
b) They are hydrophobic
c) Their oxidation mainly occurs in mitochondria
d) All of these

69. Glycogen has
a) β-1, 4-linkage b) α-1, 6-linkage
c) α-1, 4 and α-1, 6-linkage d) α-1, 4-linkage

70. Which pair of amino acid will have the highest absorbance at 280 nm?
a) Thr and His b) Phe and Pro
c) Trp and Tyr d) Phe and His

71. Which of the following is the most abundant membrane lipid in biosphere?
a) Glycerophospholipid b) Sphingolipid
c) Galactolipid d) Glycolipid

72. If a reaction is at equilibrium, the free energy G change is
a) 1 b) 0.1
c) 10 d) 0

[CSIR (NET/JRF) Exam. Dec 2003]

73. In a chemical reaction
a) The rate depends on the value of ΔG
b) The rate depends on the activation energy
c) The rate activation energy depends on the value of ΔG
d) The change in free energy depends on the activation energy

74. In a polypeptide if alanine is replaced by proline then
    a) It tends to form α-helix increases
    b) It tends to form β-sheets increases
    c) The hydrophobicity of chain decreases
    d) There would be no effect

[CSIR (NET/JRF) Exam. June 2006]

75. In all enzymes the active site
    a) Contains the substrate binding site
    b) Contains a metal ion as a prosthetic group
    c) Contains the amino acid side chains involved in catalyzing the reaction.
    d) Is contiguous with the substrate binding site in the primary sequence.

76. In Michaelis-Menton model of enzymatic catalysis, the reaction velocity is independent of substrate concentration, when
    a) The concentration of substrate is very small
    b) The enzyme is fully saturated with substrate
    c) The active sites are unoccupied by substrate
    d) A competitive inhibitor is present.

[CSIR (NET/JRF) Exam. June 2006]

77. In the Line weaver - Burk plot which of the following is y intercept?
    a) $-1/K_m$ b) $1/V_{max}$
    c) K_m/V_{max} d) $1/V$

78. In the study of enzymes, a sigmoidal plot of substrate concentration ([S]) versus the reaction velocity [V] indicates
    a) Michaelis-Menton kinetics   b) Competitive inhibition
    c) Cooperative binding   d) Non-competitve inhibition

79. Inulin is polymer of
    a) Glucose   b) Fructose
    c) Galactose   d) Glucose and Fructose

80. Iodoacetamide irreversibly inhibits few enzymes by reacting with the amino acid residue at the active site having the functional group-
    a) -NH2   b) -OH
    c) -COOH   d) -SH

[CSIR (NET/JRF) Exam. Dec 2002]

81. K_m of an enzyme is
    a) One-half of the V_{max}
    b) Dissociation constant
    c) The normal physiological substrate concentration
    d) The substrate concentration that gives half maximal velocity

82. Left-handed α-helices are commonly not found in proteins because they are less stable. The reason behind it is that
   a) Amino acids found in proteins are L-amino acids
   b) Amino acids found in proteins are D-amino acids
   c) Left-handed α-helices are glycine and proline rich
   d) Left-handed α-helices are rich in disulphide bonds

83. Mehler reaction results in the production of
   a) Hydroxyl ion b) Hydroxyl free radical
   c) Superoxide d) Hydrogen peroxide

84. Mercaptoethanol can cleave reversibly
   a) Hydrophobic bonds in a protein
   b) Disulphide bonds in a protein
   c) Ionic bonds in a protein
   d) Hydrogen bonds in a protein

85. NMP Kinases can enhance the rate of reaction by
   a) Acid base catalysis b) Substrate strain
   c) Covalent catalysis d) Entropy effect

86. Osmotic potential in plant cell is maintained by
   a) Proline and glycine betaine b) Histidine
   c) Lysine d) Glycine

87. Pernicious anemia is caused by deficiency of
   a) Vitamin B_2 b) Vitamin B_{12}
   c) Vitamin B_6 d) Vitamin B_1

88. PLP acts as a coenzyme in which of the following
   a) Transamination reactions only.
   b) Transamination and decarboxylation reactions only
   c) Transamination, decarboxylation and racemization reactions.
   d) Transamination and racemization reactions only.

[CSIR (NET/JRF) Exam. Dec 2001]

89. Proteins showing cooperativity effect must have
   a) alpha helix
   b) low content of hydrophilic amino acids.
   c) high content of hydrophilic amino acids.
   d) quarternary structure

90. Pyridoxal phosphate is the prosthetic group for many enzymes that catalyze
   a) Carboxylation
   b) Acyl group transfer
   c) Alkylation
   d) Transamination

91. Replacement of alanine by proline in polypeptide would favour?
    a) Increase in a helical content
    b) Greater rigidity of polypeptide
    c) Increase in β-sheet structure
    d) Decrease in hydrophobisity of polypeptide

[CSIR (NET/JRF) Exam. June 2006]

92. Serine proteases catalyze a reaction by
    a) Substrate strain mechanism b) Covalent catalysis
    c) Proximity effect d) Transition state stabilization

93. Steady-state kinetics defines
    a) Where enzyme is present at very small molar concentration compared with substrate acted upon
    b) Where enzymes present at very high molar concentration compared with substrate acted upon
    c) Where enzyme and substrate is present at equimolar concentration
    d) None of the above

94. Suicide inhibitors are kept under
    a) Competitive inhibitors b) Uncompetitive inhibitors
    c) Non competitive inhibitors d) None of the above

95. The best definition of ATP is that it is
    a) A molecule stored for food use
    b) A molecule that supplies energy to do work
    c) A molecule stored for an energy reserve
    d) A molecule used as a source of phosphate

96. The best example of regulation of enzyme by reversible covalent modification is
    a) Acetylation b) Proteolytic cleavage
    c) Glycosylation d) Phosphorylation

97. The bonding which is responsible for holding two β-sheets together is
    a) Disulphide bond b) Covalent bond
    c) Hydrogen bond d) Hydrophobic interation

98. The catalytic efficiency of two different enzymes can be compared by the
    a) Km value b) Optimum pH value
    c) Formation of the product d) Molecular size of the enzyme

99. The coenzymes involved in transfer of carboxyl group is
    a) NADH b) Biotin
    c) S-Adenosyl methionine d) Coenzymes-A

[CSIR (NET/JRF) Exam. Dec 2001]

100. The degree of inhibition for non-competitive inhibition of an enzyme catalyzed reaction
   a) Increases with increase in substrate concentration
   b) Reaches a maximum with increase in substrate concentration and then decreases
   c) Decreases with increase in substrate concentration
   d) None of these

101. The difference between the energy levels of ground state and transition state is called
   a) Excitation energy b) Orbital energy
   c) Transition energy d) Activation energy

102. The double-reciprocal transformation of the Michaelis-Menton equation, also called the Lineweaver-Burk plot, is given by 1/Vo = Km/Vmax [S] + 1/Vmax. To determine Km from double reciprocal plot, you would-
   a) Take the X-axis intercept where V_0= Vmax
   b) Multiply the reciprocal of X-axis intercept by-1
   c) Take the reciprocal of the X-axis intercept
   d) Take the reciprocal of the Y-axis intercept

103. The entropy of reaction refers to
   a) The heat given off by the reaction
   b) The tendency of the system to move toward maximal randomness
   c) The energy of the transition state
   d) The effect of temperature on the rate of the reaction

104. The enzymes which catalyze the transfer of a functional group from one position to another in the same molecule are grouped under
   a) Enolase b) Mutase
   c) Transferase d) Lyase

105. The essential amino acids - phenylalanine, tyrosine and tryptophan can not be synthesized by animals because they lack
   a) Glycolytic pathway b) Shikimic acid pathway
   c) Aminotransferases d) Nitrogenase

106. The folded states of globular proteins found in aquous solution are stabilized by
   a) Formation of peptide bonds
   b) Formation of disulfide bonds
   c) Hydrophobic interactions
   d) Formation of ionic bonds

107. The intercept on the X-axis of Lineweaver-Burk plot is equal to
a) $1/V_{max}$ b) K_m
c) K_m/V_{max} d) $-1/K_m$

108. Hyaluronic acid is a component of vitrous humor of eye and of the lubricatng fluid of joints. It is a
a) Derivative of amino acid b) Oxidized sugar
c) Glycoconjugate d) Glycosaminoglycan

109. The maximum possible available energy of substance is termed as
a) Free energy b) Entropy
c) Enthalpy d) Chemical potential

110. The Michaelis-Menton hypothesis
a) Enables to calculate the isoelectric point of an enzyme
b) Postulate that all enzymes are proteins
c) States that the rate of enzymatic reaction may be independent of substrate concentration.
d) Postulates the formation of an enzyme-substrate complex.

111. The most abundant protein in human body is
a) Albumin b) Keratin
c) Hemoglobin d) Collagen

112. The most efficient substrate of an enzyme would have
a) Largest Km b) Largest Vmax
c) Largest Vmax/Km d) Smallest Vmax/Km

113. The number of different pentapeptides that are possible with 20 naturally occurring amino acid is
a) 20 b) 100
c) 5^{20} d) 20^5

114. The number of high-energy phosphate bonds in ATP is
a) 1 b) 2
c) 3 d) 0

[CSIR (NET/JRF) Exam. Dec 2001]

115. The presence of histidine in active site of an enzyme can be confirmed by treating with
a) Iodoacetamide b) Phenylglyoxal
c) Diethylpyrocarbonate d) Iodine

[CSIR (NET/JRF) Exam. Dec 2001]

116. The secondary structure of proteins is stabilized by
a) Ionic bonds b) Hydrogen bonds
c) Hydrophobic bonds d) Disulphide bonds

117. The steady state hypothesis for enzyme suggest that
   a) Rate of formation of ES complex by substrates is equal to rate of break down of ES complex into products
   b) Rate of formation of ES complex is equal to rate of formation of products
   c) Rate of formation of ES complex and its dissociation into E and S are equal
   d) Enzymes are steadily consumed in the reaction

118. The weak, short-range forces between non-polar groups are called
   a) H-bonds b) Covalent bonds
   c) Ionic bonds d) van der Waals forces

119. What are the units for the Michaelis constant Km?
   a) Time, in seconds or minutes
   b) Moles/sec.
   c) Moles/Lit - Sec.
   d) Moles/Liter. **[CSIR (NET/JRF) Exam. Dec 2001]**

120. Amino acids are usually more soluble at pH extremes than they are at neutral pH because
   a) They have a net charge at neutral pH
   b) They have a net charge at pH extremes, and the molecules tend to repel each other
   c) pKa values are maximum at pH extremes
   d) pKa values are minimum at pH extremes

121. What is the coenzyme associated with the enzyme acetyl-CoA carboxylase?
   a) FAD b) NADP+
   c) Biotin d) FMN

122. What is the number of residues per turn in an alfa-helix?
   a) 3.6 b) 3.0
   c) 5.4 d) 1.5

123. What stabilize the higher order structure of biological macromolecules?
   a) Covalent forces b) Gravity
   c) Non covalent interactions d) Electromagnetic forces

124. What would happen if 2, 3-BPG (2,3-bisphosphoglycerate) were not present in blood?
   a) Very much oxygen would be released in the capillaries
   b) Very less oxygen would be released in the capillaries
   c) Haemoglobin would follow Michaelis-Menton kinetics
   d) RBCs would be sickled

125. Which amino acid is usually found in the folds and turns of -helix?
a) Proline
b) Glycine
c) Tryptophan
d) Alanine

[CSIR (NET/JRF) Exam. June 2007]

126. Which bond can not usually be observed between enzyme and substrate?
a) Hydrophobic bond
b) Hydrogen bond
c) Covalent bond
d) Ionic bond

127. Which enzyme is involved in detoxification reaction?
a) Glutathione oxidase
b) Catalase
c) Topoisomerase
d) Restriction enzymes

128. Pectin is an important polysaccharide found in plant cells. It is a polymer of
a) D-glucitol
b) Galactose
c) Glucuronic acid
d) Galacturonic acid

129. Which of the following amino acid has only one genetic code?
a) Tryptophan
b) Tyrosine
c) Isoleusine
d) Phenylalanine

130. Which of the following amino acid is a precursor of nitric oxide?
a) Asparagine
b) Arginine
c) Glutamine
d) Histidine

131. Which of the following amino acid is likely to be found on the surface of a globular protein?
a) Alanine
b) Serine
c) Valine
d) Leucine

132. Which of the following amino acid is not found in histones?
a) Proline
b) Tryptophan
c) Valine
d) Histidine

133. Woolen clothing shrinks when washed in hot water, but items made of silk do not because
a) Wool consists largely of the protein keratin and its disulphide bonds are broken down
b) Of α-helical conformation
c) β-sheet conformation of wool changes into α-conformation
d) Non colvalent bonds are very sensitive to hot water

134. Which of the following coenzymes can not function as cosubstrate?
a) Coenzyme A
b) Tetrahydrofolate
c) Ubiquinone
d) Lipoamide

135. Which one of the following thermodynamic properties determines the feasibility of a chemical reaction?
a) ΔS b) ΔH
c) ΔT d) ΔG

136. Which of the following inhibitor type can be expected to change the V_{max} of an enzyme but not the Km?
a) Competitive b) Non-competitive
c) Allosteric d) Irreversible

137. Which of the following inhibitor type can be expected to change the Km of an enzyme but not the V_{max}?
a) Competitive b) Non-competitive
c) Allosteric d) Irreversible

138. Which one of the following reagents is used to irreversibly modify sulfhydryl groups in a protein?
a) Iodoacetic acid b) Dithiothreitol
c) 2-mercaptoethanol d) Diethylpyrocarbonate

[CSIR (NET/JRF) Exam. June 2006]

139. Which of the following is analogous to the Km of an enzyme for a respiratory pigment?
a) p50 b) pCO_2
c) pH d) pO_2

140. Which of the following is not a characteristic feature of allosteric enzymes?
a) They are usually oligomeric proteins
b) They show co-operativity effect
c) Their substrate Vs velocity plot is sigmoid
d) None of the above

141. Which of the following is the most abundant enzyme on Earth next to Rubisco?
a) Carbonic anhydrase b) Catalase
c) Nitrogenase d) Nitrite reductase

142. Which one of the following is the least important factor as far as protein folding is concerned?
a) Hydrophobic effect b) Hydrogen bonding
c) Electrostatic interactions d) Quaternary association

143. β-carotene is precurosr of
a) Vitamin B b) Vitamin C
c) Vitamin E d) Vitamin A

144. Which of the following pairs of a chemical reaction is certain to result in spontaneous reactions?
a) Exothermic and decreasing disorder
b) Endothermic and increasing disorder
c) Exothermic and increasing disorder
d) Endothermic and decreasing disorder

145. Which one of the following interactions plays no role is stabilizing native conformation of proteins?
a) Electrostatic interactions b) Covalent interactions
c) π–π interactions d) Co-ordinate bonding

146. Which of the following statement is not true regarding the action of an allosteric enzyme?
a) Binding of an initial S molecule makes it easier to bind a second S molecule
b) Low concentration of competitive inhibitors appear to act as activators.
c) The enzyme has quaternary structure.
d) Enzyme displays hyperbolic kinetics.

147. Which of the following statement is correct for α-helix of a protein?
a) It has H-bonding in two or more parallel running chains
b) There is intrachain H-bonding in single helix
c) No H-bonding is seen
d) It is tertiary structure

148. Which of the following statement regarding enzyme inhibition is correct?
a) Non-competitive inhibition of an enzyme can be overcome by adding large amount of substrate.
b) Competitive inhibition is seen when substrate competes with an enzyme for binding to an inhibitor protein.
c) Competitive inhibition is seen when the substrate and inhibitor compete for the active site on the enzyme.
d) Non-competitive inhibitors often bind to the enzyme irreversibly.

149. Which one of the following amino acid can function as compatible substance?
a) Histidine b) Tryptophan
c) Proline d) Phenylalanine

150. Which one of the following amino acid is a precursor of the biological pigment melanin?
a) Phenylalanine b) Tryptophan
c) Tyrosine d) Arginine

151. During biochemical evolution the polyphosphate group of nucleotides was selected as a biological condensing agent because polyphosphates are
a) Kinetically stable and thermodynamically unstable
b) Kinetically unstable and thermodynamically stable
c) Thermodynamically and kinetically stable
d) Thermodynamically and kinetically unstable

152. Which of the following pairs of vitamins used by humans is metabolic product of bacteria?
a) Vitamin A and vitamin B_{12}
b) Vitamin B_{12} and vitamin K
c) Vitamin B_6 and vitamin B_{12}
d) Vitamin A and vitamin D

153. Oligosaccharides moiety containing sialic acid are present in
a) Animals
b) Plants
c) Archeabacteria and animals
d) Both (a) and (b)

154. Plasmalogens are present in
a) Liver b) Kideny
c) Heart d) All of the above

155. Aromatic amino acids are formed in
a) Shikimic acid pathway b) Mevalonate pathway
c) Hatch-Slack pathway d) Salvage pathway

156. Which of the following lipid molecule decides the blood group of an organism
a) Glycerophospholipid b) Glycosphingolipid
c) Glucosylcerebroside d) Galactosylcerebroside

157. Which of the following is essential in the diet of animal
a) Linoleic acid b) Omega-3 fatty acid
c) Omega-6 fatty acid d) All of the above

158. Pellagra disease is caused by the deficiency of
a) Thiamin b) Niacin
c) Riboflavin d) Biotin

159. Which is correct for chylomicron
a) It is a derivative of triglycerides
b) Transported through lymph
c) Extracted by the liver
d) All of the above

160. In a chemical reaction catalyzed by enzyme following the Michaelis-Menton equation what will be concentration of substrate when the velocity of the reaction is 90% of the maximum velocity
   a) 18 km
   b) 9 km
   c) 5 km
   d) 1 km

161. Which of the following is not a property of an enzyme?
   a) Form complex with substrate
   b) Decrease activation energy
   c) Decrease Gibb's free energy
   d) Increases rate of reaction

162. Which of the following is a carbohydrate binding protein?
   a) Spectrin
   b) Selectin
   c) Glycophorin
   d) Ankyrin

163. Which of the following is the most important protein structure of the soluble globular proteins?
   a) α-helix
   b) β-pleated sheet
   c) α-turn-a motif
   d) All of the above

164. Sulpholipids are the major constituent of
   a) E R cisternae
   b) Golgi cisternae
   c) Thylakoid membrane
   d) Mitochondrial inner membrane

165. Which of the following sugar alchohol is component of FMN and FAD?
   a) Mannitol
   b) Ribitol
   c) Sorbitol
   d) Erythritol

166. Ramachandran plot shows the α-helix and β-conformation fall within a relatively restricted range of sterically allowed region. The left-handed α-helix fall within
   a) Positive left side
   b) Positive right side
   c) Negative left side
   d) Negative right side

167. When hair is exposed to moist heat, then what would happen?
   a) α-keratin of hair are stretched out until they arrive at the fully extended β-conformation.
   b) The hair to be waved or curled is first bent around a form of appropriate shape.
   c) The moist heat breaks hydrogen bonds and causes the a-helical structure of the polypeptide chains to uncoil.
   d) All of the above.

168. The first intermediate with a complete purine ring in *de novo* synthesis is
   a) UMP (Uridylate)   b) IMP (Inosinate)
   c) AMP (Adenylate)   d) XMP (Xanthylate)

169. Glutamine is a primary amino acid which is used in the purine nucleotide biosynthesis. It is formed from
   a) 3-phosphoglycerate   b) α-ketogluterate
   c) Phosphoenolpyruvate   d) Oxaloacetate

170. Pyrethroids are neurotoxins that interfere with Na^+ ion channel. It is
   a) Monoterpene   b) Sesquiterpene
   c) Diterpene   d) Polyterpene

171. Which of the following is incorrect?
   a) The lower the value of pKa for an acid, to form H^+ ion.
   b) Detergents can be used to break ionic bond.
   c) Helical path of twisting in α-helix is left-handed super helix.
   d) Spider web contains β-helix.

172. Which of the following is incorrect for dextran?
   a) It is formed by the bacteria and yeast.
   b) It is polysaccharide of D-glucose linked with α-1,6 linkage with no branching.
   c) It is an extracellular adhesive molecule.
   d) Synthetic form of dextran used in the fractionation of proteins by size-exclusion chromatography.

173. α-1,4 linkage is not present in
   a) Glycogen   b) Amylose
   c) Trehalose   d) Amylopectin

174. In K-class of allosteric enzymes, double reciprocal plots are obtained and it is similar to
   a) Competitive inhibition   b) Noncompetitive inhibition
   c) Uncompetitive   d) No similarity

175. Which of the following is not the characteristic feature of water?
   a) Has sp3 hybridization.
   b) Has a high dielectric constant.
   c) Has a high heat of vaporization and low specific heat.
   d) Show proton hopping.

176. 6-N-Methyl lysine is a non-standard amino acid present in
   a) Elastin   b) Myosin
   c) Prothrombin   d) All of the above

177. Which of the following protein recognizes carbohydrates linked to protein and lipids on the cell surface?
   a) Glycoproteins b) Lipoproteins
   c) Lectins d) Sulphoproteins

178. The spatial arrangement of backbone atoms in proteins results in
   a) Primary structures b) Secondary structures
   c) Tertiary structures d) Quaternary structures

179. Which of the following HSP utilizes ATP during correct folding of proteins?
   a) HSP 70 b) HSP 90
   c) sm-HSP d) Ubiquitin

180. CoA is a cofactor of
   a) Carboxylases b) Dehydrogenases
   c) Histone acetyltransferases d) Reductases

181. Which of the following amino acid is particularly useful in mediating acid-base catalysis?
   a) Aspartic acid b) Tyrosine
   c) Histidine d) Serine

182. Methotrexate is a competitive inhibitor of
   a) Succinate dehydrogenase b) Dihydrofolate reductase
   c) Isocitrate dehydrogenase d) Pyruvate dehydrogenase

183. Defect in the enzyme glucocerebrosidase causes
   a) Tay-Sachs disease b) Gaucher's disease
   c) Niemann-Pick disease d) Sandhoff's disease.

184. Which statement is not correct for water
   a) Water is a universal solvent due to high dielectric constant
   b) H-O-H bond angle is 104.5°
   c) Maintained body temperature due to high specific heat
   d) Non-polar gases are more soluble in water

185. Desmosine is an uncommon amino acid present in
   a) Elastin b) Myosin
   c) Collagen d) Prothrombin

186. Silk fibroin is
   a) α-Keratin b) β-Keratin
   c) Collagen d) Both α- and β-Keratin

187. Which type of bond is present in amylopectin
   a) α-1,4 - linkage b) α-1,4 and α-1,6-linkage
   c) β-1,4 - linkage d) α-1,1- linkage

188. Guanidino group is present in
   a) Arginine b) Tryptophan
   c) Histidine d) Asparagine

189. Taxol is a
   a) Monoterpene b) Diterpene
   c) Triterpene d) Polyterpene

190. Molybdenom is the main metal cofactor of
   a) Nitrite reductase b) Urease
   c) Superoxide dismutase d) Glutamate mutase

191. Maximum possible pKa values of an amino acid are
   a) 2 b) 3
   c) 4 d) 6

192. Isoionic point (pI) of an amino acid can be obtained by
   a) (pKa1 + pKa2)/2 b) (pKa1 + pKa2)
   c) 2(pKa1 + pKa2) d) 2 pKa

193. Protomers are
   a) Nascent polypeptide chains
   b) Two nonidentical polypeptide chains
   c) Proteins containing more than one polypeptide chains
   d) Two identical polypeptide chains

194. Fat obtained from milk is rich in
   a) Saturated fatty acids
   b) Unsaturated fatty acids
   c) Equally rich in both saturated and unsaturated fatty acid
   d) None of the above

195. Snake venom has enzymes known as phospholipases which can break the membrane lipids. The target lipid is/are
   a) Phosphatidyl choline
   b) Phosphatidyl ethanolamine
   c) Phosphatidyl serine
   d) All of the above

196. Eicosanoids are derived from
   a) Linoleic acid b) Linolenic acid
   c) Oleic acid d) Arachidonic acid

197. Enantiomers are stereoisomers that are
   a) Nonsuperimposable mirror images of each other
   b) Superimposable mirror images of each other

c) Not mirror images of each other
d) None of the above

198. Isozymes are
a) Different molecular form that catalyze the same reaction
b) Identical molecular form that catalyze the different reactions
c) More than two subunits of one enzyme which act independently
d) Regulatory enzymes which regulate different metabolic reactions

199. Which of the following statement is correct?
a) Enzymes change the thermodynamics of the reaction
b) Enzymes determine the ratio of products to reaction at equilibrium.
c) Phosphorylation is the most common method of reversible covalent modification
d) Suicide enzymes are not used in the reaction.

200. Which of the following enzyme has the maximum turn over number
a) Catalase b) Carbonic anhydrase
c) Acetylcholine esterase d) DNA Polymerase - I

201. In a reaction, we add a chemical compound which increases the Km, if we apply more substrate the reaction goes normally and nullify the additional chemical effect. It is an example of
a) Competitive inhibition b) Uncompetitive inhibition
c) Noncompetitive inhibition d) Both (a) and (b)

202. Which of the following statement is incorrect?
a) Classical enzymes follow hyperbolic kinetics.
b) In steady-state kinetics the concentration of ES remains constant because the rate of formation equals the rate of its break down.
c) Enzymes affinity with transition state is less than the ground state of substrate
d) Enzymes lower the activation energy of reaction.

203. Which of the following is not a helical molecule
a) Agarose b) Glycogen
c) Starch d) Sucrose

204. Chylomicrons are used to transport
a) Lipids b) Proteins
c) Glycoproteins d) Sugars

205. Which of the following statement is not correct for α-helix
a) They are stabilized by hydrogen bonds between back bone atoms
b) Alanine is frequently found in α-helix
c) Each α-helical turn has 3.6 amino acid residues
d) Sulfhydril groups of cysteine residues are involved in disulphide bonds

in α-helix

206. Which of the following statement is not correct?
a) Peptide bonds in proteins are more stable in *trans*-configuration
b) Iodoacetamide can break ionic bonds in proteins
c) Rotation around C_α–C=O is not restricted
d) Quaternary structure of proteins is mainly stabilized by hydrophobic interactions.

207. Sialic acid is a derivative of
a) Sugars b) Lipids
c) Proteins d) Nucleic acids

208. ABA is a plant stress hormone, it is
a) Monoterpene b) Diterpene
c) Triterpene d) Sesquiterpene

209. Lipid synthesis is mediated by
a) ATP b) GTP
c) CTP d) UTP

210. Fish living in the subzero waters of the antarctic and arctic are protected from freezing by the presence of
a) ABA b) AFGP
c) DMSP d) PEG

211. Which of the following amino acids are frequently in short supply in plant proteins?
a) Lysine and arginine b) Methionine and cystein
c) Serine and tyrosine d) Lysine and methionine

212. The widely used broad-spectrum herbicide glyphosate inhibits EPSP synthase that is key enzyme in biosynthesis of aromatic amino acid. It is
a) Competitive inhibitor b) Noncompetitive inhibitor
c) Uncompetitive inhibitor d) Irreversible inhibitor

213. When enzyme-catalysed reactions are occurring under conditions of high substrate concentrations [S], the velocity of the reaction becomes nearly independent of [S] because
a) Substrate molecules begin acting like inhibitor molecules
b) Active sites of all enzyme molecules are bound with substrate
c) The reverse reaction becomes more important
d) Enzyme molecules become denatured

214. From intestinal epithelial cells glucose passes into the blood via a specific transporter called GLUT 2. If Na^+ - K^+ ATPase of epithelial cells has lost its activity then what would happen?
   a) Concentration of glucose increases in the blood
   b) Concentration of glucose decreases in the blood
   c) Glucose remains stored in intestinal epithelial cells.
   d) Glycogen synthesis increases

215. On the molar scale which of the following interaction in a non-polar environment provides highest contribution to the biomolecule?
   a) van der Waals interaction   b) Hydrogen bonding
   c) Salt bridge   d) Hydrophobic interaction

[CSIR (NET-JRF) Exam. Dec. 2011]

216. Michaelis and Menten derived their equation using which of the following assumption?
   a) Rate limiting step in the reaction is the breakdown of ES complex to product and free enzyme
   b) Rate limiting step in the reaction is the formation of ES complex
   c) Concentration of the substrate can be ignored
   d) Non-enzymatic degradation of the substrate is the major step

[CSIR (NET-JRF) Exam. Dec. 2011]

217. The attraction of water molecule to other water molecules is
   a) Cohesion   b) Adhesion
   c) Capillary action   d) Surface tension

218. The free energy ΔG of a dissolved solute
   a) increases with solute concentration.
   b) decreases with solute concentration.
   c) is independent of solute concentration.
   d) depends only on temperature. **[CSIR (NET/JRF) Exam. June 2011]**

219. The area of allowed regions in the Ramachandran map will be least for
   a) Gly.   b) L-Ala.
   c) L-Prol.   d) α- methyl L- valine.

[CSIR (NET/JRF) Exam. June 2011]

220. The mode of action of the anticancer drug methotrexate is through its strong competitive inhibition on
   a) dihydrofolate reductase.   b) thymidine synthase.
   c) thymidine kinase.   d) adenylate cyclase.

[CSIR Model Paper 2011]

Part C

1. Which of the following statements is correct regarding fatty acids?
   a) Most fatty acids in nature have odd number of carbon atoms, with 16- and 18- carbon fatty acids being the most common in the cells of plants and animals.
   b) Most fatty acids in nature have an even number of carbon atoms, with 18- and 20-carbon fatty acids being the most common in the cells of plant and animals.
   c) Most fatty acids in nature have an even number of carbon atoms, with 16- and 18-carbon fatty acids being the most common in the cells of plants and animals.
   d) Most fatty acids found in the cells of plants and animals may equally have odd an even carbon atoms.

2. The most usual conformation of amylose is a helix with 6 residues per turn. Iodine molecules can fit to form starch-iodine complex, which has a characteristic dark-blue colour. To form this characteristic colour
   a) 36 turns of the helix containing 1296 glycosyl residues are required.
   b) 7 turns of the helix containg 49 glycosyl residues are required.
   c) 6 turns of the heix containg 36 glycosyl residues are required.
   d) 12 turns of the helix containg 144 glycosyl residues are required.

3. Amylopectin and glycogen are brached polymer of glucose but glycogen is more highly branched in comparison to amylopectin. Which of the following is not a significance of this more branching?
   a) more branching in glycogen makes it more water soluble.
   b) because of the branching the glycogen molecule gives rise a number of available glucose molecule at a time when it is being hydrolyzed to provide energy.
   c) The glycogen phosphorylase will have more potential target if there are more branch
   d) Glycogen is found primarily in liver and muscles.

4. The half life of cytoplasmic protein is determined to a large extent by its amino-terminal residues. It is refered to as the N-terminal rule or N-terminal degron. The following statements are related with protein degradation
   (A) A specific sequence of amino acids, termed degron, indicates that a protein should be degraded by lysosomes
   (B) Cyclin destruction boxes, and PEST sequences are examples of degrons that are found in many proteins

(C) E3 enzymes are the readers of N-terminal residues
(D) Proteasome is strictly essential to read degron by E3 enzymes
Which of the following combination is correct?

a) A and B   b) B and C
c) A and C   d) B and D

5. Equilibrium constant (K) of noncovalent interaction between two non-bonded atoms of two different groups was measured at 27°C. It was observed that K=100M-1. The strength of this noncovalent interaction in terms of Gibbs free energy change is:

a) 2746 kcal/mole   b) -2746 kcal/mole
c) 247 kcal/mole.   d) -247 kcal/mole

[CSIR (NET-JRF) Exam. Dec. 2011]

6. Biosynthesis of tyrosine is detailed below:

Shikimic acid $\xrightarrow{A}$ shikimic acid-5-phosphate $\xrightarrow{B}$ C ⟶ chorismic acid ⟶ prephenic acid D $\xrightarrow{\text{transaminase}}$ (NAD^+ → NADH, CO_2) ⟶ tyrosine. Identify A, B, C and D.

a) ATP, phosphoenolpyruvic acid, 3-enolpyruyl shikimic acid-5-phosphate, p-hydroxyphenylpyruvic acid.
b) GTP, pyridoxal phosphate, 3-enolpyruvyl shikimic acid-5-phosphate, phenylpyruvic acid.
c) NADP, 3-phosphohydroxypyruvic acid, 3-enolpyruvyl shikimic acid-5-phosphate, p-hydroxyphenylpyruvic acid.
d) ATP, 3-phosphohydroxypyruvic acid, 3-enolpyruvyl shikimic acid-5-phosphate, pyridoxylphosphate

[CSIR (NET-JRF) Exam. Dec. 2011]

7. If van der Waals interaction is described by the following relation,

$$\Delta G_{Van} = \frac{A}{r^{12}} - \frac{B}{r^6} + \frac{q_1 q_2}{r}$$

where GVan is the free energy of the van der Waals interaction, A and B are constants, r is the distance between two nonbonded atoms 1 and 2, and q1 and q2 are partial charges on the dipoles 1 and 2. In this relation, the parameter A describes

a) electron shell attraction   b) electron shell repulsion
c) dipole-dipole attraction   d) dipole-dipole repulsion

[CSIR (NET-JRF) Exam. Dec. 2011]

8. The pH of blood of a healthy person is maintained at 7.40 ± 0.05. Assuming that this pH is maintained entirely by the bicarbonate buffer (pKa1 and pKa2 of carbonic acid are 6.1 and 10.3, respectively), the molar ratio of [bicarbonate]/[carbonic acid]in the blood is
   a) 0.05 b) 1
   c) 10 d) 20

   [CSIR (NET-JRF) Exam. Dec. 2011]

9. The hydrolysis of pyrophosphate to orthophosphate is important for several biosynthetic reactions. In E.coli, the molecular mass of the enzyme pyrophosphatase is 120 kD, and it consists of six identical subunits. The enzyme activity is defined as the amount of enzyme that hydrolyzes 10 μmol of pyrophosphate in 15 minutes at 37°C under standard assay condition, The purified enzyme has a Vmax of 2800 units per milligram of the enzyme. How many moles of the substrate are hydrolysed per second per milligram of the enzyme when the substrate concentration is much greater than Km?
   a) 0.05 μmol b) 62 μmol
   c) 31.1 μmol d) 1 μmol

   [CSIR (NET-JRF) Exam. Dec. 2011]

10. An experiment was done to determine the effect of compound Y on the biochemical reaction A + B → C. It was found that in the presence of Y, very little if any, product C was formed however, on increasing the concentration of A, C could be detected. Some of the explanations are given
    (A) Y, is a competitive inhibitor of A
    (B) A, is an enzyme as well as substrate
    (C) Y, is an structural analogue of A
    (D) Y, is an uncompetitive inhibitor of B
    Which of the following is most appropriate?
    (a) A only (b) D only
    (c) A and C (d) B only

11. A mutation that changes an alanine residue in a protein to an isoleucine leads to a loss of activity. Activity is recognized when a further mutation at the same site changes the isoleucine to a glycine. This is because
    a) Isoleucine has larger side chain and there is not enough room in the native conformation.
    b) The pKa values of alanine and glycine are same.
    c) Glycine is usually found at the ends of polypeptide chains.
    d) Glycine always over comes negative effects of isoleucine in proteins.

12. You have isolate and purified an unknown protein from an insect. Its amino acid composition was determined often acid catalyzed hydrolysis: Gly 45%,

Ala 30%, Serine 12%, Tyr 5%, Val 2% and others 6%. Which of the following is probably not true for this protein?

a) It would be expected to be primarily β-sheet.
b) It would be expected to be globular protein.
c) It would be water insoluble.
d) It probably plays a structural role.

13. The diversity and complexity of the carbohydrate units and the variety of ways in which they can be joined in oligosaccharides and polysaccharides suggest that they are functionally important. It is now clear that these carbohydrate structures are the recognition sites for a special class of proteins, termed glycan-binding proteins (lectins) which bind specific carbohydrate structures on neighboring cell surfaces. Following statements relate to some characteristic features of these lectins.

(A) They are ubiquitous and no living organisms have been found that lack these key proteins.
(B) The chief function of lectins is to facilitate cell-cell contact.
(C) C type lectins are found in animals and they require calcium for protein-sugar interaction.
(D) Influenza virus recognizes sialic acid residues linked to galactose residues that are present on cell surface glycoproteins. The viral glycan-binding protein that binds to these sugars is called hemagglutinin.

Which of the following combinations is correct?

a) A and D　　b) C and D
c) A, B and D　　d) A, B, C and D

14. A protein in 100 mM KCl solution was heated and the observed Tm (mid-point of unfolding) was 60°C. When the same protein solution in 500 mM KCL washeated, the observed Tm was 65°C. What is the most probable reason for this increase in Tm?

a) Hydrophobic interaction is increased and electrostatic repulsion is decreased.
b) Hydrophobic interaction is decreased and electrostatic repulsion is increased.
c) Hydrogen-bonding is increased.
d) van der Waals interaction is increased

[CSIR (NET/JRF) Exam. June 2011]

15. Am amino acid contains no ionizable group in its side chain (R). It is titrated from pH 0 to 14. Which of the follwing ionizable state is not observed during the entiretitration in the pH range 0-14?

a) $H_3\overset{+}{N} - \underset{}{\overset{R}{\overset{|}{C}}}H - COO^-$

b) $H_3\overset{+}{N} - \overset{R}{\overset{|}{C}}H - COOH$

c) $H_2N - \overset{R}{\overset{|}{C}}H - COO^-$

d) $H_2N - \overset{R}{\overset{|}{C}}H - COOH$

[CSIR (NET/JRF) Exam. June 2011]

16. A researcher has isolated a restriction endonuclease that cleaves at only one specific 10 base pair site.
   A. Would this enzyme be useful in protecting cells from viral infections, given that a typical viral genome is 5×10^4 base pairs long?
   B. Restriction endonucleases are slow enzymes with turnover number of 1^{s-1}. Suppose the isolated endonuclease was faster with turnover numbers similar to those for carbonic anhydrase (106^{S-1}), would this increased rate be beneficial to host cells, assuming that the fast enzymes have similar levels of specificity?

The correct combination of answer is
a) (A) : No(B) : Yes
b) (A) : No (B) : No
c) (A) : Yes (B) : No
d) (A) : Yes (B) : Yes

[CSIR (NET/JRF) Exam. June 2011]

17. An α-helix in a peptide or protein is characterized by hydrogen bonds and characteristic dihedral angles. Choose the right combination.
a) Hydrogen bonding between the amide CO of residue i and amide NH of residue i+4. Dihedral angles in the region $\phi \sim -50^0, \Psi \sim -60^0$.
b) Hydrogen bonding between the amide NH of residue i and amide CO of residue i+4. Dihedral angles in the region of $\phi \sim -50^0, \Psi \sim -60^0$.
c) Hydrogen bonding between the amide CO of residue i and amide NH of residue i+4. Dihedral angles in the region of $\phi \sim -50^0, \Psi \sim +60^0$.
d) Hydrogen bonding between the amide CO of residue i and amide NH of residue i+3. Dihedral angles in the region of $\phi \sim -50^0, \Psi \sim -60^0$.

[CSIR (NET/JRF) Exam. June 2011]

18. Precursors of the atoms in the purine skeleton are

6 C, 7 N, 5 C, 1N, C8, 2C, 4 C, N 9, N 3

a) N1, Asp; C2 and C8, formate; N3 and N9, guanidine of Arg; C4, C5 and N7, Gly; C6, CO_2.
b) N1, Asp; C2 and C8, citrate; N3 and N9, amide nitrogen of Gln; C4, C5 and N7; Gly; C6, CO_2.
c) N1, Asp; C2 and C8, formate; N3 and N9, amide nitrogen of Gln; C4, C5 and N7, Gly; C6, CO_2.
d) N1, Glu; C and C8, acetate; N3 and N9, amide nitrogen of Asn; C4, C5 and N7, Gly; C6, CO_2.

[CSIR (NET/JRF) Exam. June 2011]

19. A typical animal cell (nucleated) membrane contains glycolipids and glycoproteins in the plasma membrane. To determine its topological distribution, lectin is used as a probe.
The following interactions may be the basis of the probing method:
(A) Protein-protein interaction (B) Protein-sugar interaction
(C) Protein-lipid interaction (D) Protein-sterol interaction.
The appropriate answer is
a) Only (A).
b) Only (B).
c) All of (A), (B) and (C).
d) Only (D).

[CSIR Model Paper 2011]

Answer Sheet

Part B

1.	c	2.	d	3.	a	4.	d	5.	b	6.	b
7.	d	8.	c	9.	b	10.	c	11.	d	12.	c
13.	c	14.	c	15.	d	16.	d	17.	a	18.	d
19.	b	20.	b	21.	a	22.	c	23.	d	24.	a
25.	a	26.	c	27.	d	28.	c	29.	b	30.	c
31.	d	32.	d	33.	d	34.	c	35.	b	36.	d
37.	d	38.	d	39.	b	40.	c	41.	d	42.	d
43.	d	44.	c	45.	c	46.	c	47.	b	48.	b
49.	a	50.	b	51.	b	52.	c	53.	d	54.	c
55.	d	56.	a	57.	a	58.	d	59.	c	60.	a
61.	b	62.	c	63.	a	64.	d	65.	c	66.	d
67.	a	68.	d	69.	c	70.	c	71.	c	72.	d
73.	c	74.	b	75.	c	76.	b	77.	b	78.	c
79.	b	80.	d	81.	d	82.	a	83.	c	84.	b
85.	d	86.	a	87.	b	88.	c	89.	d	90.	d
91.	c	92.	b	93.	a	94.	d	95.	b	96.	d
97.	c	98.	a	99.	b	100.	d	101.	d	102.	c
103.	b	104.	b	105.	b	106.	c	107.	d	108.	d
109.	a	110.	d	111.	d	112.	c	113.	d	114.	b
115.	c	116.	b	117.	a	118.	d	119.	d	120.	b
121.	c	122.	a	123.	c	124.	b	125.	d	126.	c
127.	b	128.	d	129.	a	130.	b	131.	b	132.	b
133.	b	134.	d	135.	d	136.	b	137.	a	138.	a
139.	a	140.	d	141.	c	142.	d	143.	d	144.	c
145.	d	146.	d	147.	b	148.	c	149.	c	150.	c
151.	a	152.	b	153.	a	154.	c	155.	a	156.	b
157.	a	158.	b	159.	d	160.	b	161.	c	162.	b
163.	b	164.	c	165.	b	166.	b	167.	d	168.	b
169.	b	170.	a	171.	b	172.	b	173.	c	174.	a
175.	c	176.	b	177.	c	178.	b	179.	a	180.	c
181.	c	182.	b	183.	b	184.	d	185.	a	186.	b
187.	b	188.	d	189.	b	190.	a	191.	b	192.	a
193.	d	194.	a	195.	d	196.	d	197.	a	198.	a
199.	c	200.	a	201.	a	202.	c	203.	d	204.	a
205.	d	206.	b	207.	a	208.	d	209.	c	210.	b

211.	d	212.	a	213.	b	214.	b	215.	b	216.	a
217.	a	218.	b	219.	d	220.	a				

Part – C

1.	c	2.	c	3.	d	4.	b	5.	b	6.	a
7.	b	8.	d	9.	c	10.	c	11.	a	12.	b
13.	d	14.	a	15.	d	16.	b	17.	b	18.	c
19.	b										

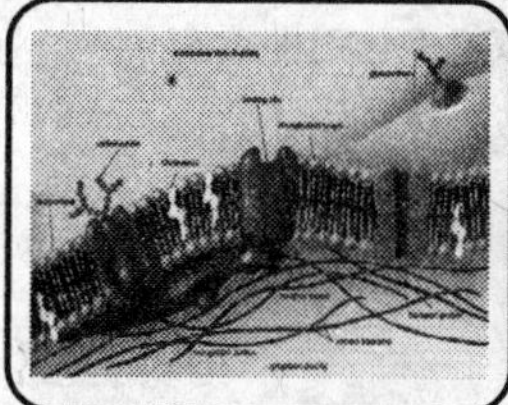

Chapter 2
Cell Biology

Part B

1. Vertebrates cells internalize insulin through
   a) Simple diffusion
   b) Facilitated diffusion
   c) Receptor mediated endocytosis
   d) Carriers
2. The function of detoxification of drugs in the cells, is perfomed by
   a) Lysosomes b) Peroxisomes
   c) Smooth ER d) Rough ER
3. Which of the following is not a component of endomembrane system of eukaryotic cells?
   a) Endoplasmic reticulum b) Golgi complex
   c) Lysosomes d) Peroxisomes
4. In genetic engineering the gene encoding for the enzyme luciferase is usually used as reporter gene. This enzyme is found in
   a) Mitochondria b) Plastids
   c) Lysosomes d) Peroxisomes
5. A Barr body is
   a) A result of primary non-disjunction
   b) Inactive Y-chromosome
   c) Gene that plays a key role in male development
   d) Inactive X chromosome
6. A cell has four DNA molecules. At metaphase stage it will have
   a) Four DNA molecules b) Eight DNA molecules
   c) Six DNA molecules d) Two DNA molecules
7. A fast-acting cellular signal would probably
   a) Travel through the blood stream
   b) Affect nearby cells
   c) Be long- lived
   d) Affect distant cells

8. A functional chromosome must have all of the following except
   a) Replication origins b) Centromere
   c) Telomere d) Telomerase

9. A large multisubunit protease complex which degrades proteins is called
   a) Proteasome b) Protome
   c) Proteogenome d) Hydrogenosome

10. A mediated transport system would be expected to
    a) Show a continuously increasing initial rate of transport with increasing substrate concentration
    b) Exhibit structural and /or stereospecificity for the substrate transported
    c) Be fast than that of a simple diffusion system
    d) Establish a concentration gradient across the membrane

11. According to the second law of thermodynamics, molecules spontaneously move from region of higher concentration to one of lower concentration. However, Na^+ are present at 143mM outside the cell and 14mM inside the cell. Yet Na^+ cannot pass through the plasma membrane. Transport of Na^+ into the cell is achieved by
    a) Facilitated diffusion b) Release of acetylcholine
    c) Release of norepinephrine d) Na^+ transporter

12. Acetylcholine receptor is
    a) Na^+ channel b) Ca^{2+} channel
    c) K^+ channel d) Cl^- channel

13. Addition of manose-6-phosphate to a protein results in its localisation in
    a) Nuclei b) Plasma membrane
    c) Lysosome d) Golgi body

    [CSIR (NET/JRF) Exam. Dec 2005]

14. Amino acids are translocated by intestinal epithelial cells by
    a) Facilitated diffusion
    b) H^+/amino acid co-transporters
    c) Na^+/amino acid co-transporters
    d) Amino acid/glucose anti-porters

15. Among closely lying cells signal are communicated by
    a) Neurotransmitters b) Hormones
    c) Gap junction d) Cell membrane proteins

16. Among the following which ion is not used in active transport?
    a) Na^+ b) K^+
    c) Ca^{++} d) Cl^-

17. Among the following which is not involved in cell communication?
a) Cadherins b) Selectins
c) Integrins d) None of the above

18. Among the following which muscle protein has affinity to bind with Ca^{2+} ions
a) Tropomyosin b) Troponin
c) Actin d) Myosin

19. An example of a cell which is devoid of nuclear membrane and mitochondria is a -
a) Bacterial cell b) Protozoan cell
c) Spong cell d) Sperm cell

20. Anastral mitosis is characteristic of
a) Higher plants b) Higher animals
c) All living organsims d) Lower animals

21. At the time of cell division sister chromatids are joined together with the help of
a) Centromere b) Cohesin protein
c) Separin d) Kinetochore

22. At which of the following stage sister chromatids separate and move towards poles ?
a) Prophase b) Metaphase
c) Anaphase d) Telophase

[C.S.I.R. (NET-J.R.F.) Exam. June 2008]

23. Biological membranes are associated with all of the following except
a) Prevention of free diffusion of ionic solutes
b) Specific systems for the transport of uncharged molecules
c) Sites for biochemical reactions
d) Free movement of proteins and nucleic acids across the membrane

24. Button like points of intercellular contact that serve as anchoring sites of intermediate filaments and help to hold adjacent cells together are called-
a) gap junctions b) connections
c) cadherins d) desmosomes

25. Which one of the following is not an example of active transport?
a) Transport through ion channel
b) Transport through ABC transporter
c) Transcytosis
d) Transport of mRNA from nucleus to cytosol

26. Ca^{2+} - ATPase transports
    a) Two Ca^{2+} from the inside of cells to the outside while returning two H^+ from outside per ATP
    b) Two Ca^{2+} from the inside of cells to the outside per ATP
    c) One Ca^{2+} from the inside of cells to the outside while returning one H^+ from outside per ATP
    d) One Ca^{2+} from the inside of cells to the outside per ATP

27. Ca^{++}-binding protein is
    a) Tropomysosin b) Actin
    c) Myosin d) Troponin

[C.S.I.R (NET-JRF) Exam. Dec 2005]

28. Calmodulin, a calcium binding protein, is found in living organisms except
    a) Plants b) Animals
    c) Prokaryotes d) Both animals and prokaryotes

29. cAMP has
    a) always positive control on *lac* operon
    b) always negative control on *lac* operon
    c) no role in operon control
    d) both positive and negative control

30. cAMP is directly involved in regulation of
    a) Adenylate cyclase b) Protein kinase A
    c) PFK d) ATP

31. Caspases are involved in apoptosis. They are found in
    a) Mitochondria b) ER lumen
    c) Cytosol d) Plasma membrane

32. Cdc2 in cell cycle acts at
    a) S-Phase b) G1-phase
    c) G2-phase d) M-phase

[CSIR (NET/JRF) Exam. June 2005]

33. Cdk is a kinase which is important for
    a) Cell division b) Signal transduction
    c) Transcription d) Genetic Engineering

34. Cdk1 with cyclin B acts at
    a) G1 phase b) G2 phase
    c) S phase d) M phase

35. Cdk-1/cyclin A complex acts at
    a) G1 to S transition point b) S to G2 transition point
    c) RESTRICTION POINT d) G2 to M transition point

36. Cell division is primarily regulated at
   a) G1 - stage b) S - stage
   c) G2 - stage d) G0 - stage

37. Cell membrane is
   a) A lipid bilayer
   b) A lipid bilayer sandwiched between two protein layers
   c) A protein bilayer sandwiched between two lipid layers
   d) Protein in lipid is mosaic mixture

38. Cell size is determined by
   a) Volume: weight ratio b) Volume: surface area ratio
   c) Surface area : volume ratio d) Surface area : weight ratio

39. Cell-cell recognition is achieved by
   a) Glycolipids b) Glycoproteins
   c) Phosphatidates d) Peripheral proteins

40. Cells uptake iron through
   a) Phagocytosis b) Transcytosis
   c) Exocytosis d) Receptor mediated endocytosis

41. Cellular proteins are degraded by
   a) Lysosomes b) Proteasomes
   c) Cyclosomes d) Chymotripsins

42. Cellulose and hemicellulose, which are the constituents of cell wall, are synthesized by
   a) lysosome b) microbodies
   c) smooth ER d) Golgi body

43. Chiasmata are formed in meiosis
   a) before metaphase I b) after metaphase I
   c) during prophase II d) during metaphase II

[CSIR (NET/JRF) Exam. Dec 2001]

44. Cholera toxin causes diarrhea because it
   a) Inhibits adenylate cyclase
   b) Blocks conformational change in trimeric G-protein.
   c) Activates cAMP phosphodiesterase
   d) Inhibits GTPase activity of $G\alpha_s$ by ADP ribosylation

45. Cholesterol occurs in most of the membranes of organelles, except
   a) outer membrane of mitochondria and chloroplast
   b) Inner membrane of mitochondria and chloroplast
   c) Endoplasmic reticulum
   d) Golgi body

46. Chromosomal translocation and inversions are readily detectable in
    a) Lampbrush chromosomes b) Polytene chromosomes
    c) B-chromosomes d) All of the above

47. Clathrin coated vesicles are usually involved in the
    a) Transport of cargo from trans-Golgi to Lysosomes
    b) Endocytosis
    c) Transport of cargo from ER to Golgi complex
    d) Both a and b

48. Clathrin is a
    a) Variable coat protein b) conserved coat protein
    c) virus coat protein d) None of the above

49. Coated vesicles in the cell gives rise to
    a) Endosome b) Microsome
    c) Ribosome d) Episome

50. Colchicine treated cells are arrested in
    a) S phase b) Prophase
    c) G1 phase d) Metaphase

51. COP II vesicles transport proteins from
    a) Rough ER to the Golgi
    b) From the cis Golgi to the rough ER
    c) From plasma membrance and the trans Golgi to late endosomes
    d) From trans golgi to the lysosome

52. Crossing-over occurs at
    a) Leptotene b) Zygotene
    c) Pachytene d) Diplotene
    [CSIR (NET/JRF) Exam. June 2005]

53. C-value enigma explains
    a) C- value paradox b) Junk DNA in eukaryotes
    c) Cot curve d) Genome complexity

54. C-value paradox is
    a) Correct correlation between genome size and complexity
    b) Lack of correlation between genome size and complexity
    c) Percentage of junk DNA in eukaryotes
    d) None of the above **[CSIR (NET/JRF] Exam. June 2007]**

55. C-value refers to
    a) Haploid level of DNA b) Diploid level of DNA
    c) Triploidy d) Polyploidy

56. Cytoplasmic streaming is associated with
a) Microfilaments b) Microtubules
c) Intermediate filaments d) All of the above

57. Cytoplasmic streaming results into mobility of substances and organelles. It involves interaction of
a) Tubulin, kinesin b) Tubulin, myosin
c) Actin, kinesin d) Actin, myosin
[CSIR (NET/JRF] Exam. Dec 2008]

58. You have isolated a motile, Gram positive cell with no visible nucleus, you can assume this cell has
a) Mitochondria b) Ribosome
c) Golgi complex d) ER

59. DNA in the form of minicircles and maxicircles is found in
a) Mitochondrial genome b) Chloroplast genome
c) Kinetoplast d) Apicoplast

60. During cell division the transition of the cell into the S phase is controlled by?
a) CDK4/CDK6 b) CDK1
c) CDK2 d) CDK25

61. During chromatid separation microtubules attach to the
a) Centromere b) Kinetochore
c) Telomere d) Secondary constriction

62. During glycosylation of proteins the oligosaccharide groups are modified by
a) proteases b) glycosyl transferases
c) mutases d) None of the above

63. During meiosis centromere divides at
a) Metaphase b) Anaphase
c) Anaphase II d) Interkinesis

64. During meiosis cohesin protein is broken down at
a) Metaphase b) Anaphase-I
c) Anaphase-II d) Telophase

65. During programmed cell death usually which one of the following gives "eat me" signal?
a) Phosphatidyl choline b) Phosphatidyl inositol
c) Phosphatidyl serine d) Sphingomyelin

66. Effect of release of IP_3 during signal transduction pathway is
    a) Closure of Ca^{2+} channel in ER
    b) Increase in intracellular Ca^{2+} level
    c) Increase of extra cellular Ca^{2+} level
    d) Inactivation of calmodulin proteins.

67. Endoreduplication can be seen in
    a) Lampbrush chromosomes
    b) B-chromosomes
    c) Salivary gland chromosomes
    d) Maligant cells

68. Epinephrine plays its role in glycogenolysis through
    a) Activating phophorylase kinase
    b) Activating glycogen synthase.
    c) Inactivating phosphorylase kinase.
    d) Inactivating adenylyl cyclase.

69. Eukaryotic cells communicate through
    a) Gap junction
    b) Synapses
    c) Neurotransmitters
    d) Desmosomes

[CSIR (NET/JRF) Exam. June 2008]

70. Eukaryotic chromosomes are transcriptionally most active during
    a) Prophase
    b) Metaphase
    c) Anaphase
    d) Interphase

71. Fever occurs due to change in membrane potential of neurons of hypothalamus. which of the following ion channel is responsible for this physiological phenomenon?
    a) Cl^- ion channel
    b) Na^+ ion channel
    c) K^+ ion channel
    d) Ca^{2+} ion channel

72. Flippases helps in the movement of phospholipids of plasma membrane from extra cellular monolayer to cytosolic inner monolayer. These are
    a) Carriers
    b) Direct redox coupled transporter
    c) P-type ATPases
    d) ABC transporters

73. For every molecule of ATP hydrolysed, Na^+/ K^+ ATPase Transport
    a) One Na^+ into cell and one K+ out of the cell
    b) Two Na^+ out of the cell and one K^+ into the cell
    c) Two Na^+ out of the cell and two K^+ into the cell
    d) Three Na^+ out of the cell and two K^+ into the cell

74. Gaucher's disease occurs due to accumulation of cerebrosides. Which of the following cell organelle become defective in this case?
   a) Mitochondria
   b) Endoplasmic reticulum
   c) Golgi body
   d) Lysosome

[CSIR (NET/JRF) Exam. June 2008]

75. Genes for cytoplasmic male sterility in plants are generally located in
   a) Mitochondrial genome
   b) Cytosol
   c) Chloroplast genome
   d) Nuclear genome

76. Glycoconjugates on proteins in intracellular membranes are oriented toward
   a) Cytoplasmic face
   b) Lumen side
   c) Embedded in membrane
   d) on both sides

[CSIR (NET/JRF] Exam. June 2007]

77. Glycolipids in plasma membrane functions as "finger prints of the cell" because they are involved in
   a) Cell recognition
   b) Tissue recognition
   c) Organ recognition
   d) All of the above

78. Goblet cells are present in
   a) Liver
   b) Intestinal villi
   c) Duodenum
   d) Kidney

[CSIR (NET/JRF] Exam. June 2005]

79. Gram-negative bacteria are typically less susceptible to penicillin than are gram positive bacteria because
   a) They lack a transport system for penicillin
   b) They lack teichoic acid in the cell wall
   c) Their peptidoglycan is chemically modified to be resistant to attack by penicillin
   d) Their outer membrane is an effective permeability barrier

80. Growth factor receptors are
   a) G protein linked
   b) Receptor tyrosine kinases
   c) Ion channel linked
   d) Cytosolic

81. Histones are replaced by protamines in
   a) Nerve cells
   b) muscle cells
   c) Heart cells
   d) sperms

82. Holocentric chromosomes are found in
   a) *Luzula*
   b) Man
   c) Chimpanzee
   d) Birds

83. Hopanoids are sterol like-molecules which are found in the plasma membrane of
    a) Certain bacteria and cyanobacteria
    b) Fungi
    c) Mycoplasma
    d) Archaebacteria

84. How many kinetochores are present in a human cell?
    a) 48 b) 23
    c) 46 d) 92

85. Hydrolytic enzymes are stored in
    a) Lysosomes b) Peroxisomes
    c) Golgi complex d) Glyoxysomes

86. Hydrophobic drug transporters found in plasma membrane are kept under
    a) Channels b) Pumps
    c) Group translocators d) ABC transporters

87. If there is mutation in cdk/cyclin, the key molecule in regulating the cell cycle, then
    a) There would be uncontrolled growth
    b) Cell will not pass to S phase
    c) The level of cdk/cyclins will enhance
    d) Cells will arrest to Go phase

88. In a cell if acidity of lysosome is lost, it can cause loss of
    a) Phagocytosis of invading bacteria
    b) Elevated phosphatase level
    c) Glycogen degradation
    d) No major effect

89. In a normal resting cell chromosome exists as fibre of
    a) 10 nm. b) 30 nm.
    c) 300 nm. d) 700 nm.

90. In cell - cycle centrioles replicate in
    a) G1-phase b) S-Phase
    c) G2-Phase d) M- Phase

91. In comparison to their natural environments biologically active cells are
    a) Isotonic b) Hypotonic
    c) Hypertonic d) Vary from condition to condition

92. In DNA the histone responsible for higher order chromatin structures is
    a) H2A b) H2B
    c) H3 and H4 d) H1

93. In eukaryotes facultative heterochromatin can be observed in
   a) Telomere b) Centromere
   c) Barr body d) All of the above

94. In human cells, sacroplamic reticulum is specialized for
   a) storage and rapid release of Ca^{++}
   b) Storage and rapid release of lipids
   c) Secretion of proteins
   d) None of the above

95. In mammals, G protein coupled receptors play a major role in mediating effects of various hormones not through
   a) Activation of adenylate cyclase
   b) Activation of protein kinase A
   c) Activation of tyrosine kinase activity
   d) Inactivation of adenylate cyclase

96. In meiosis the maximum shortening and thickening of chromosomes takes place during
   a) Pachytene b) Diplotene
   c) Metaphase-I d) Diakinesis

97. In mesokaryotes well organized chromosomes are not present due to absence of
   a) DNA b) Histones
   c) Centromere d) None of the above

98. In nucleosome core DNA wound around the histone octamer in a
   a) Right handed superhelix
   b) Left- handed superhelix
   c) Both left-handed and right-handed superhelix
   d) None of these

99. In programmed cell death formation of apoptosome is induced by
   a) Endogenous instructions b) Stress effects
   c) Cell-mediated cytotoxicity d) Complement proteins

100. In the chromosome chromatids are joined at
   a) Synaptonemal complex b) Centromere
   c) Telomere d) Nucleolar organizer

[CSIR (NET/JRF) Exam. June 2008]

101. In trimeric G proteins GTPase activity is found in
   a) G_s b) $G_s\alpha$
   c) $G_s\gamma$ d) $G_s\beta\gamma$

102. In yeasts and plant cells lysosomes are not found. The functions of lysosomes in these cells are assumed by
a) Golgi complex
b) Endosome
c) Vacuole
d) Peroxisome

103. Insulin receptor is
a) Trans membrane serine/tyrosine kinase
b) Serine/threonine kinase
c) Tyrosine kinase found in the cytosol
d) Transmembrane tyrosine kinase

104. Intercellular tansport of solutes through plasmodesmata is called
a) Apoplastic transport
b) Symplastic transport
c) Periplamsic transport
d) Intracellular transport

105. Intracellular negative potential and extra cellular positive potential occurs in
a) Liver cells
b) Neurons
c) Kidney cells
d) In all cells

[CSIR (NET/JRF] Exam. Dec 2008]

106. Ionophores are used as antibiotics because they
a) inhibit transcription
b) are competitive inhibitor of pyruvate dehydrogenase
c) equilibriate concentration gradient across the membrane for a particular solute
d) cause ionization of enzymes involved in metabolic reactions

107. JAK-STAT pathway is governed by
a) Heterotrimeric G-protein linked receptor
b) Monomeric G-protein linked reception
c) Tyrosine kinase receptor
d) Ion channel linked receptor

108. Kinetochore is a proteinaceous structure of centromere. It is important for cell division because
a) It causes disappearance of nucleolus
b) It causes spindle formation
c) Microtubules attach to kinetochore during separation of chromosomes
d) It is involved in cytokinesis.

109. Which one the following ion channels is an example of second messenger gated ion channel?
a) Na^+ channel
b) Cl^- channel
c) K^+ channel
d) Ca^{2+} channel

110. Lipid bilayers can be formed by phospholipids which have variable head groups and fatty chains. The fluidity of the membrane will depend on
   a) Length and degree of unsaturation of fatty acid chains
   b) Only unsaturation irrespective of the length of the fatty acid chains.
   c) Only the nature of head groups
   d) Only the length of the fatty acid chains irrespective of the extent of unsaturation

111. Lipid-bilayer-fluid-mosaic model is not applicable to the plasma membranes of
   a) Mitochondria b) Bacteria
   c) Oleosomes d) Lysosomes

112. Low pH of the lysosomal compartment is maintained by
   a) electron transport b) H^+ ATPase at the membrane
   c) luminal acid production d) glycolysis

113. Which one of the following transporters enables eukaryotic cells to pump out a large number of different drugs and other foreign compounds?
   a) H^+ pumps b) Na^+/K^+ pumps
   c) ABC transporters d) Aquaporins

114. Lysozyme has no effect on archaeal cell because
   a) it works on outer membrane and archaeal cell lacks outer membrane
   b) it works on cell wall and archael cell lacks it.
   c) it works on β-1,3 glycosidic bond and this bond is not found in archael cell wall
   d) it works on β-1,4 linkage and archaeal cell lacks it.

115. Mad2 protein acts at mitotic spindle assembly check point of cell cycle. It attaches at
   a) Telomeric region of chromosomes
   b) Centromeric region of chromosomes
   c) Randomly any region of chromosomes
   d) Secondary constriction

116. Mannose-6-phosphate receptor is found in
   a) ER b) Lysosome
   c) cis Golgi network d) trans Golgi network

[CSIR (NET/JRF] Exam. June 2007]

117. Membrane channels
   a) Have a large aqueous area in the protein structures so are not very selective
   b) Commonly contain amphipathic α-helices

c) Are opened or closed only as a result of a change in the transmembrane potential
d) Allow substrates to flow only from outside to inside the cell

118. Membrane potential is controlled by
a) Ligand-gated ion channels
b) Voltage-gated ion channels
c) Second messenger-gated ion channels
d) Pressure sensitive ion channels

119. Membranes of which of the following organelles are continuous
a) ER and Golgi
b) Nucleus and ER
c) Golgi and plasma membrane
d) Golgi and lysosome

120. Mesokaryotic cells have
a) nucleus without nuclear membrane
b) genetic material with histones but lacks nuclear membrane
c) nucleus with nuclear membrane but lacks histones
d) nuclear membrane and histones.

121. Methotrexate is used as anticancer drug because
a) It blocks mitosis
b) It blocks cytokinesis
c) It inhibits synthesis of dNTPs
d) It stabilizes cells in Go phase

122. Mitochondria is involved in all of the following except?
a) ATP production
b) Fatty acid biosynthesis
c) TCA cycle
d) Apoptosis

123. Mitosis promoting factor is
a) Complex of cyclin proteins
b) Cyclin dependent protein kinase
c) Cyclin independent protein kinase
d) Complex of securin and proteasome

124. Movement of solute through the cell membrane against the concentration gradient is termed active transport and occurs when
a) It is transported with a carrier protein
b) Energy is utilized for this purpose
c) A metal ion, Ca^{++} is bound to it
d) Facilitated by hydrolysis of ATP

125. Multidrug resistance transporter protein is an example of
a) P-type ATPase b) V-type ATPase
c) G-type ATPase d) ABC-transporter

126. Na^+/K^+ pump is an example of
a) Symporter b) Uniporter
c) Antiporter d) None of these
[CSIR (NET/JRF) Exam. June 2005]

127. Nieman-Pick disease and Gaucher syndrome occurs due to loss of enzymes from
a) Microbodies b) Endosomes
c) Lysosomes d) Proteasomes

128. Nitric oxide receptor is
a) Membrane bound and ion channel linked
b) Membrane bound and enzyme linked
c) Membrane bound and G-protein linked
d) Cytosolic

129. Nucleosome consists of
a) H2A, H2B, H3, H4 and 200bp
b) Two H2A, H2B, H3, H4 and 200bp
c) Two H2A, H2B, H3, H4, H1 and 200bp
d) Two H2A, H2B, H3, H4, non-histone protein and 200bp
[CSIR (NET/JRF] Exam. June 2007]

130. O-linked glycosylation of proteins occurs in
a) Cytosol b) Endoplasmsic reticulum
c) Golgi body d) Lysosome

131. Which one of the following transport mechanism across the membrane is not an active process?
a) Uptake of glucose by intestinal epithelial cells
b) Uptake of fructose by intestinal epithelial cells
c) Entry of pyruvate into mitochondria
d) Uptake of glucose by erythrocytes

132. One of the major transmembrane proteins in a "tight junction" is
a) Integrin b) Lectin
c) Claudin d) Adherin

133. Oubain is a potent inhibitor of
a) Na^+ ion channel b) H^+ pump
c) Na^+/K^+ pump d) Na^+/Ca^{2+} antiporter

134. Parietal cells are found in
   a) Stomach   b) Liver
   c) Pancreas   d) Heart

135. Pemphigoid is an autoimmune disease in which the patient develops antibodies against proteins in
   a) Desmosomes   b) Hemidesmosomes
   c) Na^+ ion channel   d) Cl^- ion channel

136. Which one of the following statement is true for prokaryotic cells?
   a) Their endomembrane system consists only of ER and mesosomes
   b) Their cytoskeleton consists only of microtubules
   c) They always divide mitotically
   d) Their signaling system involves two component system

137. Pertusis toxin causes
   a) Ceasation of GTPase activity of $G_S\alpha$
   b) ADP-ribosylation of $G_S\alpha$
   c) ADP-ribosylation of Giα
   d) Hydrolysis of cAMP

138. Phagocytes kill harmful bacteria by
   a) endocytosis   b) complement
   c) T-cell stimulation   d) inflammation

139. Phosphatidyl serine is usually found in
   a) Outer leaflet of lipid bilayer
   b) Inner leaflet of lipid bilayer
   c) It is randomly distributed in both leaflets of lipid bilayer
   d) Its presence in the membrane is matter of cell signaling

140. Phospholipase-C is found in
   a) Outer membrane of mitochondria
   b) ER membrane
   c) Tonoplast
   d) Plasma membrane of an eukaryotic cell

141. Plant cells communicate through
   a) Gap junctions   b) Cell wall
   c) Plasmodesmata   d) Desmosomes

142. Plasmodesmata of plant cells are similar to the animal's
   a) Tight junctions   b) Gap junctions
   c) Adherens junctions   d) Desmosomes

[CSIR (NET/JRF] Exam. Dec 2007]

143. Podophyllotoxin is used to treat cancer. It prevents cell division by inhibiting
   a) Cdks
   b) Cyclin synthesis
   c) Polymerization of microtubules
   d) Cohesin breakdown

144. Primary and secondary active transport both.
   a) Are based on passive movement of sodium ions.
   b) Include the passive movement of glucose molecules.
   c) Use ATP directly.
   d) Can move solutes against their concentration gradients.

145. Prokaryotes lack the membranous subcellular organelles characteristic of eukaryotes, but their plasma membranes may be enfolded to form
   a) Endosomes b) Lysosomes
   c) Plasmosomes d) Mesosomes

146. Protein present in coated pits involved in receptor mediated endocytosis is
   a) Adopter b) Clathrin
   c) Coatamer d) Diamine

147. Proteins can not be synthesized in
   a) WBCs b) Nerve fibres
   c) Sieve tubes d) None of these above

148. Proteins synthesized on ER-bound ribosomes can not be transported into
   a) ER b) Golgi complex
   c) Lysosome d) Peroxisome

149. Quorum sensing in bacteria involves
   a) Cell signaling cascading mediated by cAMP
   b) Cell signaling cascading mediated by cGMP
   c) Histidine phosphorylation
   d) Tyrosine phosphorylation

150. Quorum sensing in gram positive bacteria occurs through
   a) Stringent response b) One component system
   c) Two component system d) G-protein coupled signaling

151. Which one of the following statement is not correct?
   a) Oubain can inhibit Na^+/K^+ pump
   b) Transport through channels is always passive
   c) Group translocator change chemical property of solute during transport process
   d) Transport through symporter is fast than ion channels

152. Which one of the following statement is not correct?
   a) Fatty acids in the plasma membrane are saturated and unsaturated
   b) Unsaturated fatty acids in the plasma membrane have cis-double bonds
   c) Unsaturated fatty acids in the plasma membrane have trans-double bonds
   d) Sphingolipids are usually found in the outer monolayer of plasma membrane

153. Replicate copies of each chromosome are called ______ and are joined at the ______.
   a) Homologus/centromere
   b) Sister chromatids/kinetochore
   c) Sister chromatids/centromere
   d) Homologus/kinetochore

154. Ribophorin proteins are found in the membrane of
   a) Chloroplast
   b) Golgi body
   c) Ribosome
   d) Endoplasmic reticulum

155. Ribosomal subunits are assembled in
   a) Cytoplasm
   b) Nucleolus
   c) Nucleus
   d) Endoplasmic reticulum

156. Ribosomes are attached to endoplasmic reticulum through
   a) Ribophorins
   b) r-RNA
   c) t-RNA
   d) Hydrophobic interaction

157. Which one of the following statement is not correct?
   a) Exocytosis and endocytosis are energy consuming processes
   b) Rab proteins are trimeric G-proteins that are involved in vesicle fusion
   c) Tetrodotoxin blocks Na^+ channels
   d) DAG is a membrane derived second messenger

158. Secondary metabolites in plant cells accumulate in
   a) Lysosomes
   b) Glyoxysomes
   c) Vacuoles
   d) Oleosomes

159. Secretary proteins are mainly modified in
   a) Nucleus
   b) Ribosome
   c) ER lumen
   d) Golgi apparatus

160. Siderophores are
   a) Calcium binding proteins
   b) Iron binding proteins
   c) Magnesium binding proteins
   d) Phosphorus binding proteins.

161. Signal hypothesis is associated with
a) Transport of mRNA from nucleus
b) Transport of ribosomes from nucleus
c) Synthesis of secretary proteins
d) Anterograde transport

162. Signaling process mediated by insulin and epidermal growth factors occur through
a) Ion channel linked receptors
b) G-protein linked receptors
c) Tyrosine kinase linked receptors
d) Cell adhesion molecules

163. Smooth ER is the site of synthesis and metabolism of
a) Proteins b) Fatty acids and phospholipids
c) Carbohydrates d) Glycogen

164. Somatic pairing is often seen in
a) Polytene chromosome
b) Lampbrush chromosomes
c) Chromosomes of somatic cells
d) During meiosis in germ cells

[CSIR (NET/JRF) Exam. Dec. 2007]

165. Spectrin is integral membrane protein of
a) Epithelial cells b) RBCs
c) Macrophages d) Endosomes

166. Steroid receptors are
a) G-protein linked b) Ion-channel linked
c) Intracellular d) Integral membrane protein kinases

167. Structural component of a metaphase chromosome which anchor 30 nm chromatin loop is called
a) Scafold b) Centromere
c) Telomere d) Synaptonemal complex

[CSIR (NET/JRF) Exam. June 2008]

168. Structural unit of chromatin is
a) 10 nm b) 30 nm
c) 300 nm d) 700 nm

169. Synaptonemal complex is formed in
a) Pachytene b) Diplotene
c) Zygotene d) Diakinesis

170. Synthesis of sugar from fatty acids occurs in
a) Sphaerosome b) Glyoxysome
c) Peroxisome d) Cytosol

171. Taxol an anticancer drug prevents cell division because it
a) Inhibits microtubule polymerization
b) Stabilizes microtubules
c) Inhibits DNA replication
d) Inhibits cytokinesis

[C.S.I.R. (NET-J.R.F.) Exam. Dec. 2007]

172. Which one of the following small G-protein regulates cytoskeleton?
a) Ran b) Rab
c) Rho d) Arf

173. Telomeric DNA is made up of
a) Single copy of unique sequences
b) AT-rich sequences
c) Nucleolar organizing regions
d) Short repeat sequences

174. Tetrodoxin inhibits
a) Na^+ channels b) K^+ channels
c) Na^+/K^+ pump d) H^+ pump

175. The 10 nm thick fibre of chromatin is called
a) Nucleolus b) Nucleosome
c) Chromosome d) Solenoid

176. The acidic environment of lysosomes is regulated by?
a) P-type ATPase b) V-type ATPase
c) F-type ATPase d) ABC-Cassettes

177. Which one of the following is not a second messenger?
a) Ca^{2+} b) cAMP
c) Mn^{2+} d) PIP_3

178. Which one of the following is not the component of extracellular matrix?
a) Collagen b) Proteoglycans
c) Glycoproteins d) Major histocompatibility complexes

179. The basic structural unit of the metaphase chromosome is
a) 10 nm filament b) 30 nm filament
c) 300 nm filament d) 600 nm filament

180. The biologically active proteasome is
   a) 19S b) 20S
   c) 26S d) 39S

181. The cytoskeleton consists of
   a) Microfilaments, cilia and flagella
   b) Microtubules, cilia and microfilaments
   c) Intermediate filaments, microtubules and cilia
   d) Intermediate filaments, microfilaments and microtubules

182. The enzyme protein kinase - G is activated by
   a) cAMP b) IP_3
   c) DAG d) cGMP

183. The epithelial cells that line our intestine uptake glucose by
   a) Facilitated diffusion b) H^+/glucose symporter
   c) Na^+/glucose symporter d) Na^+/glucose antiporter

184. The Golgi apparatus
   a) Is found only in animals.
   b) Is found in prokaryotes.
   c) Packages and modifies proteins.
   d) Is the appendage that moves a cell around in its environment.

185. The inner side of plasma membrane is negatively charged. The reason behind it is
   a) Donann Equillibrium b) Simple diffusion
   c) Facilitate diffusion d) Active transport

[CSIR (NET/JRF) Exam. June 2008]

186. The internal system of protein fibres that contributes to a eukaryotic cell's structure and allows movement is called
   a) Endomembrane system b) Lysosomal system
   c) Cytoskeleton d) Extracellular matrix

187. The major constituent of the cell organelle centriole is
   a) Actin b) Myosin
   c) Tubulin d) Intermediate filaments

188. The major function of nucleolus in a nucleus concern
   a) Organisation of chromosomes
   b) Replication of DNA
   c) Synthesis of Ribosomes
   d) Chromatid separation

189. The mechanism for transporting components of surrounding medium into cytoplasm is:
a) Phagocytosis b) Exocytosis
c) Transduction d) Endocytosis

190. The membrane proteins of RBCs which are responsible for transport of glucose into them functions as
a) Receptor b) Ion channel
c) Carrier d) Pump

191. The molecular motor that is involved in chromosome movement during cell division comprises
a) Microtubules and actin b) Kinesin and microtubules
c) Troponin and dynein d) Kinesins and dyneins

192. The most important point in the regulation of cell cycle occurs in the
a) G1 phase b) S phase
c) G2 phase d) M phase

193. The movement of material from the ER through the Golgi complex toward the plasma membrane is called
a) Anterograde transport b) Retrograde transport
c) Bulk flow d) Facilitated diffusion

194. The Na^+/K^+ pump is found in
a) Plants b) Bacteria
c) Animals d) All of the above

195. The normal intracellular concentration of free Ca^{2+} is
a) 10^{-5}M b) 10^{-7}M
c) 10^{-6}M d) 10^{-9}M

196. Which one of the following is not a characteristic feature of cancer cells?
a) Their cytoskeleton structure is changed
b) They avoid programmed cell death
c) Glycosyl transferases becomes more active
d) Cell-cycle check points are failed

197. The procces by which a cell secretes macromolecules by fusing a vesicle to the plasma membrane is called
a) Endocytosis b) Exocytosis
c) Pinocytosis d) Phagocytosis

198. Which one of the following is not a characteristic feature of cancerous cells?
a) They accumulate lactate
b) Their cell surface markers remains unchanged
c) They have increased blood vessels
d) Their monomeric G-protein Rho is mutated

199. The protein of Golgi complex which contain irregular cisternae and tubules is known as
a) Cis Golgi b) Trans Golgi
c) Medial Golgi d) Intercisternal Golgi

200. The shortening of eukaryotic chromosome during replication is prevented by
a) Ligase b) Reverse transcriptase
c) Telomerase d) RNA polymerase

[CSIR (NET/JRF) Exam. June 2008]

201. Which one of the following hormone binds to intracellular receptors?
a) Growth hormone b) Glucagon
c) Insulin d) Estrogen

202. The type of intercellular signalling in which one cell can communicate with another over long distances is called
a) Autocrine b) Paracrine
c) Juxtacrine d) Endocrine

203. The uptake of cholesterol by mammalian cells can be explained by
a) Phagocytosis
b) Pinocytosis
c) Receptor-mediated endocytosis
d) Transcytosis

204. To achieve active conformation calmodulin protein binds minimum
a) Two Ca^{2+} ions b) Three Ca^{2+} ions
c) Four Ca^{2+} ions d) Six Ca^{2+} ions

205. Tonofilaments are the structural unit of
a) Microtubules b) Microfilaments
c) Intermediate filaments d) Flagella

206. Which one of the following component of the plasma membrane of eukaryotic cells is not found in the membrane of prokaryotes?
a) Glycerophospholipids b) Sphingolipids
c) Cholesterol d) Glycoproteins

207. Transport of molecules through channel protein present in the plasma membrane is?
a) Always passive b) May be active or passive
c) Always active d) None of the above

208. Transport of sodium ions from outer side to the inner side of an eukaryotic cell is
a) Simple diffusion b) Facilitated diffusion
c) Primary active d) Secondary active

209. Transport vesicles involved in retrograde transport are coated with

a) Clathrin b) COP I
c) COP II d) Caveolin

210. Two sisters chromatids are separated at anaphase by the action of

a) Cohesin b) Separin
c) APC d) MAD2

211. Tyrosine kinase is activated by

a) Phosphorylation b) Acetylation
c) Dephosphorylation d) Methylation

[CSIR (NET/JRF] Exam. June 2007]

212. Ubiquitination of proteins is marked for all of the following except

a) Endocytosis b) Chromatin remodeling
c) Protein degradation d) Correct folding of proteins

213. Vacular ATPases are

a) H^+ pumps b) K^+/H^+ pumps
c) Ca^{2+} pumps d) Na^+/K^+ pumps

214. Viagra is used in treatment of erectile dysfunction because it

a) Stimulates nitric oxide systhesis.
b) Inhibits diesterase
c) Increase half-life of guanylyl cyclase
d) Inhibits NO synthase.

215. *Vibrio cholerae* causes diahorrea by

a) Opening ion channels
b) Constitutive expression of adenylate cyclase
c) Closing absorption of water from gut epithelium
d) Destroys cells of intestinal lining

216. Vinblastin is used as anticancerous drug because it

a) Blocks cell division and functions as antimitotic drug.
b) Causes cell death.
c) Promotes cell growth.
d) Stimulates DNA synthesis.

[CSIR (NET/JRF) Exam. Dec. 2005]

217. Virus encoded 'ras' oncogene transforms normal mammalian cells into cancer cells. Viral Ras protein differs from its normal counterpart by

a) Diminished GTPase activity
b) Increased GTPase activity
c) Diminished ATPase activity
d) Increased ATPase activity

218. Viruses can cross biological membranes with the help of
   a) Glycocalyx b) Integral membrane proteins
   c) Lipid bilayer d) Pores

219. What cellular connection is "leak-proof"?
   a) Anchoring junction b) Plasmodesmata
   c) Tight junction d) Gap junction

220. What happens to the Cdk-cycA complex at metaphase?
   a) Both cyclin A and Cdk are degraded
   b) Only cyclin A is degraded
   c) Both cyclin A and Cdk remain undegraded
   d) Only Cdk is degraded

221. When a cell expands energy to move a solute across its membrane against a concentration gradient, the process is called
   a) Diffusion b) Facilitated diffusion
   c) Active transport d) Osmosis

222. When *bcl*-2 gene is mutated it results in tumor, like chronic lymphoblastic leukemia (CLL). Normally this gene regulates
   a) Cell division b) Cell differentiation
   c) Synthesis of growth factors d) Programmed cell death.

223. Which group of bacteria on sporulation show cell-coordination and social behaviour?
   a) Archaebacteria b) *Bacillus* species
   c) Actinobacteria d) Myxobacteria

[CSIR (NET/JRF) Exam. Dec. 2005]

224. Which GTPase regulate intracellular transport in mammalian cells through vesicle fusion?
   a) Rab b) Ran
   c) Ras d) Rho

225. Which is responsible for cytoplasmic streaming?
   a) Microfilaments b) Intermediate filaments
   c) Microtubules d) Endoplasmic reticulum

226. Which is true for gap junction?
   a) It is made of connexon protein
   b) Allows free movement of large molecules across cells
   c) Made up of two subunit of connexons
   d) None of the above

227. Which one of the following component of cytoskeleton plays a crucial role in vesicular transport?
a) Microfilaments
b) Intermediate filaments
c) Microtubules
d) Molecular motors

228. Which of the following are not true cells?
a) Phagocytes
b) Basophils
c) Platelets
d) Lymphocytes

229. Which of the following biomolecule crosses nuclear membrane?
a) RNA
b) Carbohydrate
c) Lipid
d) Glycoprotein

[CSIR (NET/JRF] Exam. June 2007]

230. Which of the following cell junctions are very commonly found in uterus and bladder?
a) Gap junctions
b) Tight junctions
c) Spot desmosome
d) Hemidesmosome

231. Which one of the following cells can not divide?
a) Liver cells
b) Lymphocytes
c) RBCs
d) Stem cells

232. Which of the following cell organelle is involved in fatty acid oxidation?
a) Glycosome
b) Peroxisome
c) Chloroplast
d) Glyoxysome

233. Which of the following cell organelle has half unit membrane?
a) Ribosome
b) Sphaerosome
c) Lysosome
d) Peroxisome

234. Which of the following cell organelle is involved in apoptosis?
a) Mitochondria
b) Peroxisome
c) ER
d) Golgi complex

235. Which of the following cell organelle is not found in pollen grains?
a) Ribosome
b) ER
c) Mitochondria
d) Chloroplast

236. Which of the following cell organelles lacks DNA?
a) Mitochondria
b) Hydrogenosome
c) Chloroplast
d) None of the above

237. Which of the following cellular process can never occur without input of energy
a) Water uptake
b) Glucose uptake by RBCs
c) Protein secretion
d) Solute transport

238. Which of the following cellular process is not governed by p53 protein?
a) Apoptosis b) DNA repair
c) Inhibition of angiogenesis d) Promotion of lactate sysnthesis

239. Which of the following component of electron transport system of mitochondria can induce programmed cell death?
a) FMN b) CoQ
c) Cytochrome a/a3 d) Cytochrome c

240. Which of the following cyclin-dependent kinase is responsible for S to G2 transition?
a) Cdk1/cyc B b) Cdk1/cyc A
c) Cdk4/cyc D d) Cdk2/cyc A

241. Which of the following function as "fluidity buffer" in membranes?
a) Integral proteins b) Peripheral proteins
c) Sterols d) Fatty acids chains of phospholipids.

242. Which of the following is a channel forming ionophore?
a) Gramicidin A b) Actinomycin
c) Valinomycin d) Nicin

243. Which of the following is a hydrophobic second messenger?
a) cAMP b) IP_3
c) Ca^{++} d) DAG

244. Which of the following is a membrane derived second messenger?
a) Prostaglandins b) Thromboxanes
c) DAG d) All of the above

245. Which of the following is a membrane derived second messenger?
a) Ca^{2+} b) cAMP
c) IP_3 d) cGMP

246. Which of the following is a most common fine control mechanism of cellular metabolic activities?
a) ADP-ribosylation of target proteins
b) Methylation of target proteins
c) Phosphorylation of target proteins
d) Acetylation of target proteins

247. Which of the following is an energy-requiring transport across the membrane?
a) Simple diffusion b) Facilitated diffusion
c) Osmosis d) Transcytosis

248. Which of the following is an example of pressure sensitive ion channel?
a) Cl^- ion channel
b) K^+ ion channel
c) Aquaporins
d) Mg^{2+} ion chennel

249. Which of the following is commonly called as the "digestive system" of cells
a) Golgi complex
b) Peroxisomes
c) Lysosomes
d) Glyoxysomes

250. Which of the following is not a calcium binding protein.
a) Troponin
b) Calmodulin
c) Calsequestrin
d) None of these

251. Which of the following is not a characteristic feature of cancerous cell?
a) Change in surface markers
b) Increase in cell size
c) High oxygen demand
d) Normal Bcl2 protein in the outer membrane of mitochondria

252. Which of the following is not a component of extracellular matrix (ECM) of animals?
a) Collagens
b) Elastins
c) Proteoglycans
d) Extensins

253. Which of the following is not a function of Golgi body?
a) Golgi body plays major role in glycosylation
b) It is responsible for the synthesis of fatty acids and lipids
c) It appears to be involved in addition of sulphate to carbohydrate moiety of the glycoproteins.
d) It is responsible for acrosome formation

254. Which of the following is not a lysosomal storage disease?
a) Tay-sachs disease
b) Gaucher's disease
c) Niemann-Pick disease
d) Cystic fibrosis disease

255. Which of the following is not a property of plasma membrane?
a) Self sealing ability
b) Selective permeability
c) Three dimensional structure
d) Lipid bilayer

256. Which of the following is not a protooncogene?
a) ras
b) fos
c) myc
d) None of above

257. Which of the following is not a second messenger?
a) Ca^{2+} b) cGMP
c) DAG d) AMP

258. Which of the following is not an event of meiosis-I?
a) Crossing-over b) Reduction division
c) Centromere division d) Chiasmata formation

259. Which of the following is not considered as a component of nucleosome?
a) H1 b) H2 A
c) H2 B d) H3

260. Which of the following is not naturally found in biological membranes of eukaryotes?
a) cis-fatty acids b) Transmembrane proteins
c) Sterols d) Trans-fatty acids

261. Which of the following is precursor for humoral hormones?
a) Cholesterol b) Arachidonic acid
c) Biotin d) PIP_2

262. Which of the following is centre of post-translational modification of proteins?
a) Endoplasmic reticulum b) Lysosome
c) Golgi body d) Endosome

263. Which of the following kind of movement is not thermodynamically favourable in membrane lipid bilayer?
a) Rotational movement of lipid
b) Lateral movement of lipid
c) Transverse movement of lipid
d) All of the above

264. Which of the following level of chromatin organization is the substrate for several nuclear processes like DNA replication, repair, recombination, and transcription?
a) Nucleosome b) 30 nm fibre
c) Radial loops d) Metaphase chromosome

265. Which of the following lipid is involved in cell signalling?
a) Phosphatidyl enthanolamine
b) Phosphatidyl serine
c) Phosphatidyl choline
d) Phosphatidyl inositiol-4, 5-bisphophate

266. Which of the following lipid is not found in membranes?
 a) Glycerophospholipids b) Sphingolipids
 c) Triacylglycerol d) PIP_2

267. Which of the following mammalian cells usually does not divide in adult life?
 a) Liver Cells b) Osteoblast cells
 c) Epithelial cells in lung d) Nerve cells in brain

268. Which of the following memnrane derived messenger regulates intracellular Ca^{2+} ion concentration?
 a) DAG b) Ceramide
 c) Sphingosine d) IP_3

269. Which of the following monomeric G-proteins is involved in vesicle fusion during exocytosis and endocytosis?
 a) Ran b) Arf
 c) Rab d) Ras

270. Which one of the following cell-cell junction of animal cells can permit free movement of small water soluble molecules?
 a) Tight junction b) Anchoring junction
 c) Gap junction d) Pores

271. Which of the following organelles are thought to have arisen from primitive prokaryotes
 a) ER and nucleus
 b) Golgi apparatus and lysosomes
 c) Chloroplast and mitochondria
 d) Vacuoles and transport vesicles

272. Which of the following organelle is similar to bacteria
 a) Lysosome b) Endoplasmic reticulum
 c) Nucleus d) Mitochondria

[CSIR (NET/JRF] Exam. Dec. 2006]

273. Which of the following property of biological membrane can not be explained by fluid-mosaic model?
 a) Two dimensional structure b) Selective permeability
 c) Fluidity d) Membrane potential

274. Which of the following protein functions as 'molecular motor' and causes movement of chromosomes at anaphase
 a) Cohesion b) Kinetochore
 c) Kinesin d) Securin

275. Which one is the main function of Golgi complex
   a) Protein synthesis b) Protein sorting
   c) Detoxification d) Phagocytosis

276. Which of the following stage of the cell cycle is most variant?
   a) G_o b) M
   c) G_1 d) G_2

[CSIR (NET/JRF] Exam. Dec. 2006]

277. Which of the following statement is not correct?
   a) In plant plasma membranes, the direction of H^+/Ca^{++} pump is outward
   b) Ion pumps can be either electrogenic or electroneutral
   c) Bacteria use F-type ATPases to pumpout toxic heavy metal ions
   d) Membrane transport is usually a physical rather than a chemical process

278. Which of the following statement is not correct?
   a) Na^+ ion gradient is the major source of energy for active transport of glucose in intestinal cells
   b) Na^+ ion gradient is the major source of energy for active transport of glucose in RBCs
   c) Extra cellular Na^+ ion concentration is always high.
   d) Na^+ ions can pass across the membrane through facilitated diffusion.

279. Which of the following statement about ion channels is not correct?
   a) Transport through channels is extremely rapid
   b) Ion channels are highly selective because narrow pores in the channels restrict passage to ions of the appropriate size and charge
   c) Most ion channels are permanently open
   d) In ion channels conformational change do not occur during transport of ions across the membrane

280. Which of the following statement is not correct?
   a) Facilitated diffusion is mediated
   b) Facilitative transporters are specific for the molecules they transport
   c) Facilitative transporters obey saturation kinetics
   d) Intestinal epithetical cells absorb glucose through facilitated diffusion

281. Which of the following statement is not correct?
   a) Transmembrane proteins are always either α-helix or β-sheets
   b) cAMP is involved in the regulation of pore size of gap junctions
   c) Valinomycin is a carrier former ionophore
   d) Colchicine induces polymerization of microtubules.

282. Which of the following translocation system of plasma membrane changes chemical nature of solutes during translocation process?
a) Active transporters
b) Aquaporins
c) Ion channels
d) Group translocators

283. Which of the following tumour suppressor gene causes apoptosis
a) Rb
b) p53
c) NF-1
d) MTS-1

284. Which of the following will be more prominent in the inner monolayer of biological membrane?
a) Glycolipids
b) Glycoproteins
c) Phosphatidylinositol
d) Peripheral proteins

285. All our cells contain protooncogenes, which can change into cancer-causing genes. Why do cells possess such potential time-bombs?
a) Protooncogenes are unavoidable environmental carcinogenes
b) Protooncogenes are necessary for normal control of cell division
c) Protooncogenes are genetic junk that has not been eliminated by natural selection
d) Proto oncogenes protect cells from infection by cancer-causing viruses

286. Animals uptake fructose from the lumen into the intestinal absorptive cells (enterocytes) through
a) Transcytosis
b) Na^+/fructose cotransporter
c) Facilitated diffusion
d) H^+/fructose antiporter

287. Cancer cells provoke angiogenesis in
a) WBC
b) Platelets
c) Endothelial cells
d) All of these

[CSIR (NET/JRF) Exam. Dec. 2005]

288. Cold resistant animals in their plasma membrane have more
a) Cholesterol
b) Short chain fatty acids
c) Saturated fatty acids
d) Unsaturated fatty acids

289. Deficiency of glycosyltransferases have been seen in malignant cells. This causes
a) Uncontrolled cell division
b) Changes in the surface markers
c) Changes in cytoskeleton
d) All of the above

290. In many tumours, there is a growth of blood vessels in the direction of tumours. The phenomenon is known as
a) Necrosis
b) Carcinogenesis
c) Angiogenesis
d) Morphogenesis

[CSIR (NET/JRF) Exam. Dec 2002]

291. Methotrexate is used to treat cancer because it
   a) Inhibits spindle formation and prevents mitosis.
   b) Is a competitive inhibitor of an enzyme which is involved in the synthesis of purines and pyrimidines
   c) It is irreversible inhibitor of the enzyme dihydrofolate reductase.
   d) Causes programmed cell death.

292. The ability of a malignant cell to detach itself from a tumour and establish a new tumour at another site within the host is called
   a) Anaplasia b) Metastasis
   c) Hyperplasia d) Metaplasia

293. The action potential results from
   a) Decrease in negative charge inside the nerve fibre
   b) Increased in positive charge outside the nerve fibre
   c) Opening of voltage gated Na^+ channels
   d) Activation of the Na^+/K^+ pump

294. The antibiotic amphothericin-B disrupts plasma membranes by combining with sterol, it will affect all of the following cells except
   a) Bacterial cells b) Mycoplasma cells
   c) Fungal cells d) Plant cells

295. The phase of the cell cycle during which the chromosomal material separates after duplication is known as
   a) G_1-Phase b) G_2- Phase
   c) S-Phase d) M-Phase

296. The special channels found in plasma membrane for water transport are
   a) Porins b) Aquaproins
   c) Permeases d) Pumps

297. The stored seed oils are converted to carbohydrates in
   a) Peroxisome b) Cytosol
   c) Glyoxysome d) Sphaerosome

[CSIR (NET/JRF) Exam. Dec 2005]

298. The fluid-mosaic model of plasma membrane was proposed by Singer and Nicholson. Their model was published in the journal.
   a) Science b) Nature
   c) Cell d) Structural Biology

299. Which of the following is an actin-binding protein?
   a) Calmodulin b) Troponin
   c) Caldesmon d) Calsequestrin

300. Which of the following is involved in the majority of the ATP dependent cytosolic degradation of proteins in eukaryotes?
   a) Cathepsins b) Calpains
   c) 20 S proteasomes d) 26 S proteasomes

301. Which of the following second messenger was first to be discovered?
   a) cGMP b) cAMP
   c) IP_3 d) Ca^{2+}

302. Which of the following statement is not correct?
   a) In plants cAMP-dependent protein kinases are absent
   b) Plants have jasmonic acid instead of steroid hormones
   c) G-proteins and tyrosine kinases are much less prominent in plants
   d) Microorganisms have two-component system for signalling

303. Which of the following statements is not correct ?
   a) Almost all of the prokaryotes have a single circular chromosome
   b) Almost all of the prokaryotes have cell wall
   c) All prokaryotes have plasmid
   d) The genetic material in prokaryotes is not enclosed in any structure surrounded by membranes.

304. Among the following which is characteristic feature of Meiosis-I?
   a) Separation of homologous chromosomes
   b) Separation of chromatids
   c) Doubling of DNA content
   d) Movement of chromosome towards poles

305. Bacterial genome is prevented by its own endonucleases by
   a) Immune mechanism
   b) Nuclease resistant genome
   c) Methylation at restriction sites
   d) Are not much effective on bacterial genome

[CSIR (NET/JRF) Exam. Dec 2006]

306. What would happen if a chromosome lacks a centromere?
   a) The DNA replication is not possible
   b) The DNA will replicate but the chromosome will not segregate properly to the progeny cells
   c) Neither DNA replication nor chromosome segregation possible
   d) Transcription and translation are inhibited

307. V type ATPases are found in intracellular membranes. Which of the following cells have V type ATPases in its plasma membranes?
   a) Liver cells b) Heart cells
   c) Kidney cells d) Nerve cells

308. Insulin like growth factors are secreted from
  a) Pancreas b) Liver
  c) Kidney d) Heart

309. Plants uptake NH^{4+} from soil through
  a) Simple diffusion
  b) NH^{4+} - H^{+} symporter
  c) Facilitated diffusion mediated by a carrier
  d) NH^{4+} - H^{+} antiporter

310. Which of the following is not a second messenger?
  a) IP_3 b) cAMP
  c) Sphingosine-1-phosphate d) PIP_2

311. Which of the following statement is not correct?
  a) cAMP acts as a type of hormone in *Dictyostelium* during its development.
  b) Ethylene is synthesized from methionine.
  c) Insulin regulates GLUT-5
  d) Bacteria have two component syetem for signaling.

312. Which of the following does not regulate fluidity in the membrane?
  a) Cholesterol
  b) Length of fatty acid chain.
  c) Degree of saturation in fatty acids.
  d) Asymmetric distribution of lipids between lipid bilayer.

313. Cyclin-dependent protein kinases are
  a) Tyrosine kinases b) Serine kinases
  c) Threonine kinases d) Serine/threonine kinases

314. In the intrinsic pathway of apoptosis which of the following protein is not released from mitochondria which promotes cell death?
  a) Cytochrome C b) Apoptosis-inducing factor
  c) p53 protein d) Endonuclease G

315. Which of the following is not a component of extracellular matrix?
  a) Collagen b) Proteoglycans
  c) Fibronectin and laminin d) Cadherins

316. Cell wall is absent in
  a) Synchitrium b) *E. coli*
  c) Sacchromyces cerevaceae d) Cynobacteria

317. Animal cells are connected to the extracellular matrix through
  a) Glycoprotein b) Fibronectin
  c) Integrin d) Collagen

318. Which of the following is incorrect?
   a) Gap junction is made up of an identical hexamer of connexon protein.
   b) Transport through channel is always passive but all the anions are taken up actively into the cytosol.
   c) α-bungarotoxin blocks the voltage gated Potassium channel.
   d) V-type ATPases are specifically inhibited by high concentration of nitrate.

319. Which of the following is incorrect?
   a) Movement of transport vesicles from the golgi to the ER is assisted by COP-I and Arf proteins.
   b) Raf-effectors proteins facilitate vesicle transport, membrane tethering and fusion.
   c) Intermediate filament serves to organize metabolism and intracellular transport in the non-dividing cell.
   d) Vandate is a potent inhibitor of ABC-transporters.

320. ω-oxidation occurs only when β-oxidation is defective. It occurs only in
   a) Peroxisome b) Mitochondria
   c) ER of liver and kidney d) All of the above

321. Phosphodiesterase-II is the marker enzyme of
   a) Lysosome
   b) Golgi complex
   c) Mitochondria (inner membrane)
   d) Chloroplast (inner membrane)

322. Tight junction is made up of
   a) Innexins b) Pannexins
   c) Cadherins d) Claudin

323. Which of the following is incorrect for peroxisome?
   a) Detoxification of harmful compounds.
   b) Catabolism of xenobiotics.
   c) Reduction of fatty acids.
   d) Metabolism of nitrogen - containing compounds.

324. Smooth movement of bacteria during chemotaxis is due to
   a) Tumbling
   b) Dephosphorylation of Che Y
   c) Movement of H+ across plasma membrane.
   d) Phosphorylation of Che A

325. Retinoblastoma is one of the important proteins involved in cancer. The function of Rb is to hold the protein involved in

a) G1 arrest b) G1/S promotion
c) DNA repair d) Apoptosis

326. Centromeres contain a histone H3 variant called
a) CENP-A b) H3FA3
c) H3FT d) H2A-Bbd

327. Homologous chromosomes remain paired with one another throughout the mitotic cell cycle in
a) Zebra fish b) *C. elegans*
c) Maize d) *Drosophila*

328. In animal cells cytokinesis is mediated by a contractile ring which is made of
a) Actin filaments b) Intermediate filaments
c) Microtubules d) Phragmoplast

329. Chromocenter is a unique feature of chromosomal arrangement in
a) *C. elegans* b) *Arabidopsis*
c) *Neurospora* d) Fruit fly

330. Which statement is correct regarding meiosis?
a) There is two round of replication and two round of cell division
b) There is one round of replication and one round of cell division
c) There is one round of replication and two round of cell division
d) There is two round of replication and one round of cell division

331. Activation of replication origins in S phase is triggered by phosphorylation of the pre-replicative complex, which is carried out by S phase Cdks with assistance from another protein kinase,
a) Cdc 9 b) Cdc 7
c) Cdc 16 d) Cdc 27

332. *Caulobacter crescentus* emerged as a powerful model organism for cell cycle studies in bacteria because of
a) It divides very fast
b) It has several clearly visible structures and the appearance and disappearance of thesc structures is tightly linked to cell cycle events
c) Its DNA is very small
d) It has overlapping replication cycles

333. Which of the following is the only DNA repair pathway available in G1 phase?
a) Direct repair b) NHEJ repair
c) Homology-directed repair d) Excision repair

334. The global regulator kinase ATR is recruited to the DNA damage which subsequently initiates the DNA damage response in mammals. Which of the following is not correct for this kinase?
   a) It is recruited to double-strand breaks.
   b) It activates check point kinase CHK 1.
   c) It regulates Cdc 25 phosphatase.
   d) It slows the movement of replication fork when DNA damage occurs.

335. Chi sequences are present in
   a) Yeast genome
   b) *E. coli* genome
   c) Mammals genome
   d) Mitochondrial genome

336. P450 cytochromes are heme-containing monooxygenases. They are involved in metabolism of an unusually wide range of endogenous and exogenous substances. In eukaryotic cells they are found in
   a) Mitochondrial inner membrane
   b) ER membrane
   c) Lysosomal membrane
   d) Both (a) and (b)

337. Transport of anions such as arsenate, in archaea is mediated by
   a) P-type ATPases
   b) ZIP transporter
   c) A-type ATPases
   d) ABC transporter

338. Which of the following statement is not correct?
   a) All ABC transporters have two nucleotide-binding domains and two membrane domains.
   b) Na^+-K^+ pump consists of α and β subunits, with ion-binding sites and catalytic site on the α-subunit.
   c) Many of the ABC transporters in humans have medical significance.
   d) Phosphorylated form of Na^+-K^+ pump shows high affinity for Na^+ ions.

339. Mitochondria evolved from
   a) Gram positive bacteria
   b) Gram negative bacteria
   c) Archaebacteria
   d) Cyanobacteria

340. In bacteria which of the following is homologous of tubulin that is involved in cytokinesis?
   a) FtsZ
   b) Par M
   c) Crescentin
   d) Mbl

341. Glanzmann's disease is the result of defect in
   a) Cadherin
   b) Integrin
   c) Connexin
   d) Claudins

342. Phosphoaminolipids are transported from outer leaflet of plasma membrane towards inner leaflet of plasma membrane by
a) Flippase b) Floppase
c) Scrumblase d) Carrier proteins

343. Glutamate receptor channels in plants induce
a) Uptake of Nitrate b) Uptake of calcium ions
c) Uptake of potassium ions d) Uptake of ammonium

344. In which of the following cellular components H+-pyrophosphatase is found?
a) Lysosome b) Endoplasmic reticulum
c) Golgi apparatus d) Endosomes

345. Which of the following monomeric G-protein is involved in vesicle formation?
a) Rab b) Rho
c) Arf d) Ras

346. Which of the following region of nuclear receptors contain sequences responsible for the localization of the receptor to the nucleus?
a) A/B domain b) C-domain
c) D-domain d) E-domain

347. Which of the following component of Na+/K+ pump binds digitalin?
a) α-subunit b) β-subunit
c) α/β dimer d) Glycoprotein of outer monolayer

348. Cholera toxin causes ADP-ribosylation of Gs α at
a) Cystein residue b) Arginin residue
c) Aspartate residue d) Histidine residue

349. Plant shaker channels are specific for the transport of
a) Na^+ b) K^+
c) NO_3^- d) Ca^{2+}

350. Hybrid and non-hybrid kinases are groups of
a) Serine/threonine kinases b) Receptor tyrosine kinases
c) Cytosolic tyrosine kinases d) Histidine kinases

351. Purinoceptors are found in
a) *Drosophila* b) *Caenorhabditis elegans*
c) *Arabidopsis* d) *Dictyostelium*

352. Lactose permease which transports lactose across the plasma membrane of *E. coli* is
a) Na^+-driven antiporter b) H^+-driven antiporter
c) Na^+-driven symporter d) H^+-driven symporter

353. Which of the following glucose transporter is expressed usually only in neurons?
a) GLUT 1 b) GLUT 3
c) GLUT 4 d) GLUT 5

354. The molecular motor myosin uses the molecular track which is a polymeric form of
a) Tubulin b) Actin
c) Glycoproteins d) Collagen

355. When a repellant binds to receptor in the plasma membrane of bacteria it
a) Increases concentration of phosphorylated Che Y
b) Decreases concentration of phosphorylated Che Y
c) Inactivates Che A
d) Causes smooth swimming

356. Which of the following is NOT a peripheral protein of RBC
a) Ankyrin b) Spectrin
c) Glycophorin d) Demantin

357. The venom of black Mamba snake interferes with
a) Na^+-ion channels b) K^+ -ion channels
c) Na^+/K^+-pump d) Ca^{2+}-pump

358. Antibiotic rifampicin inhibits the transcription of bacterial RNA. It especially
a) Prevents binding of RNA polymerase to the promoter
b) Inhibits initiation of transcription
c) Inhibits elongation of transcription
d) Inhibits backtracking of RNA polymerase that is very important for proofreading

359. Which of the following enzyme is NOT essential for the activation of M phase kinase?
a) CAK b) Weel Kinase
c) Cdc25 phosphatase d) ATM kinase

360. Which of the following monomeric G-protein is involved in anaphase to telophase progression during cell division?
a) Rac b) Rho
c) Tem1 d) Ras

361. Telomerase is an enzyme that is involved in the end replication of eukaryotic chromosomes. It is a
a) Template independent RNA polymerase
b) Template independent DNA polymerase
c) Template dependent RNA polymerase
d) Template dependent DNA polymerase

362. When cells divide newly synthesized S phase histones H3 and H4 are marked by
a) Methylation b) Acetylation
c) ADP-ribosylation d) Phosphorylation

363. Caspases are proteolytic enzymes which are involved in programmed cell death. Their active sites contain
a) Serine residue b) Cystein residue
c) Cystein-histidine dyad d) Arginine residue

364. CENP-A is a histone protein which is found in the nucleosomes of the centromeric region of humans. Cells that lack CENP-A fails to recruit most known kinetochore components to the kinetochore. CENP-A is a
a) Histon H2A variant b) Histone H3 variant
c) Histone H1variant d) Histone H4 variant

365. Which of the following amino acid in the histone tails are the most common targets of covalent modification during chromatin remodeling?
a) Lysine b) Arginine
c) Serine d) Threonine

366. Genes for which of the following protein complexes are found in the chloroplast genome?
a) Photosystem protein complexes
b) Small ribosomal subunit
c) Light harvesting complex
d) None of the above

367. Cholera toxin molecule binds with
a) GM1 ganglioside b) GM2 ganglioside
c) GM3 ganglioside d) Ceramide

368. Which of the following does not correctly matched
a) Arf - vesicle trafficking
b) Rab - vesicle budding, vesicle targeting and vesicle fusion
c) Rho - cytoskeleton regulation
d) Ran - Cdc42 signaling

369. Adenylate cyclase is a transmembrane enzyme but it is also present in the cytosol of
a) Eggs b) Sperms
c) Muscle cells d) Cancer cells

370. How many molecules of cAMP are required to activate PKA?
a) 1 b) 2
c) 4 d) 8

371. Chloroplast membrane consists of
a) Sulpholipid
b) Galactolipid
c) Glyceroglycolipid
d) All of the above

372. Phospholipids and sphingolipids are degraded by
a) Lysosome
b) Vacuole
c) Proteasome
d) Both (a) and (b)

373. Which of the following is incorrect?
a) PKC is a membrane bound enzyme activated by DAG and Ca^{++}.
b) Somatostatin receptor leads to activation of stimulatory G protein.
c) Cholera toxin has ADP ribosyltransferase activity which inhibit the $Gs\alpha$ subunit.
d) Growth hormones act via tyrosine kinase associated receptors.

374. Protein disulphide isomerase is located in
a) ER lumen
b) ER membrane
c) Golgi body membrane
d) Golgi body lumen

375. Which is not true for vesicle transport?
a) Arf proteins are responsible for COP I and clathrin coat assembly at golgi membranes.
b) Sar 1 proteins are responsible for COP II coat assembly at the ER membrane.
c) Vesicular transport specificity is maintained by Rab proteins.
d) Sar 1 proteins are responsible for the COP II and clathrin coat assembly at the ER membrane.

376. Which is not the characteristic feature of CAK?
a) Phosphorylates threonine-161
b) Made up of Cdk 7 and cyclin H
c) Involved in the transcription coupled DNA repair
d) None of the above

377. Cohesin proteins are proteolytically cleaved by
a) APC
b) Securin
c) Separase
d) Proteasome

378. Mitogen associated protein kinase is a
a) G protein linked kinase
b) Tyrosine kinase
c) Serine/threonine kinase
d) Histidine associated kinase

379. If Fms protein is mutated it causes cancer. This proteins is
a) Epidermal growth factor
b) Epidermal growth factor receptor
c) Nerve growth factor receptor
d) Fibroblast growth factor receptor

380. Which of the following is the mode of action of Maspin
   a) It inhibits angiogenesis
   b) It inhibits cell cycle
   c) It activates DNA repair pathway
   d) All of the above

381. BCl2 gene mutation causes
   a) Restriction of cytochrome C transportation
   b) Inhibition of APAF-1
   c) Formation of Bax and Bid
   d) All of the above

382. Phospholipase A is secreted in
   a) Tears b) Sweat
   c) Urine d) All of the above

383. Pemphigus is a autoimmune disease in which the patient has developed anti-bodies against
   a) Integrin b) Cadherin
   c) Catenin d) Aggregin

384. Saxitoxin blocks
   a) Na^+ channel b) Na^+/K^+ pump
   c) K^+ channel d) H+ pump

385. Allolactose is a inducer which activates lac operon. It is formed by the enzyme
   a) β-galactosidase b) β-galactoside permease
   c) Galactoside transacetylase d) Imported from outside of the cell

386. Selfish DNA is
   a) Nuclear DNA b) mtDNA
   c) cpDNA d) Transposons

387. Proteins having NLS sequence are destined for
   a) Mitochondria b) Chloroplast
   c) Nucleus d) ER

388. Protamines are present in
   a) Chick embryo b) Sperm
   c) *Arabidopsis thaliana* d) *Sacchromyces pombi*

389. Cyclosome is
   a) Anaphase promoting complex
   b) Proteasomal assembly
   c) Phagolysosome
   d) Apoptosome assembly

390. Spindle assembly checkpoint works at
   a) G2/M transition
   b) Metaphase to anaphase transition
   c) Anaphase to telophase transition
   d) Restriction point

391. MAD2 protein inhibits
   a) Microtubule attachment   b) Cyclin protein
   c) CAK   d) APC

392. In sea urchin block to polyspermy signaling is mediated by
   a) cAMP   b) PIP2
   c) Histidine kinase   d) Tyrosine kinase

393. Ca^{++} binding protein is/are
   a) Troponin   b) Selectins
   c) Recoverin   d) All of the above

394. Signaling of olfaction in vertebrate is mediated by
   a) Transducin   b) Gustducin
   c) Arrestin   d) Recoverin

395. Integrin plays important role in
   a) Blood clotting   b) Angiogenesis
   c) Tumor metastasis   d) All of the above

396. Cystic fibrosis is a hereditary disease of humans, in this disease defect occurs in
   a) Na^{+} channel   b) K^{+} channel
   c) Ca^{++} channel   d) Cl^{-} channel

397. Adenine nucleotide antiporter is located in
   a) Nuclear membrane
   b) Mitochondrial outer membrane
   c) Mitochondrial inner membrane
   d) All of the above

398. The molecular motor myosins move along
   a) Microfilaments   b) Intermediate filaments
   c) Microtubules   d) Kinesins and dyneins

399. CDKs are controlled through
   a) Cyclin protein degradation
   b) Phosphorylation and dephosphorylation
   c) Binding of inhibitory proteins
   d) All of the above

400. Enzyme which is involved in the movement of phospholipid across the membrane down its concentration gradient are
   a) Flippases b) Floppases
   c) Scrumblases d) Both (a) and (b)

401. Ionophores are
   a) Lipid soluble molecules b) Disrupts electrochemical gradient
   c) Can act as antibiotics d) All of the above

402. p53gene product is a
   a) ATM/ATR serine kinase b) Serine - Threonine kinase
   c) Tyrosine kinase d) Histidine associated kinase

403. The enzyme which is involved in transportation of phospholipids and belongs to the P-type ATPase family is
   a) Flippase b) Floppase
   c) Scrumblase d) All of the above

404. Aurovertin inhibits
   a) ATP synthase
   b) Cytochrome oxidase
   c) Cytochrome C oxidoreductase
   d) Succinate dehydrogenase

405. Glycerol-dialkyl-glycerol tetraethers (GDGTs), are a unique membrane lipids present in
   a) Archaebacteria b) Prokaryote
   c) Eukaryote d) Archaebacteria and Eukaryote

406. NADPH-cytochrome c reductase is a marker enzyme of
   a) Endoplasmic reticulum b) Golgi body
   c) Chloroplast d) Mitochondria

407. Glyoxalate cycle occurs in
   a) Prokaryote b) Prokaryotes and plant
   c) Plant and animals d) All of the above

408. Gap junctions are made up of
   a) Connexins b) Pannexins
   c) Occludin d) Both (a) and (b)

409. ATP synthase is
   a) P type ATPase b) V type ATPase
   c) F type ATPase d) ABC transporter

410. Periplasmic space of bacteria is analogous to
a) Lysosome b) Golgi body
c) Glyoxysome d) Peroxisome

411. Dephosphorylating enzyme which activate CdK1 is
a) CAK (CdK activating kinase)
b) Wee 1
c) Myt 1
d) Cdc25C

412. The plasma membrane of altered cells is rich in
a) Na^+/K^+ pump b) Aquaporins
c) ABC transporters d) Cl^- ion channels

413. Which of the following regulates the size of gap junctions in animal cell
a) cAMP b) Ca^{++}
c) Connexins d) All of the above

414. Which cellular component is considered to be a nano?
a) Lipids b) Ribosomes
c) DNA d) mRNA

415. Which protein regulates the cell cycle by monitoring the environment of each stage and making sure the previous cycle is complete?
a) Cyclin-dependent kinases b) E2F
c) Cyclins d) p53

416. Sister chromatids separate during anaphase of mitosis, when the separase enzyme proteolytically cleaved the cohesin subunit
a) Smc1 b) Smc 3
c) Scc 3 d) α-klesin subunit (Scc1)

417. Cohesin is essential for sister chromatid cohesion. A loss of function in Scc1 results in.
a) Premature sister separation.
b) Sister chromatid not separated
c) Don't cause defect because the α-kleisin Rec 8 replaces Scc1 in meiotic cohesion complexes.
d) Don't cause defect because Scc3 replaces Scc1.

418. Separase enzyme is
a) Tyrosine protease b) Serine protease
c) Cysteine protease d) Aspartate protease

419. Microtubule nucleation is regulated by the γ-tubulin ring complex (γTuRC). Which of the following protein bind or activate γ-tubulin complexes
a) pericentrin b) ninein
c) CG-NAP and CEP 192 d) all of the above

420. Microtubule catastrophe is
   a) rapid polymerization of microtubules.
   b) rapid depolymerization of microtubules that occurs when GTP has been hydrolysed in all tubulin subunit.
   c) disassembly of TuRC.
   d) disassociation of mitotic-spindle organizing protein from a ring of tubulin 1.

421. Actin polymerization and depolymerization is meadiated by small GTPases, named
   a) Rho b) Rac
   c) Cdc-42 d) All of the above

422. Which of the following is not the cell-cell adhesion molecule?
   a) E-cadherin b) E-selectin
   c) Fibronectin d) VCAM-1

423. Measurement and mapping with spatial resolution the membrane potential of a cell, which is too small for microelectrode impalement, is done using
   a) radioisotope b) voltage-sensitive dye
   c) pH sensitive chemical d) vital dyes

[CSIR (NET/JRF) Exam. Dec. 2011]

424. In contrast with plant cells, the most distinctive feature of cell division in animal cells is
   a) control of cell cycle transitions by protein kinases
   b) enzymes responsible for DNA replication
   c) ubiquitin-dependent pathway for protein degradation
   d) pattern of chromosome movement.

[CSIR (NET/JRF) Exam. Dec. 2011]

425. The membrane lipid molecules assemble spontaneously into bilayers when placed in water and form a closed spherical structure known as
   a) lysosome b) peroxisome
   c) liposome d) endosome

[CSIR (NET/JRF) Exam. Dec. 2011]

426. Most common type of phospholipids in the cell membrane of nerve cells is
   a) phosphatidylcholine b) phosphatidylinositol
   c) phosphatidylserine d) sphingomyelin

[CSIR (NET/JRF) Exam. Dec. 2011]

427. Which of the following is not mediated by ABC transporter?
   a) Transport of inorganic ions
   b) Vitamin B_{12} transport across the membrane in bacteria

c) Biogenesis of cytochrome c enzyme
d) PO_4^{-2} transport in plant root cells

428. In estuaries, plants are generally halophytes. For maintaining their osmoticum they use
a) Na^+ - H^+ symporter
b) Na^+/K^+ pump
c) Na^+ - K^+ - $2Cl^-$ transporter
d) Na^+ - H^+ antiporter

429. The trap door mechanism model explains the gating of
a) Voltage gated ion channel
b) Mechanosensitive channels
c) Ligand gated channels
d) Aquaporis

430. Sphingosine-1-phosphate is a second messenger generated from sphingosine by sphingosine kinase which is present in
a) Plasma membrane
b) Mitochondria
c) Lysosome
d) Endoplasmic Reticulum

431. In the fission Yeast which reproduce by elongating itself and then splitting into two equal-sized cells, Cdc25 phosphatase is mutated. What result would you expect?
a) Yeast cell divides prematurely.
b) Yeast cell divides continuously.
c) Yeast cell does not divide.
d) Yeast cell does not divide but continues to grow.

432. Glycosyl transferases are the enzymes which are involved in the glycosylation of secretory proteins. If the genes encoding these enzymes are mutated and produce altered enzymes then what would not be the effect of these mutations?
a) Cell - cell interaction is affected.
b) Stability of some essential proteins is reduced.
c) Cells divide rapidly.
d) Development of embryos is affected.

433. Which of the following statement is not correct?
a) Insulin regulates GLUT-4 transporters that actively transport glucose from blood into the cells.
b) Glycine opens Cl- ion channels.
c) Proteases involved in cell death are cystein rich.
d) Sialic acid is not found in plant cell membrane.

434. Transport of water across aquaporins is regulated by the presence of which of the following sequence of three highly conserved amino acids?
a) Ala-Asn-Pro.
b) Pro-Asn-Ala.
c) Asn-Pro-Ala.
d) Pro-Ala-Asn.

[CSIR (NET/JRF) Exam. June 2011]

435. Which of the cyclin has essential functions in S-phase of cell cycle?
a) A-type. b) B-type.
c) D-type. d) Both B- and D-types.
[CSIR (NET/JRF) Exam. June 2011]

436. With which protein of Yersinia would integrin proteins of mammalian cells interact for internalization?
a) Pilin b) Fimbrin
c) Invasin d) Adherin
[CSIR (NET/JRF) Exam. June 2011]

437. G protein-linked receptors are transmembrane proteins of
a) single-pass b) three-pass
c) five-pass d) seven-pass
[CSIR (NET/JRF) Exam. June 2011]

438. Which of the following molecules is involved in Ca^{++}-dependent cell-cell adhesion?
a) Calmodulin b) Cadherin
c) N-CAM d) Calpain
[CSIR (NET/JRF) Exam. June 2011]

439. Both halophytes and glycophytes compartmentalize cytotoxic ions into the intracellular comparment or actively pump them out of the cell to the apoplasts with the help of membrane transport proteins. Among these, the Na^+-H^+ antiporter, NHX1, is localized in the
a) plasma membrane.
b) chloroplast (inner envelope).
c) mitochondria (outer membrane).
d) tonoplast. **[CSIR (NET/JRF) Exam. June 2011]**

440. Na^+-K^+ ATPase is a tetramer of 2 α and 2 β subunits. On which of the followingsubunits are the Na^+ and K^+ binding sites present?
a) both on α b) both on β
c) Na^+ on β and K^+ on α d) Na^+ on and K^+ on
[CSIR (NET/JRF) Exam. June 2011]

441. Which of the following protein acts as an energy transducer?
a) G-protein. b) Bacteriorhodopsin.
c) Hemoglobin. d) Heat shock protein.
[CSIR Model Paper 2011]

442. Which of the following predicted property of lipid bilayers would result if the phospholipids had only one hydrocarbon chain instead of two?

a) The bilayers formed would be much less fluid.
b) The diameter of the head group would be much larger than the acyl chain and would tend to form micelles rather than bilayers.
c) the bilayers formed would be much more fluid.
d) the bilayers would be more permeable to small water-soluble molecules.

[CSIR Model Paper 2011]

443. Which of the following signaling molecule enters the cell to initiate its action?

a) Transferrin b) Insulin
c) Glucagon d) Thyroxine

[CSIR Model Paper 2011]

444. Due to the presence of cellulose in the cell wall of plants, leaf shape is determined in the leaf primorida by

a) rates of cell division. b) planes of cell division.
c) cell migration. d) cell-cell interactions.

[CSIR Model Paper 2011]

Part C

1. Studies in mice and other organisms revealed that there is a significant functional overlap between the Cdks, with one Cdk being able to compensate for another that has been deleted. The exception which is essential for viability is
   a) Cdk 4 b) Cdk 2
   c) Cdk 1 d) Cdk 6
2. Bacteria growing in nutrient-rich growth media tend to be larger than those grown in nutrient-poor media. In *Bacillus subtilis*, cell division is inhibited by a metabolic pathway that senses the amount of available glucose: under rich growth conditions, where glucose is abundant, an enzyme called Ugt P localizes to cell midline and inhibits cell division, thereby forcing the cell to reach a larger size before the cell divides. Ugt P specifically inhibits the assembly of Fts Z, a protein that is needed for
   a) Cell division b) Chromosome segregation
   c) DNA supercoiling d) Multifork replication
3. Certain staining techniques cause the chromosome to have the appearance of a series of striations which are called G-bands. These G-bands are
   a) Lower in G-C content and transcriptionly active
   b) Rich in G-C content and transcriptionly active
   c) Lower in A-T content and transcriptionly active
   d) Rich in A-T content and transcriptionly active
4. Condensin and cohesin are subject to dynamic mechanisms of regulation that differ throughout the cell cycle and are regulated by post-transcriptional modifications. The following statements are related with this
   (A) Cohesin is estabilished by the acetyltransferase Eco-1, which acetylates at two lysine residues in the structural maintenance of chromosome 3 (Smc 3) head region.
   (B) Cdc5 (polo kinase)-dependent phosphorylation promote α-kleisin subunit (Scc 1/Rec 8) cleavage by separase.
   (C) Cdc2 and Aurora B kinase phosphaylate all three non-SMC (Structural maintenance protein) subunits of condensin I and are required for casdensin-I loading and super coiling of chromosome.
   (D) Aurora B kinase control the association of condensin-II with mitotic chromosome.

   Which of the following combination is correct?
   a) A and B b) A, B and C
   c) B C and D d) A, B, C and D

5. The α-tubulin and β-tubulin heterodimer is the fundamental repeating subunit of microtubules, when bound to GTP heterodimers come together. Read the following statements
   (A) Positive end of microtubule is made up of β-tubulin and negative end is made up of α-tubulin.
   (B) In 13-protofilament microtubules, a 'seam' is formed as a result of lateral α-tubulin- β-tubulin interactions.
   (C) A microtubule organizing centres (MTOCs) rely on γ-tubulin, a homologue of α-tubulin and β-tubulin, for nucleating microtubules.
   (D) γ-tubulin is nearly ubiquitous throughout the eukaryotes.
   Which of the following is correct?
   a) A and C b) A, B and C
   c) A, B and D d) A, B, C and D

6. The erythrocyte membrane cytoskeleton consists of a meshwork of proteins underlying the membrane. The principal component spectrin has , subunits which assemble to form tetramers. The cytoskeleton is anchored to the membrane through linkages with the transmembrane proteins band 3 and glycophorin C. The cytosolic domain of band 3 also serves as the binding site of glycolytic enzymes such as glyceraldehyde-3-phosphate dehydrogenase. Analysis of the blood sample of a patient with haemolytic anemia shows spherical red blood cells. The patient carries
   a) a mutation in glycophorin C.
   b) a mutant spectrin with increased tetramerization propensity.
   c) mutant β spectrin defective in αβ dimerization ability.
   d) mutant glyceraldehydes 3-phosphate dehydrogenase.

[CSIR (NET/JRF) Exam. Dec. 2011]

7. Synthesis of normal hemoglobin requires coordinated synthesis of globin globin. Thalassemias are genetic defects perturbed in this coordinated synthesis. Patients suffering from deficiency of globin chains (β-thalassemia) could also be due to mutations affecting the biosynthesis of β globin mRNA.

   The following statements describe the genesis of non-functional globin leading to β-thalassemia.
   A. Mutation in the promoter region of the β globin gene.
   B. Mutation in the splice junction of the β globin gene.
   C. Mutation in the intron I of the β globin gene.
   D. Mutation towards the 3' end of the β globin gene that codes for polyadenylation site.
   Which of the following combinations is correct?
   a) A, B and D b) A, B and C
   c) B, C and D d) C, D and A

[CSIR (NET/JRF) Exam. Dec. 2011]

8. Maturation-promoting factor (MPF) controls the initiation of mitosis in eukaryotic cells. MPF kinase activity requires cyclin B. Cyclin B is required for chromosome condensation and breakdown of the nuclear envelope into vesicles. Cyclin B degradation is followed by chromosome decondensation, nuclear envelope reformation and exit from mitosis. This requires ubiquitination of a cyclin destruction box motif in cyclin B. RNase-treated Xenopus egg extracts and sperm chromatin were mixed. MPF activity increased with chromosome condensation and nuclear envelope breakdown. However, this was not followed by chromosome decondensation and nuclear envelope reformation because
   a) RNase contamination persisted in the system
   b) cyclin B was missing from the system.
   c) ubiquitin ligase had been overexpressed.
   d) cyclin B lacking the cyclin destruction box had been overexpressed.

[CSIR (NET/JRF) Exam. Dec. 2011]

9. The bacterial flagellar motor is a multi-protein complex. Rotation of the flagellum requires movement of protons across the membrane facilitated by a multi-protein complex. The flagellar motor proteins combine to create a proton channel that drives mechanical rotation. In a screen for mutants, some non-motile ones were selected. These could have
   a) mutations in tubulin and actin proteins
   b) mutations in kinesin proteins
   c) mutated H+-ATPase.
   d) mutations in the charged residues lining the ridge of the FliG subunit.

[CSIR (NET/JRF) Exam. Dec. 2011]

10. Intracellular transport and cytoskeletal organization of a cell is regulated by nucleotide exchange of different small molecular weight GTPases of Ras super family. Overexpression of which of the following GTPase modulates the actin-cytoskeleton of HeLa cells?
   a) Ran in GDP bound form
   b) Ran in GTP bound form
   c) Rho in GTP bound form
   d) Rho in GDP bound form **[CSIR (NET/JRF) Exam. Dec. 2011]**

11. Tumor cells were isolated from a breast cancer patient. These cells were injected into nude mice and they were divided into four groups. Group 1 received EGF receptor-conjugated with methotrexate; Group 2 received transferrin receptor-conjugated with methotrexate; Group 3 received mannose receptor-conjugated with methotrexate; Group 4 received same amount of the free drug. In which of the following cases tumorigenic index would be minimum?

a) Free drug
b) EGF receptor-conjugated drug
c) Transferrin receptor-conjugated drug
d) Mannose receptor-conjugated drug

[CSIR (NET/JRF) Exam. Dec. 2011]

12. Proteins imported into mitochondria are usually taken up from the cytosol within seconds or minutes of their release from ribosomes. Which of the following statements is NOT correct:
    a) The signal sequences that direct precursor proteins into the mitochondrial matrix space form an amphiphilic a helix rather than the precise amino acid sequence of the signal sequence.
    b) The TOM complex transfers proteins across the outer membrane.
    c) TIM complexes transfer proteins across the inner membrane and it uses ATP.
    d) The TOM complex is required for the import of all nucleus-encoded mitochondrial proteins.

13. The lipid bilayer provides the basic structure for all cell membranes. Following statements relate to some characteristic features of plasma membrane of a living cell.
    (A) They are thought of as two two-dimensional fluids because the lipids, along with other molecules in the membrane, can diffuse quite rapidly within each plane of the bilayer.
    (B) Lipid asymmetry is functionally important, especially in converting extracellular signals into intracellular ones.
    (C) Animal exploit the phospholipid asymmetry of their plasma membrane to distinguish between live and dead cells.
    (D) Like most membrane lipids, membrane proteins can flip-flop across the lipid bilayer.

    Which of the following is NOT correct?
    a) A and C   b) Only C
    c) B and D   d) Only D

14. ABC transporters constitute the largest family of membrane transport proteins. Following are some of the statements regarding ABC transporters.
    (A) They contain two transmembrane domains and two ATP binding domains.
    (B) ATP binding leads to dimerization of the two ATP binding domains.
    (C) Most ABC transporters are unidirectional. But, both importing and exporting ABC transporters are found in eukaryotes.
    (D) The stoichiometry of ABC pumps is about one ATP hydrolyzed per molecule of substrate transported.

Which one of following conbinations of above statements is true?

a) A and D b) B and C
c) A and B d) C and D

15. The SCF ubiquitin ligase complex catalyzes ubiquitination of proteins that regulates the transition from G1 into S phase whereas APC ubiquitin ligase catalyzes the ubiquitination of proteins that drives anaphase and mitotic exit. SCF and APC ligases are involved in proteasome-mediated protein degradation. The protein destruction properties of these ligases differ in relation to
    (A) The SCF ubiquitin ligase complex catalyses ubiquitination of phosphorylated proteins.
    (B) The APC ligase requires F-box protein which determines the substrate specificity.
    (C) SCF ligases have RING domain while APC ligases do not have.
    (D) Substrate specificity of APC ligase is determined by its activator subunits Cdc20 and Cdh1.

    The correct statements are
    a) A and C b) B an D
    c) A, B and D d) A and D

16. Epinephrin signaling begins with ligand binding to a protein called the ß-adrenergic receptor which is an example of GPCR. Following are some statements for GPCR.
    (A) They constitute the second largest class of cell-surface receptors.
    (B) The N- terminal end of these receptors is on the exterior face of the plasma membrane, whereas the C-terminal end is on the inside.
    (C) Receptor phosphorylation on their C-terminal domain creates a binding site for the protein Arrestin.
    (D) Phosphorylated receptor is sensitized even while the signal is absent.

    Which one of the following combinations of the above statements is true?
    a) A and D b) A and C
    c) B and C d) B and D

17. During receptor-mediated endocytosis, apolipoprotein B on the surface of a LDL particle binds to the LDL-receptor present in coated pits containing clathrin. The receptor-LDL complex is internalized by endocytosis, trafficked to lysosomes and the LDL-receptor is finally recycled. A patient reports with familial hypercholesterolemia. This could be due to
    a) mutation in the LDL molecule.
    b) defect in LDL-receptor recycling.
    c) mutation in the LDL-receptor.
    d) defect in cholesterol binding with its receptor.

[CSIR (NET/JRF) Exam. June 2011]

18. Eukaryotic genomes are organized into chromosomes and can be visualized at mitosis by staining with specific dyes. Heat denaturation followed by staining with Giemsa produced alternate dark and light bands. The dark bands obtained by this process are mainly
   a) AT-rich and gene rich regions.
   b) AT-rich and gene desert regions.
   c) GC-rich and gene rich regions.
   d) GC-rich and gene desert regions. **[CSIR (NET/JRF) Exam. June 2011]**

19. Budding yeast cells that are deficient for Mad2, a component of the spindle-attachment-check point, are killed by treatment with benomyl, which causes microtubles to depolymerise. In the absence of benomyl, however, the cells are perfectly viable. Which explanation out of the following is able to justify this observation?
   a) In the absence of benomyl, the majority of spindles form normally and the spindle-attachment checkpoint (Mad2) plays no role.
   b) In the presence of benomyl, the majority of spindles form normally and Mad2 plays critical role in cell survival.
   c) Other than the role in cell survival, microtuble depolymerization affects oxidative phosphorylation in the absence of Mad2.
   d) Benomyl also affects protein synthesis in the absence of Mad2.
   [CSIR (NET/JRF) Exam. June 2011]

20. Cancer causing gene can be functionally classified into mainly three types: (i) genes that induce cellular proliferation, (ii) tumor suppressor genes, (iii) genes that regulate apoptotic pathway.
   Epstein-Barr virus that causes cancer by modulating apoptotic pathway, con tainsa gene having sequence homology with which of the following genes?
   a) bax
   b) bcl-2
   c) p53
   d) caspase-3
   [CSIR (NET/JRF) Exam. June 2011]

21. Based on the structural regions of a nuclear receptor shown in the diagram, the following predictions were made.

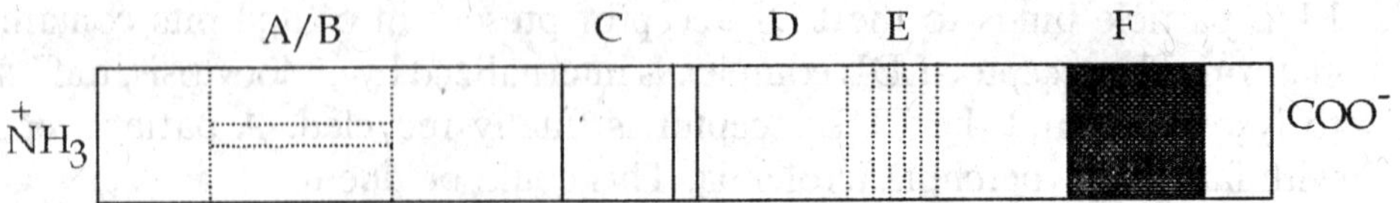

   A. Region F is responsible for binding to ligands and contains two zinc-finger-like binding motifs.

B. Receptors with A/B domains generally associate with chaperones and do not bind to DNA.
C. Region E indicate that receptors associate with chaperones which protect the nuclear hormone receptors.
D. Region C contains the P-box and the D-box required for dimerization of the receptor and creates contact with DNA phosphate backbone.

Which one of the following is true?

a) A and B b) B and C
c) B and D d) C and D

[CSIR (NET/JRF) Exam. June 2011]

22. Glucose is mobilized in muscle when epinephrine activates Gs. In an experiment in which muscle cells were stimulated with epinephrine, glucose mobilization was observed even after withdrawal of epinephrine. This could be
a) due to the presence of a cAMP phosphodiesterase inhibitor.
b) very low rates of cyclic AMP formation.
c) due to the presence of a cAMP phosphodiesterase activator.
d) due to the absence of protein kinase A.

[CSIR (NET/JRF) Exam. June 2011]

23. During many important cell processes, many proteins need to undergo degradation to culminate a part of the process. For example, during cell cycle, cycling proteins need to be degraded to allow the cells to exit mitosis. This is achieved by selective ubiquitination of cyclin followed by its degradation by proteasomes. The specific protein factor that is involved in this process is called Anaphase Promoting Complex (APC). APC is possibly a protein which is known as
a) El enzyme. b) E2 enzyme.
c) E3 enzyme. d) Protease. **[CSIR Model Paper 2011]**

24. Two protein kinases, Kl and K2 function sequentially in regulating intracellular pathway in response to extracellular signal. The following observations are made:
(i) Response is observed even in the absence of extracellular signal when a mutation permanently activates Kl.
(ii) Response is observed even in the absence of extracellular signal when Kl contains an activating mutation and K2 with inactivating mutation.
(iii) No response in the cells is detected even in the presence of extracellular signal when both kinases are inactivated by mutation.

Which one of the following is correct?

a) Kl activates K2 b) K2 activates Kl
c) Kl inhibits K2 d) K2 inhibits Kl

[CSIR Model Paper 2011]

25. When oxygen is plentiful, cells convert glucose to energy through the consecutive processes of glycolysis and oxidative respiration. However cancer cells prefer the much less efficient process of glucose fermentation of energy production even in the presence of oxygen. This seems counter-intuitive because rapid cell proliferation, which is required for tumour growth, has high energetic demands. Due to this why cancer cells under go this metabolic shift?
    A. To prevent ROS formation from oxidative respiration.
    B. Decreased catalytic activity of pyruvate kinase is associated with tumor progression and leads to activation of a pentose phosphate pathway.
    C. The glycolytic enzyme pyruvate kinase facilitates tumor growth by preventing accumulation of ROS.
    a) Only A	b) A and B
    c) A and C	d) A, B and C

26. Platelets are miniature cells without a nucleus. They circulate in the blood and help to stimulate blood clotting at sites of tissue damage, there by preventing excessive bleeding. Platelet cell secrete a signaling protein called TGF-β. Following statements correlate with TGF- β protein.
    A. inhibits the proliferation of cells either by blocking cell-cycle progression in G1 or by stimulating apoptosis.
    B. TGF-β activates NFkB protein of cancer cell surface, and make the cell more invasive.
    C. TGF-β controls organ size by inhibiting cell growth and promoting cell death.
    D. TGF-β blocks periostin protein of cancer cell, prevents metastasis.
    Which of the following combination is correct?
    a) A and B	b) A and C
    c) A, C and D	d Only B.

27. Proteins imported into mitochondria are usually taken up from the cytosol within seconds or minutes of their release from ribosomes. Some statements are given below related to mitochondrial protein transport.
    A. Proteins entering the matrix space contain a signal sequence at their N-terminus that a signal peptidase rapidly removes after import.
    B. TOM complex transfers protein across the outer membrane.
    C. TIM complex transfers protein outer membrane to inner membrane.
    D. SAM complex mediates the insertion of inner membrane proteins that are synthesized by mitochondria.
    Which of the following is correct?
    a) A and B	b) B and C
    c) B, C and D	d) A, B and C

28. Cytokine is an extracellular signal protein or peptide that acts as a local mediator in cell-cell communication. It acts through cytokine receptor present in plasma membrane.
Following statements correlate with cytokine signaling
A. Cytokine receptors are associated with Janus kinases (JAKs)
B. JAKs cis-phosphorylate each other on tyrosine.
C. STATs proteins are located in the cytosol, dimerizes when phosphorylated by JAKs.
D. STAT proteins referred to as latent gene regulatory proteins because they only migrate into the nucleus and regulate gene transcription after they are activated.
Which of the following is correct?
a) A, C and D b) B, C and D
c) A and C d) A, B, C and D

29. Endocytosis is the primary mechanism for the specific internalization of most macromolecules by eukaryotic cell. Some explanations of endocytosis are given below
A. Endocytosis regulates cell signaling most simply by controlling the number of receptors available for activation in the plasma membrane.
B. The endocytosis of many signaling receptors is stimulated by ligand induced activation.
C. b-arrestin bind to phosphatidylinositol-4,5 bis phosphate (PIP2), which promotes the plasma membrane recruitment of b-arrrestins and decreases the endocytic activity.
D. Membrane receptors are sorted to recycling and endosomal pathways in the same way as other endocytic cargo.
Which of the following is not correct?
a) A and C b) B and C
c) Only C d) A and D

30. The internalization of receptors, lipid membranes and extracellular fluid at the plasma membrane of higher eukaryotes is carried out by various endocytic trafficking pathways. Following are some statements regarding endocytosis.
A. Retrograde movement of vesicles from early endosome to endoplasmic reticulum or towards lysosome is mediated by dynein-dynactin complex.
B. The movement of early endosome from center of the cell to the cell periphery is mediated by plus-end directed myosin motor proteins.
C. COP-II coat assembly at the ER membrane is mediated by Arf monomeric GTPases proteins.
D. Rabs are small GTP-binding proteins that carry out multiple roles in endocytic trafficking, vesicle tethering, fusion, budding and motility.

Which of the following combination is true?

a) A, B and C
b) A, C and D
c) A and D
d) Only D

31. Gangliosides are glycolipids having one or more sialic acid residues in its structure, found in the plasma membrane of eukaryotic cells. However, mutant mice that are deficient in all of their complex gangliosides

A. Show no obvious abnormalities.
B. Males cannot transport testosterone normally in testes and are consequently sterile
C. Cholera toxin infects easily to intestinal epithelial cells.
D. Their absence alters the electrical field across the membrane.

Which of the following is correct?

a) A and B
b) Only A
c) C and D
d) A, B and D

32. The mitochondria-mediated pathway of apoptosis involves the alteration of mitochondrial membrane permeability and activation of the casapases. Caspases are responsible for diverse cellular function including inflammation and apoptosis.

Following are some statements regarding mitochondria-mediated apoptosis.

A. Caspases cleaves substrates on the carboxyl side of aspartate residue.
B. Initiator caspases function upstream within apoptotic signaling pathways.
C. Initiator caspases are capable of activating downstream effectors caspases either directly, through proteolysis, or indirectly via a secondary messenger mechanism.
D. Apoptosis partly depend on the decreasement of Bax/Bcl-2 protein ratio.

Which of the following combination is correct?

a) A and C
b) A, B and C
c) B, C and D
d) A, C and D

Answer Sheet

Part – B

1.	c	2.	c	3.	d	4.	d	5.	d	6.	b
7.	b	8.	d	9.	a	10.	b	11.	a	12.	a
13.	c	14.	c	15.	c	16.	d	17.	d	18.	b
19.	a	20.	a	21.	b	22.	c	23.	d	24.	d
25.	a	26.	a	27.	d	28.	c	29.	a	30.	b
31.	c	32.	d	33.	a	34.	d	35.	b	36.	a
37.	a	38.	c	39.	b	40.	d	41.	b	42.	d
43.	a	44.	d	45.	b	46.	b	47.	d	48.	b
49.	a	50.	d	51.	a	52.	c	53.	b	54.	b
55.	a	56.	a	57.	d	58.	b	59.	c	60.	c
61.	b	62.	b	63.	c	64.	c	65.	c	66.	b
67.	c	68.	a	69.	a	70.	d	71.	a	72.	c
73.	d	74.	c	75.	a	76.	b	77.	d	78.	b
79.	d	80.	b	81.	d	82.	a	83.	a	84.	c
85.	a	86.	d	87.	a	88.	c	89.	c	90.	b
91.	c	92.	d	93.	c	94.	a	95.	c	96.	c
97.	b	98.	b	99.	b	100.	b	101.	b	102.	c
103.	d	104.	b	105.	d	106.	c	107.	c	108.	c
109.	d	110.	a	111.	c	112.	b	113.	c	114.	d
115.	b	116.	d	117.	b	118.	b	119.	b	120.	c
121.	c	122.	b	123.	b	124.	b	125.	d	126.	c
127.	c	128.	d	129.	b	130.	c	131.	d	132.	c
133.	c	134.	a	135.	b	136.	d	137.	c	138.	a
139.	b	140.	d	141.	c	142.	b	143.	c	144.	d
145.	d	146.	b	147.	c	148.	d	149.	c	150.	c
151.	d	152.	c	153.	c	154.	d	155.	a	156.	a
157.	b	158.	c	159.	c	160.	b	161.	c	162.	c
163.	b	164.	a	165.	b	166.	c	167.	a	168.	a
169.	c	170.	b	171.	b	172.	c	173.	d	174.	a
175.	b	176.	b	177.	d	178.	d	179.	b	180.	c
181.	d	182.	d	183.	c	184.	c	185.	d	186.	c
187.	c	188.	c	189.	d	190.	c	191.	d	192.	a
193.	a	194.	c	195.	b	196.	c	197.	b	198.	b
199.	c	200.	c	201.	d	202.	d	203.	c	204.	b
205.	c	206.	c	207.	a	208.	b	209.	b	210.	b
211.	a	212.	d	213.	a	214.	b	215.	b	216.	a

217. a	218. a	219. c	220. b	221. c	222. d
223. b	224. a	225. a	226. a	227. c	228. c
229. a	230. b	231. c	232. b	233. b	234. a
235. c	236. b	237. c	238. d	239. d	240. b
241. c	242. a	243. d	244. d	245. c	246. c
247. d	248. a	249. c	250. d	251. d	252. d
253. b	254. d	255. c	256. d	257. d	258. c
259. a	260. d	261. b	262. a	263. c	264. b
265. d	266. c	267. d	268. d	269. c	270. c
271. c	272. d	273. d	274. c	275. b	276. c
277. c	278. b	279. c	280. d	281. d	282. d
283. b	284. c	285. b	286. b	287. c	288. d
289. b	290. c	291. b	292. b	293. c	294. a
295. d	296. b	297. c	298. a	299. c	300. d
301. b	302. c	303. c	304. a	305. c	306. b
307. c	308. b	309. c	310. d	311. c	312. d
313. d	314. c	315. d	316. a	317. c	318. c
319. a	320. c	321. a	322. d	323. c	324. b
325. b	326. a	327. d	328. a	329. d	330. c
331. b	332. b	333. b	334. a	335. b	336. d
337. c	338. d	339. b	340. a	341. d	342. a
343. b	344. c	345. c	346. c	347. b	348. b
349. b	350. d	351. d	352. d	353. b	354. b
355. a	356. c	357. b	358. b	359. d	360. c
361. b	362. b	363. c	364. b	365. a	366. a
367. a	368. d	369. b	370. c	371. d	372. d
373. b	374. b	375. d	376. a	377. c	378. b
379. c	380. a	381. a	382. a	383. b	384. a
385. a	386. d	387. c	388. b	389. a	390. b
391. d	392. b	393. d	394. b	395. d	396. d
397. c	398. a	399. d	400. c	401. d	402. a
403. a	404. a	405. a	406. a	407. b	408. d
409. c	410. a	411. d	412. c	413. d	414. b
415. d	416. d	417. c	418. c	419. d	420. b
421. d	422. c	423. b	424. d	425. c	426. d
427. d	428. d	429. b	430. d	431. d	432. c
433. a	434. c	435. a	436. c	437. d	438. b
439. d	440. a	441. b	442. b	443. d	444. b

Part – C

1.	c	2.	a	3.	c	4.	b	5.	d	6.	c
7.	c	8.	d	9.	c	10.	c	11.	c	12.	c
13.	d	14.	c	15.	d	16.	c	17.	c	18.	d
19.	a	20.	b	21.	d	22.	a	23.	c	24.	b
25.	d	26.	a	27.	a	28.	a	29.	c	30.	c
31.	a	32.	b								

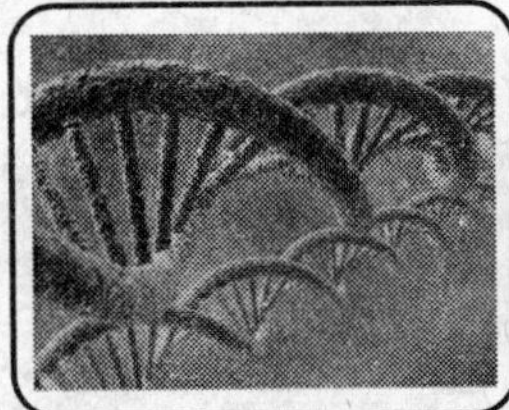

Chapter 3
Molecular Biology

Part B

1. "Alternative excision repair system" is specialized for removal of thymine dimers in
   a) *Saccharomyces pombe* b) Humans
   c) Archaea d) *Caenorhabditis elegans*
2. Which of the following statement is not correct?
   a) Okazaki fragments of eukaryotes are larger than prokaryotes
   b) Eukaryotic DNA replicates bidirectionally
   c) Licencing factors must be attached at replication origin sites in eukaryotes before replication to occur
   d) Most of the eukaryotic cells replicate in the absence of telomerase
3. 18 S RNA is synthesized by
   a) RNA polymerase I b) RNA polymerase II
   c) RNA polymerase III d) Both RNA polymerase I and III
4. 5' to 3'exonuclease activity is found in
   a) DNA polymerase I b) DNA polymerase II
   b) DNA Polymerase III d) None of these
5. A mutagen causes a base substitution leading to a change from A to T in the DNA chain. This mutation is a
   a) Deletion b) Frame-shift
   c) Transition d) None of these
6. A palindrome is a sequence of nucleotides in DNA that
   a) Is highly reiterated
   b) Is part of the introns of eukaryotic genes
   c) Has local symmetry and may serve as recognition site for various proteins
   d) Is a structural gene
7. A transition mutation
   a) Occurs when a purine is substituted from a pyrimidine or vice versa
   b) Results from insertion of one or two bases into the DNA chain

c) Always a missense mutation
d) Results from the substitution of one purine for another or of one pyrimidine for another

8. ADAR is an enzyme which plays a significant role in
a) chromatin remodeling
b) 5'-capping
c) RNA editing in eukaryotes
d) RNA editing in prokaryotes

9. All the amino acids are specified by more than one codon except
a) Phenylalanine and Tyrosine
b) Methionine and Threonine
c) Tryptophan and serine
d) Methionine and tryptophan

10. If amino acid sequence for a protein is known, we can estimate the sequence of mRNA coding that protein
a) Precisely
b) Can't be predicted
c) Precisely to certain extent if codon frequency is known
d) Data not sufficient

11. Among the following enzymes which is not involved in DNA replication process
a) Primase b) RNA polymerase
c) DNA polymerase d) Helicase

12. Among the following which mutagen induces formation of thymine dimers in DNA
a) UV Light b) Ethylmethyl sulphate
c) Nitrous oxide d) Ethydium bromide

13. An operon is inducible means
a) The operon is for catabolic process
b) The operon is for anabolic process
c) It has no relation with catabolic and anabolic processes
d) There is another operator in the system

14. Antitermination of RNA synthesis is a major mechanism of regulation in
a) Lytic phase of phage b) Lysogenic phase of ë phage
c) lac operon d) trp operon

15. Attenuation is a regulatory mechanism of gene expression. It can be explained by giving example of
a) lac operon b) trp operon
c) arabinose operon d) All of the above

16. Attenuation is a regulatory mechanism of gene expression .It is found in
    a) Prokaryotes
    b) Eukaryotes
    c) Viruses
    d) Both (a) and (b)

17. V. Ramakrishnan shared Noble Prize for chemistry in the year 2009 for describing the detailed structure of
    a) 30S ribosomal subunit
    b) 50S ribosomal subunit
    c) 60S ribosome
    d) 80S ribosome

18. Bacterial DNA polymerase I can cause nick translation. This property of the enzyme is due to
    a) 5' → 3' polymerase activity
    b) 5' → 3' exonuclease activity
    c) 3' → 5' exonuclease activity
    d) 3' → 5' polymerase activity

19. Biologically not common but sometimes playing regulatory role in gene expression, the DNA is
    a) A-form
    b) B-form
    c) Z-form
    d) None of the above

20. CAAT box and GC box are component of the promoter of
    a) Bacteria
    b) Mycoplasma
    c) Halobacteria
    d) Arabidopsis

21. Codon degeneracy has evolutionary significance because
    a) It reduces the number of t-RNA performing translation for 61 codon
    b) It creates new reading frame and promotes formation of new polypeptides
    c) It generates variations which are raw material for evolution
    d) It maintains wild-type eliminating lethal affects of mutations

22. Copy error mutation is an example of
    a) Transition
    b) Tranversion
    c) Frameshift
    d) None of these

23. Copy-error mutation is thought to occur due to
    a) UV rays
    b) Nitrous oxide
    c) Tautomeric shift
    d) DNA methylation

24. Cytoplasmic polyadenylation is a critical aspect of gene expression in
    a) Cancer cells
    b) Programmed cell death
    c) Early embryo in animals
    d) Aging

25. Degeneracy of the genetic code denotes the existence of
    a) Codons consisting of only two bases
    b) Codons that include one or more of the "unusual" bases

c) Multiple codons for a single amino acid
d) Multiple amino acids for a single codon

26. X-rays induce mutagenic changes mainly by
a) Transitions
b) Frame-shifting
c) Transversions
d) Chromosomal breakage

27. DNA gyrase is inhibited by
a) Nalidixic acid
b) Puromycin
c) Streptomycin
d) None of these

28. Wobble hypothesis explains that
a) A given amino acid can be specified by more than one nucleotide triplet
b) A single t-RNA molecule can recognize more than one codon
c) In mitochondria genetic code does not follow 'Universal rule' of genetic code
d) In some viruses and bacteria genetic code is overlapping

29. DNA replication occurs in 5' to 3' direction because
a) It enhances fidelity of the DNA
b) It is thermodynamically favourable
c) It reduces mismatch pairing
d) DNA is right handed

30. Double stranded DNA break can be repaired by
a) Nucleotide excision repair
b) Mismatch repair
c) Homologous recombination
d) Direct repair

31. During DNA replication in eukaryotes RNA primers are removed by
a) Primase
b) RNase H
c) DNA polymerase I
d) DNA polymerase

32. During DNA synthesis frame reading is from
a) 3' to 5'
b) 5' to 3'
c) Both simultaneously
d) any one direction at a time

33. During photoreactivation reaction DNA photolyase utilizes
a) Red light
b) Far-red light
c) Blue light
d) Green light

34. During RNA processing splicing is mediated by
a) SnRNA
b) mRNA
c) rRNA
d) tRNA

35. During transcription RNA polymerase holoenzyme binds to a DNA sequence and the DNA assumes a saddle-like structure at that point. What is the se-

quence called?
a) CAAT box b) GGTT box
c) TATA box d) AAAT box

36. During transcription RNA polymerase binds to
a) Operator b) promoter
c) CAP site d) regulator

37. During translation proof reading activity is performed by
a) Peptidyl transferase b) Aminoacyl transfer RNA synthetase
c) Translation factors d) Ribosome

38. Enhancers are active when they are
a) Upstream from promoter b) Downstream from promoter
c) Within the promoter d) Either upstream or downstream

39. Enhancers of eukaryotic gene may have a special form of DNA called
a) A-DNA b) B-DNA
c) Z-DNA d) C-DNA

40. Ethidium bromide causes
a) Silent mutation b) Transition
c) Transversion d) Frame shift mutation

41. The number of proteins expressed can be increased from a single eukaryotic gene through
a) Alternative protein folding b) Alternative splicing
c) Degeneracy of codons d) All of the above

42. Transcription factors for which of the following RNA polymerases an activated by mTOR?
a) RNA polymerase I and III b) RNA polymerase II and III
c) RNA polymerase I and II d) RNA polymerase I, II and III

43. Eukaryotic transcription
a) Is independent of the presence of consensus sequences upstream from the start of transcription.
b) May involve a promoter located within the region transcribed rather than upstream.
c) Requires a separate promoter region for each of the three ribosomal RNAs transcribed.
d) Is affected by enhancer sequences only if they are adjacent to the promoter.

b) Which is a part of a gene that is transcribed and persists in the mature m RNA
c) Which is located between two adjacent genes
d) Which is located at the centromere

63. Which sequence is the best target for damage by UV radiation
a) AGGCAAA b) AGGCACC
c) CTTTTGA d) GUAAAAU

64. MGMT is a "suicide enzyme". It is involved in
a) Excision DNA repair b) Mismatch DNA repair
c) Direct DNA repair d) Genetic recombination

65. Native form of DNA is called as
a) A-DNA b) B-DNA
c) Z-DNA d) All of the above

66. Neomycin in bacterial protein synthesis
a) Inhibits binding of amino-acyl t RNA to ribosome
b) Inhibits initiation of translation and causes misreading
c) Inhibits interaction between t RNA and m RNA
d) Inhibits interaction between r RNA and t RNA

67. Okazaki fragments are
a) Synthesized in the 3' to 5' direction
b) Found on the lagging strand
c) Found on the leading strand
d) Assembled as continuous replication

68. Operons are found in prokaryotes but they are also reported in an eukaryote that is
a) *Arabidopsis thaliana* b) Maize
c) *Caenorhabditis elegans* d) *Drosophila*

69. Peptidyl transferase activity is contained
a) Within the large ribosomal subunit
b) Within the small ribosomal subunit
c) Within tRNA
d) Within both large and small subunits of ribosome

70. Point mutation in which there is deletion or addition of one base pair is termed as
a) Deletion b) Transition
c) Transversion d) Frameshift mutation

71. Polyadenylation is a post-transcriptional phenomenon. It was proved after the discovery of
    a) RNA-dependent RNA polymerase
    b) Terminal sequences in template DNA
    c) AAU AAAA signal sequences in m-RNA
    d) Template independent poly (A) polymerase

72. Polyadenylation of 3'-end of mRNA is a distinguishing feature of eukaryotic transcription events. But it does not occur in
    a) mRNA for interferon proteins
    b) mRNA for histone proteins
    c) mRNA for apolipoprotein-B
    d) mRNA for tumour cells

73. Proof reading activity is performed by
    a) 3' to 5' exonuclease activity of DNA polymerases
    b) 5' to 3' exonuclease activity of DNA polymerases
    c) 3' to 5' exonuclease activity of RNA polymerases
    d) 5' to 3' exonuclease activity of RNA polymerases

74. Pyrimidine dimers are repaired by
    a) Excinuclease
    b) AP-endonuclease
    c) DNA photolyase
    d) DNA polymerase II

75. Recombination-dependent mechanism for DNA repairing is
    a) SOS repair
    b) Excision repair
    c) Post-replication repair
    d) Photoreactivation repair

76. Regarding gene expression in prokaryotes and eukaryotes, which statement is correct?
    a) mRNA and DNA are colinear
    b) mRNA and protein synthesis can occur simultaneously
    c) Processing of hnRNA yields mRNA
    d) RNA polymerase can bind to promoters situated upstream to gene

77. Reverse transcriptase is a
    a) DNA-dependent RNA polymerase
    b) RNA-dependent DNA polymerase
    c) DNA-dependent DNA polymerase
    d) RNA-dependent RNA polymerase

78. Riboswitches can regulate gene expression at
    a) Transcription level
    b) Translation level
    c) Both (a) and (b)
    d) Post translation level

79. RNA interference is an extremely effective and widely used method for
    a) Gene transfer
    b) RNA processing in vitro
    c) Regulation of gene expression at the mRNA level
    d) Interfering with transcription

80. RNA is very much susceptible to hydrolysis in alkali because
    a) It contains uracil residues in its structure
    b) Cleavage occurs in the glycosidic bonds of purine bases
    c) Its 2'-OH group participate in intramolecular cleavage of phosphodiester backbone
    d) cleavage occurs in the glycosidic bonds of pyrimidine bases

81. Some mRNA of bacteria are polyadenylated. Here polyadenylation
    a) Increases half-life of mRNA
    b) Increases rate of translation
    c) Provides polycistronic tendency
    d) Triggers degradation of mRNA

82. Sometimes the presence of introns allows the exons of a gene to be joined in different combinations resulting in the synthesis of different proteins from the same gene. Here introns play role in
    a) Trans-splicing b) cis-splicing
    c) Alternative splicing d) None of the above

83. Spliceosome removes introns from hnRNA in
    a) Mitochondria b) Chloroplast
    c) Archaebacteria d) Nucleus

84. Split genes are present in
    a) Eukaryotes b) Vertebrates only
    c) Eukaryotes and Archaea d) Eukaryotes and Eubacteria

85. srpRNA plays a role in
    a) Regulation of gene expression
    b) Transcription
    c) Targeting of secretary proteins to the ER
    d) Protein degradation

86. Stringent response in prokaryotes occurs at
    a) Transcription level b) Translation level
    c) Post translation level d) DNA replication

87. Tautomerization may result in
    a) Silent mutation b) Missense mutation
    c) Copy error mutation d) Framshift mutation

88. TBP is a component of
    a) TF II H b) RNA polymerase III
    c) TF IID d) TF IIF

89. Which one of the following is not associated with eukaryotic transcription?
    a) Histone acetyl transferase b) RNA polymerase-II
    c) RNA polymerase-III d) Poly (A) polymerase

90. The biologically predominant form of DNA is
    a) Right-handed B-DNA b) Left-handed B-DNA
    c) Right-handed A-DNA d) Left-handed A-DNA

91. The conformational variation between B and Z form of DNA is partly due to
    a) Loss of H-bond
    b) Lack of hydrophobic interactions
    c) Rotation of glycosidic bond
    d) Increase in humidity

92. The DNA molecule having no grooves and left handed is known as
    a) A-DNA b) B-DNA
    c) Z-DNA d) None of these.

93. The expression of genetic information can be regulated at the level of
    a) Replication b) Transcription
    c) Conjugation d) Cell division

94. The fastest known rate of any *in vivo* polymerization reaction is
    a) Protein synthesis b) DNA synthesis
    c) Glycogen synthesis d) Starch synthesis

95. The melting temperature Tm of DNA depends upon
    a) The length of DNA
    b) G-C content of DNA
    c) The purine content of DNA
    d) None of the above

[CSIR (NET/JRF) Exam. Dec 2000]

96. The mutation which has no effect on the phenotype is called
    a) Neutral mutation b) Missense mutation
    c) Read through mutation d) All of the above

97. The operon consists of
    a) Regulator and repressor gene

b) Regulator, structural and operator gene
c) Structural, operator and promoter gene
d) Regulator and operator gene

98. The phenomenon of reverse transcription was discovered by
a) Beadle and Tatum
b) Jacob and Monod
c) Lederberg and Hays
d) Temin and Baltimore

99. The protein complex 'dicer' is involved in
a) Proteins sorting
b) Proteins degradation
c) Gene silencing
d) Transcription

100. The region where RNA polymerase binds to promoter in prokaryotes is called
a) Pribnow box
b) Hogness box
c) Homeo box
d) Shine-Dalgarno box

101. The Z-DNA helix
a) Has fewer base pair per turn than the B-DNA
b) Is favoured by an alternating GC sequence
c) Tends to be found at the 3' end of genes
d) Is the most common conformation of DNA

102. Thymine dimers in eukaryotes are repaired by
a) Direct repair mechanism
b) Base excision repair mechanism
c) Nucleotide excision repair mechanism
d) Mismatch repair mechanism

103. Which one of the following enzyme is involved in translation step in protein biosynthesis?
a) Aminoacyl - tRNA synthetase
b) RNA polymerase
c) Ribozyme
d) Reverse transcriptase

104. Transcription coupled DNA repair is an example of
a) Direct repair
b) Excision repair
c) Mismatch repair
d) SOS response

105. Transport of mRNA from nucleus to cytosol is
a) Primary active process
b) Secondary active process
d) Facilitated diffusion
d) Simple diffusion

106. UGA is a stop codon, but in mitochondrial genome it codes for
a) Met
b) Trp
c) Tyr
d) Asp

107. UV rays usually cause
   a) Gene mutation b) Chromosome mutation
   c) Genome mutation d) Both (a) and (b)

108. When a mutation changes a termination codon into codon specifying an amino acid, it is called
   a) Back mutation b) Read through mutation
   c) Synonymous mutation d) Reverse nonsense mutation

109. When one amino acid is replaced by another owing to a mutation, it is called
   a) Synonymous mutation b) Missense mutation
   c) Silent mutation d) Frame-shift mutation

110. When release factor binds to stop codon on mRNA during translation, the synthesized peptide chain is transferred to
   a) tRNA b) Water
   c) H+ d) Amino acids
   [CSIR (NET/JRF] Exam. Dec 2008]

111. When repressor protein binds to operator of an operon which of the following process is regulated?
   a) Translation b) Transcription
   c) Replication d) None of the above
   [CSIR (NET/JRF) Exam. June 2008]

112. Which enzyme is exclusively involved in DNA repair mechanism
   a) DNA polymerase b) RNA polymerase
   c) Restriction endonuclease d) Photolyase

113. Which of the following antibiotic causes misincorporation of amino acid in synthesizing polypeptide?
   a) Polymixin-B b) Streptomycin
   c) Chloramphenicol d) Bacitracin

114. Which of the following antibiotic occasionally cause death when administered to persons who are allergic to them?
   a) Bacitracin b) Polymixin
   c) Penicillin d) Streptomycin

115. Which of the following anticancerous drugs does not act on microtubules?
   a) Colchicine b) Taxol
   c) Thiabendazole d) Methotrexate

116. Which of the following can induce SOS response in bacteria?
   a) Thymine dimers b) Hydroxylamine
   c) 5-flurouracil d) 2-Aminopurine

117. Which of the following can inhibit protein synthesis
  a) Tetracycline b) Chlorampheni
  c) Streptomycin d) Cyclohexamid

118. Which of the following DNA repair system has to
  derma pigmentosum?
  a) Direct repair c) Mismatch repa
  b) Base exicision repair d) Nucleotide exc

119. Which of the following enzymes initiate DNA replic
  a) DNA polymerase-I b) Primase
  c) DNA polymerase-II d) DNA polymera

120. Which of the following feature of genetic code has
  a) Genetic code is non-overlapping
  b) Genetic code is universal
  c) Degeneracy
  d) Codons are read in 5' to 3' direction

122. Which of the following gene regulating mechanism o
  a) Transcription b) Splicing
  c) RNA editing d) RNA interferenc

123. Which of the following interaction plays a pivotal role i
  helix DNA?
  a) Hydrogen bonding b) Phosphodiester bo
  c) β-N- glycosidic bonds d) Stacking forces

124. Which of the following is a non-antibiotic inhibitor of p
  a) Puromycin b) Neomycin
  c) Ricin d) None of these

125. Which of the following is a post transcriptional gene regu
  a) RNA interference b) Prevention of chron
  c) Prevention of 5'-capping d) Prevention of 3'-poly

126. Which of the following is a ribozyme?
  a) DNA polymerases
  b) RNA polymerases
  c) Aminoacyl t-RNA synthetases
  d) Peptidyl transferases

127. Which of the following is not a component of prokaryotic
  a) Pribnow box b) -35 consensus sequen
  c) Fis elements d) Sigma factor

g is not a post transcriptional modification?
b) RNA silencing
d) *cis* splicing

g is not used in DNA repair in prokaryotes?
I b) DNA polymerase II
d) DNA polymerase V

g is often called as error-prone repair?
b) Mismatch repair
d) SOS response

g is responsible for direct DNA repair?
III b) AP endonuclease
d) DNA Photolyases

is sometimes called as caretaker of the cell?
es b) DNA polymerases
d) p53 gene

s the most deleterious mutagen?
b) UV-light
d) Acridine orange

echanisms of DNA repair is not found in human
s?
epair b) Direct repair
d) Base excision repair

utagenic agents can induce all types of mutations,
versions, frameshift, and even chromosome aber-

b) Alkylating agents
d) X-rays

tagens are mutagenic to both replicating and non

b) Nitrous acid
d) 5-bromouracil

's no role in histone modification during tran-

b) Ubiquitination
d) GDP-ribosylation

138. Which of the following plays no role in RNA silencing?
   a) micRNA b) siRNA
   c) Dicer nuclease d) DNA polymerase

139. Which of the following process does not occur in nucleus
   a) Recombination b) Replication
   c) Transcription d) Translation

[CSIR (NET/JRF) Exam. June 2008]

140. Which of the following statement is not correct?
   a) Each chromosome contains one large molecule of DNA.
   b) In prokaryotes, nearly all the genes are single copy with the exception of rRNA and tRNA genes
   c) rRNA gene clusters do not contain any introns
   d) The most active RNA-synthesizing ability is associated with RNA polymerase III

141. Which of the following statement is not correct for eukaryotic DNA replication?
   a) Eukaryotic chromosomes have multiple sites where DNA synthesis is initiated.
   b) The rate of fork movement in eukaryotes is slower than in bacteria.
   c) In eukaryotes okazaki fragments are smaller than in bacteria.
   d) DNA replication in eukaryotes is unidirectional.

142. Which of the following statement is not correct?
   a) Okazaki fragments are larger in bacteria
   b) UV light may induce SOS response
   c) Direct repair mechanism removes thymine dimers from human genome
   d) O^6 - Methyl guanine DNA methyl transferase is a suicide enzyme because it is used in reaction

143. Which of the following statement is not correct?
   a) Polyadenylation in eukaryotic mRNAs enhances their stability
   b) poly (A) tails play an important role in transport of mRNA from the nucleus to cytoplasm
   c) Polyadenylation is achieved by template independent RNA polymerase
   d) Poly(A) tails are added with the help of DNA template dependent RNA polymerase

144. Which of the following statement is true?
   a) Shine-Dalgarno sequences are integral part of prokaryotic promoters
   b) Pribnow box is not included within core promoter of *E. coli.*
   c) AAUAAA is terminator sequence which helps in rho independent termination of transcription is prokaryotes
   d) Promoter for tRNA synthesizing gene in eukaryotes are transcribed

145. Which of the following type of mutation does not affect fitness of organism?
a) Nonsense mutation
b) Missense mutation
c) Neutral mutation
d) Frame-shift mutation

146. Which of the following type of mutation results in genetic polymorphism?
a) Frame-shift mutation
b) Non-sense mutation
c) Silent mutation
d) Missense mutation

147. Which of the following will not cause a transition mutation
a) 5-Bromouracil
b) Nitrous acid
c) 2-Aminopurine
d) None of these

148. Which of the following is absorbed by nucleic acids?
a) UV-B
b) UV-C
c) UV-A
d) All of these

149. What is the number of hydrogen bonds in a double stranded helical B-DNA structure of 100 bp with 20A and 10 T in one of the two strands.
a) 200
b) 230
c) 270
d) 300

150. The 3' ends of all eukaryotic mRNAs are modified by the addition of a tail of approximately 200 adenosine residues except
a) Those encoding protozoan histones.
b) Those encoding metazoan histones.
c) Those encoding histones of unicellular eukaryotes.
d) Those encoding histones of all eukaryotes.

151. Which of the following RNA polymerase contributes to the maximum of the total RNA synthesized in growing eukaryotic cells?
a) RNA polymerase-II
b) RNA polymerase-I and II
c) RNA polymerase-I and III
d) RNA polymerase-II and III

152. Mutations in which of the following transcription factor causes xeroderma pigmentosum?
a) TF II D
b) TF II B
c) TF II F
d) TF II H

153. Which of the following post transcriptional modification of mRNA in eukaryotes is linked to transcription termination?
a) 5'-capping
b) 3'-polyadenylation
c) RNA editing
d) Splicing

154. The group of small RNAs which primarily act to silence transposons in the germ lines of animals is called
a) siRNA
b) piRNA
c) miRNA
d) gRNA

155. Rifampicin is an antibiotic. It acts by
  a) Binding with β-subunit of RNA polymerase-II thereby blocking promoter clearance.
  b) Premature termination of polypeptide synthesis.
  c) Inhibiting peptidyl transferase activity.
  d) Inactivating 60S subunit of eukaryotic ribosome.

156. The attachment of tRNAs to its appropriate amino acid, termed tRNA charging, requires energy which is supplied by
  a) ATP b) GTP
  c) CTP d) UTP

157. TATA binding associated factor-9 (TAF-9) and TAF-6 bind with
  a) TATA box b) MTE
  c) Inr sequence d) DPE

158. Which of the following modification of histones is involved in the formation of metaphase chromosome?
  a) Acetylation b) Methylation
  c) Phosphorylation d) Ubiquitinylation

159. Which of the following subunits of RNA polymerase catalyzes the formation of phosphodiester bond?
  a) α b) β'
  c) β d) ω

160. Which of the following causes frameshift mutation?
  a) Hydroxyl amine b) Aflatoxin
  c) Alkylating agents d) All of the above

161. Which of the following is not involved in maintaining the fidelity of DNA replication?
  a) 6,4-photolyase b) DNA polymerase-δ and ε
  c) Balanced level of dNTPs d) RNase H and FEN-1

162. Which of the following have single stranded DNA molecule as a genetic material in their genome?
  a) Phage F x 174 virus b) Minute virus
  c) Parvo virus d) All of the above

163. SP6 RNA polymerase is found in
  a) Bacteria b) Bacteriophage
  c) Yeast d) Primitive eukaryotes

164. Nuclear import and export pathways are mediated by a family of soluble receptors referred to as importins or exportins. These receptors are commonly called as
a) Nuclear export and import factors
b) Nuclear localization systems
c) Karyopherins
d) Nuclear localization proteins

165. The base-paired secondary structure of RNA primarily adopts a right-handed A-type double helix because
a) RNA has ribose sugar
b) It has a deep, narrow major groove
c) It has 11 bp per turn
d) It is formed from a single strand of polynucleotide chain

166. DNA polymerases cannot initiate DNA synthesis *de novo* except
a) DNA polymerase ε b) DNA polymerase η
c) DNA polymerase α d) DNA polymerase λ

167. Chloroplast and mitochondrial DNA has
a) Single DNA replication origin site
b) Two DNA replication origin site
c) Chloroplast has single but mitochondria has two origin sites
d) Multiple origin sites like nuclear DNA

168. FG repeats are found in nucleoporins. If this repeat is mutated what would be the effect on nuclear transport?
a) Nuclear pore complex (NPC) is locked
b) Non-nuclear proteins diffuse through the NPC
c) Diffusion of nuclear proteins is fast
d) Proteins containing NLS cannot diffuse

169. Cdc6 and Cdt 1 proteins work at G1 phase of cell cycle during cell division, where assembles pre-replication complexes, these proteins are
a) Cyclin-dependent protein kinases
b) Helicase-loading proteins
c) Involved in chromatin remodeling
d) DNA unwinding proteins

170. Which of the following is the unique post-translational modification of small GTP-binding proteins?
a) Acetylation b) Prenylation
c) Glycosylation d) Phosphorylation

171. Which of the following post-transcriptional modification in mRNA is least significant to exit from nucleus?
   a) 5'-capping b) 3'-polyadenylation
   c) Splicing d) Editing

172. Trans-translation occurs of those mRNAs which
   a) Lack termination codons b) Are alternatively spliced
   c) Are polycistronic d) Lack initiation codon

173. In eukaryotes regulatory promoters contain
   a) TATA box b) CCAAT box and GC box
   c) Enhancers d) Motif ten elements

174. When DNA replication occurs replication fork is formed. Single strand binding proteins (SSB) attach to the template to prevent reannealing. In E.coli these SSBs are
   a) Trimeric b) Tetrameric
   c) Hexameric d) Diad

175. Which of the following transcription factor plays a crucial role in recognizing RNA polymerase I to its promoter?
   a) TFIID b) TFIIH
   c) SL1 d) UBF

176. Which of the following transcription elongation factor contains CDK9 kinase activity that act on the CTD of RNA polymerase II to phosphorylate it?
   a) p-TEFb b) Elongins ABC
   c) TFIIS d) Elongator complex

177. If point mutation occurs in the Shine-Dalgarno Sequence of bacterial mRNA then what would happen?
   a) mRNA is not translated b) mRNA is not completely translated
   c) Translation is not effected d) mRNA becomes monocistronic

178. Which of the following eukaryotic translation initiation factor works as a guanine nucleotide exchange factor (GEF) during translation initiation?
   a) eIF2 b) eIF4G
   c) eIF2B d) eIF3

179. Which of the following is a regulator RNA of bacteria?
   a) sRNA b) miRNA
   c) piRNA d) rasiRNA

180. Which of the following is responsible for promoter specificity in bacteria?
   a) Pribnow box b) Sigma factor
   c) -35 consensus sequence d) β subunit of RNA polymerase

181. Which protein act as a primer synthesizing protein in bacteria
   a) Dna C   b) Dna G
   c) Dna B   d) Dna A

182. Primosome is present in
   a) Eukaryote
   b) Prokaryote
   c) Eukaryote and Archea bacteria
   d) All of the above

183. Which is not correct for eukaryotic DNA replication
   a) DNA polymerase δ replicates lagging strand and DNA polymerase ε replicates leading strand
   b) Primer is removed by RNase H and FEN-1
   c) Proofreading activity is maintained by DNA polymerase δ and ε
   d) DNA polymerase α is involved in mitochondrial DNA replication

184. σ54 factor recognizes promoter of the gene which is involved in
   a) Nitrogen starvation   b) Environmental stress
   c) Housekeeping function   d) All of the above

185. Adapter molecule is
   a) tRNA   b) mRNA
   c) rRNA   d) SnRNA

186. Splicing is a removal of noncoding sequences. It occurs in
   a) Prokaryotes   b) Eukaryotes and Archaea
   c) Eukaryotes only   d) All of the above

187. Enzyme that is involved in the 5' - capping of mRNA is/are
   a) Phosphohydrolase
   b) Guanylyl transferase
   c) Guanine-7-methyltransferase
   d) All of the above.

187. Phosphorylation of CTD domain of RNA polymerase II is achieved by the activity of
   a) TFII H   b) TFII D
   c) TFII B   d) TFII F

188. Amino acid binds to the tRNA with
   a) N-terminal of amino acid   b) C-terminal of amino acid
   c) Side chains of amino acid   d) Elsewhere of the amino acid

189. Translocation of ribosome is facilitated by
   a) EF-Tu   b) EF-Ts and GTP
   c) EF-G and GTP   d) Both (a) and (b)

190. Kozak sequences are present in
   a) mRNA of eukaryote b) mRNA of prokaryote
   c) 30 S subunit of ribosome d) 40 S subunit of ribosome

191. Which of the following is not correct?
   a) Eukaryotic translation initiation involves two GTP hydrolysis event.
   b) eIF-4A have ATP dependent helicase activity
   c) eIF-4F binds at the cap to initiate translation
   d) eIF-5-GTP binds the large subunit of ribosome.

192. Which part of the RISC complex catalyzes RNA hydrolysis
   a) DCR2 b) R2D2
   c) AGO d) Dicer

193. Novobiocin is a competitive inhibitor, it acts on
   a) Gyr A unit of DNA Gyrase
   b) Gyr B unit of DNA Gyrase
   c) Topoisomerase I
   d) None of the above

194. A single-strand nick in the parental DNA helix just ahead of a replication fork causes the replication fork to break. Recovery from this calamity requires
   a) DNA ligase
   b) DNA primase
   c) site-specific recombination
   d) homologous recombination **[CSIR (NET/JRF) Exam. Dec. 2011]**

195. In which form of DNA, the number of base pairs per helical turn is 10.5?
   a) A b) B
   c) X d) Z
   [CSIR (NET/JRF) Exam. Dec. 2011]

196. α-amanitin inhibits
   a) only RNA polymerase I b) only RNA polymerase II
   c) only RNA polymerase III d) all RNA polymerases
   [CSIR (NET/JRF) Exam. Dec. 2011]

197. Reverse transcriptase has both ribonuclease and polymerase activities. Ribonuclease activity is required for
   a) the synthesis of new RNA strand
   b) the degradation of RNA strand
   c) the synthesis of new DNA strand
   d) the degradation of DNA strand **[CSIR (NET/JRF) Exam. Dec. 2011]**

198. In gene regulation, Open Reading Frame (ORF) implies
   a) intervening nucleotide sequence in between two genes
   b) a series of triplet codons not interrupted by a stop codon
   c) a series of triplet codons that begins with a start codon and ends with a stop codon.
   d) the exonic sequence of a gene that corresponds to the 5'UTR of the mRNA and thus does not code for the protein

[CSIR (NET/JRF) Exam. Dec. 2011]

199. While replicating DNA, the rate of mis-incorporation by DNA polymerase is 1 in 105 nucleotides. However, the actual error rate in the replicated DNA is 1 in 109 nucleotides incorporated. This is achieved mainly due to
   a) spontaneous excision of misincorporated nucleotides
   b) 3' 5' proof reading activity of DNA polymerase
   c) termination of DNA polymerase at misincorporated sites
   d) 5' 3' proof reading activity **[CSIR (NET/JRF) Exam. Dec. 2011]**

200. Amino acid selenocysteine (Sec) is incorporated into polypeptide chain during translation by
   a) charging of Sec into tRNAser followed by incorporation through serine codon
   b) charging of serine into tRNAser followed by modification of serine into selenocysteine and then incorporation through serine codon
   c) charging of Sec into tRNAsec and then incorporation through selenocysteine codon
   d) charging of serine into tRNAser, modification of serine into selenocysteine and then incorporation through a specially placed stop codon **[CSIR (NET/JRF) Exam. Dec. 2011]**

201. The base analog 2-aminopurine pairs with thymine, and can occasionally pair with cytosine. The type of mutation induced by 2-aminopurine is
   a) transversion   b) transition
   c) deletion   d) nonsense

[CSIR (NET/JRF) Exam. Dec. 2011]

202. A merozygote resulting from recombination of two *E. coli* lac mutants produces half maximal level of β-galactosidase with inducer. The genotype of merozygote is
   a) $O^+ I^- Z^- / O^+ I^+ Z^+$ b) $O^c I^+ Z^- / O^+ I^+ Z^+$
   c) $O^c I^- Z^+ / O^+ I^+ Z^+$ d) $O^c I^+ Z^- / O^+ I^- Z^+$

203. The enzyme responsible for conversion of negatively supercoiled DNA into a relaxed circular DNA is
   a) DNA Gyrase   b) DNA topoisomerase I
   c) DNA topoisomerase II   d) DNA helicase

204. Replication of full lenth chromosome of *E.coli*
   a) takes exactly as long as it takes *E.coli* to divide.
   b) takes longer than it takes *E.coli* to divide.
   c) takes lesser time than it takes to divide.
   d) depends on the use of N^{15} and N^{14} nitrogen source of medium.

205. A deletion of three consecutive bases in the coding region of a gene cannot result in
   a) deletion of a single amino acid without any other change in the protein.
   b) replacement of two adjacent amino acids by a single amino acid.
   c) replacement of a single amino acid by another without any other change in sequence of the protein.
   d) production of a truncated protein.

206. Which type of mutation is the most common?
   a) Insertion of one or more bases
   b) Deletion of one or more bases
   c) Base substitutions
   d) Inversion of DNA segments

207. Change from purine to pyrimidine or pyrimidine to purine is
   a) Transitition b) Transversion
   c) Frame-shift d) Reversion

208. Lactose operon is both negatively and positively regulated, this means that lactose is used
   a) Preferentialy
   b) Along with glucose
   c) After glucose has been used
   d) None of the above

209. Mutation which changes a triplet is called
   a) Silent mutation b) Missense mutation
   c) Nonsense mutation d) Neutral mutation

210. Which of the following statement is not correct?
   a) In eukaryotes DNA replication occurs bidirectionaly
   b) Theta replication model is true for phages
   c) DNA of *E. coli* replicates with only one origin site
   d) Eukaryotes have many origin sites

211. The catalytic sites of RNA polymerases include
   a) Mg^{++} b) Zn^{++}
   c) Mn^{++} d) K^{+}

212. Which of the following DNA repair pathway functions throughout the cell cycle in mammalian cells?
 a) Mismatch repair
 b) Homologous recombination
 c) Nonhomologous end joining (NHEJ)
 d) Excision repair

213. In mammals double strand DNA break is mostly repaired by
 a) Homologous recombination
 b) Direct repair
 c) Nucleotide excision repair
 d) Nonhomologous end joining

214. Lac operon is
 a) Inducible and catabolic b) Repressible and catabolic
 c) Inducible and anabolic d) Repressible and anabolic

215. Which of the following statement is not correct?
 a) The aminoacyl-tRNA-EFTu-GTP ternary complex interacts with the ribosome to ensure high accuracy during translation.
 b) Programmed frameshifting is triggered by local mRNA elements which can control gene expression in bacterial, mammalian, and viral systems.
 c) Cell cycle checkpoints in bacteria are similar to that of eukaryotic cell cycle checkpoint.
 d) Trans splicing joins exons from two separate RNA transcripts.

216. Small RNAs with internally complementary sequences that form hairpin-like structure, synthesized as precursor RNAs and cleaved by endonucleases to form short duplexes are called
 a) snRNA. b) mRNA.
 c) tRNA. d) miRNA.
 [CSIR (NET/JRF) Exam. June 2011]

217. The 5' cap of RNA is required for the
 a) stability of RNA only.
 b) stability and transport of RNA
 c) transport of RNA only.
 d) methylation of RNA. **[CSIR (NET/JRF) Exam. June 2011]**

218. The fidelity of replicative base selection can be reduced by a factor of 102 when the repair of DNA synthesis involves
 a) AP endonuclease.

b) ABC exonuclease.
c) DNA photolyase.
d) TLS DNA polymerase. **[CSIR (NET/JRF) Exam. June 2011]**

219. What is the minimum number of NTPs required for the formation of one peptide bond during protein synthesis?
a) One
b) Two
c) Four
d) Six

[CSIR (NET/JRF) Exam. June 2011]

220. If the ratio of the number of nonsynonymous to synonymous substitutions per site in protein coding gene is greater than one, it is an evidence of selection that is
a) positive.
b) negative.
c) neutral.
d) random.

[CSIR (NET/JRF) Exam. June 2011]

221. The conformation of a nucleotide in DNA is affected by rotation about how many bonds?
a) 4
b) 6
c) 7
d) 3 **[CSIR Model Paper 2011]**

222. Which of the following processes does not take place in the 5'→3' direction?
a) DNA replication
b) Transcription
c) Nick translation
d) RNA editing

[CSIR Model Paper 2011]

223. Deletion of the leader sequence of trp operon of *E. coli* would result in
a) decreased transcription of trp operon.
b) increased transcription of trp operon.
c) no effect on transcription.
d decreased transcription of trp operon in the presence of tryptophan.

[CSIR Model Paper 2011]

Part C

1. The RNA polymerase II core enzyme is catalytically active but requires the Rpb4/7 complex and the general transcription factors for initiation from promoter DNA. Which of the following function is affected if Rpb4/7 is not associated with RNA polymerase II?
   a) mRNA nuclear export and transcription-coupled DNA repair
   b) Splicing of the transcript
   c) End modification of RNA
   d) Promoter clearance
2. Many eukaryotic transcription factors contain both a site-specific DNA-binding domain and a transcriptional activation domain that recruits the transcriptional machinery. The binding domain and activation domain do not necessarily have to be on the same polypeptide. If proteins with only a DNA binding domain are provided to the cells lacking transcription factors, but proteins containing an activation domain are present, then
   a) Transcription occurs normally
   b) Transcription efficiency slows down
   c) Transcription does not occur
   d) Transcription occurs randomly
3. Bacteriophage λ has two modes in its life cycle, lytic and lysogenic. In the lysogenic mode, the expression of all the phage genes are repressed while the expression of repressor gene switches between on and off position depending on the concentration of repressor. The following statements are made:
   A. Repressor may act both as a positive regulator and a negative regulator
   B. Expression of repressor gene, cI is independent of the expression of cII and cIII genes.
   C. Mutation of cI gene will cause it to form clear plaques on both wild type E.coli and E. coli (+).
   D. Mutation at operators, OL and OR will allow the phage to act as a virulent phage.

   The correct statements are

   a) A and B b) B and C
   c) C and D d) D and A

   [CSIR (NET/JRF) Exam. Dec. 2011]
4. Pre-mRNAs are rapidly bound by snRNPs which carry out dual steps of RNA splicing, that removes the intron and joins the upstream and downstream exons.

The following statements describe some facts related to this event.

A. Almost all introns begin with GU and end with AG sequences and hence all the GU or AG sequences are spliced out of RNA.

B. U2 RNA recognizes important sequences at the 3'acceptor end of the intron.

C. The spliceosome uses ATP to carry out accurate removal of intron.

D. An unusual linkage with 2' OH group of guanosine within the intron form a 'Lariat' structure.

Which of the following combinations is correct?

a) A and B
b) B and C
c) C and D
d) D and A

[CSIR (NET/JRF) Exam. Dec. 2011]

5. In human, protein coding genes are mainly organized as "exons" and "introns". There are intergenic regions that transcribe into various type of non-coding RNA (not translating into protein). Some introns may harbor also transcription units, which are

a) always other protein coding genes.
b) protein coding gene and RNA coding genes.
c) always RNA coding genes
d) pseudo genes

[CSIR (NET/JRF) Exam. Dec. 2011]

6. Many cancers carry mutant p53 genes, while some cancers have normal p53 genes. p53 activates p21 (Wafl) which inhibits G1/S-Cdks and phosphorylation of the retinoblastoma protein (Rb). Cancers with normal p53 genes could

a) express non-phosphorylatable form of Rb.
b) express high levels of p53-deubiquitinases.
c) express inactive forms of G1/S-cdks.
d) express inactive forms of G1/S cyclins.

[CSIR (NET/JRF) Exam. Dec. 2011]

7. Insulin and other growth factors stimulate a pathway involving a protein kinase mTOR, which in its turn augments proteins synthesis. mTOR essentially modifies protein(s) which in their unmodified form act as inhibitors of protein sysnthesis. The following proteins are possible candidates :

A. eEF-1
B. eIF-4E-BP1
C. eIF-4E
D. PHAS-1

Which of the following sets is correct?

a) A and B
b) B and D
c) A and C
d) B and C

[CSIR (NET/JRF) Exam. Dec. 2011]

8. For continuation of protein synthesis in bacteria, ribosomes need to be released from the mRNA as well as to dissociate into subunits. These processes do not occur spontaneously. They need the following possible conditions:
   A. RRF and EF-G aid in this process.
   B. An intrinsic activity of ribosomes and an uncharged tRNA are required.
   C. IF-1 promotes dissociation of ribosomes.
   D. IF-3 and IF-1 promote dissociation of ribosomes.

   Which of the following sets is correct?
   a) A and D b) A and B
   c) A and C d) B and D

   [CSIR (NET/JRF) Exam. Dec. 2011]

9. A method of post transcriptional control is the selective degradation of mRNA transcripts. A transcript encoding a growth factor contains the terminal sequence AAGCUUGAAU and has a half -life of 40 minutes. Another transcript that encodes an immunoglobulin has a terminal sequence of GGAUCGCCAGG and has a half life of about 2 hours. The half life is related to the rate of degradation by the equation $t1/2 = 0.693/k$ where $t1/2$ is the half life and k is the rate of degradation. Some of the explanation given were
   (A) The terminal sequence of immunoglobulin has more C and G nucleotides so the rate of degradation is slow in this mRNA.
   (B) A sequence of A and U nucleotide near 31 poly A tail of transcripts promotes the removal of tail which destablize the mRNA.
   (C) The short half lives of mRNA transcripts of many regulatory genes are critical to function of those genes because they enable the level of regulatory proteins in the cells to be altered rapidly
   (D) The degradation rate of Growth factor transcripts will be faster in the comparision of immunoglobulin transcripts

   Which of the following combination is correct.
   (a) A, B, C and D (b) B, C and D
   (c) A, C and D (d) A, B and D

10. Glucose repression is mediated by an activator protein known as catabolic activator protien which stimulates the transcription of all the proteins necessary for the catabolism of sugars. The catabolic activator protein is an allosteric protein whose binding is controlled by an effector, in this case cAMP. Which of the following sequence of events occurs when E.coli are released from catabolite repression by transfer to low glucose medium?
    (a) cAMP levels rise, cAmp binds to CAP, cAMP-CAP complex binds to a site on DNA and activate the transcription.

(b) cAMP level rise, cAmp binds to CAP, cAMP and CAP complex binds to a site on DNA and repress transcription
(c) cAMP rises, cAmp binds to CAP, cAMP-CAP complex is removed from a site on DNA and activates transcription
(d) cAMP levels falls cAmp is removed from CAP, CAP binds to a site on DNA and represses transcription.

11. One of the most acting activators is a protein called CRP activator that controls the activity of a large sets of operons in E. coli. The protein is postive control factor. CRP is active only in the presence of cyclie AMP. which behaves as a classic small molecule inducer for positive control. A loss of function mutation in the gene that encodes the catabolic acitvator protein would have which effect on expression of lac operon.
a) Expression would be very high in the presence of lactose and stoped in its absence regardless of the presence or absence of glucose.
b) Expression would be low in the presence of lactose and stoped in its absence, regardless of presence and absence of glucose.
c) Expression would be low in the pressure of glucose and very high in its absence regardless of presence or absence of glucose.
d) Expression would be off in the presence of glucose and low in it absence, regardless of the presence or absence of lactose.

12. Tryptophan operon is a repressible operon because this operon regulate enzymes involved in an anabolic pathway. This operon is turned off allosterically usually by an effector. The trp operon consists of genes coding for enzyme that catalyses reactions involved in tryptophan biosynthesis as well as DNA sequences necessary to regulate the production of these enzymes The following statements are related with trp open
(A) When trp is short in supply the leader sequence containing the operator can not be passed and staled ribosome, modifies the mRNA so that the structural genes are transcribed.
(B) The catabolic activator protein plays a role as a co-repressor.
(C) Tryptophan operon has two kinds of regulation one by an operator and the other by an attenuator
(D) The repressor complexes with the corepressor on binding to operator blocks transcription.

Which of the following combination is correct?

a) A, B, C and D b) A, B and D
c) A, C and D d) B, C and D

13. In bacterial cells synthesis of tryptophan depends upon the absence of tryptophan in environment. When the environment lacks the tryptophan there is nothing to activate the repressor so the repressor can not prevent RNA

polymerase from binding to trp operon promoter. The tryptophan genes are transcribed and cells proceeds to manufacture tryptophan from other molecules. Now in a laboratory an E.coli bacterium mutated in such a way that synthesize greater tryptophan synthesizing enzyme than normal level in the absence of tryptophan. Which of the following mutation might result in observed phenotype.

a) deletion in trp promotor
b) deletion just after the promotor-operator region
c) deletion just before the coding sequence for trp enzymes.
d) deletion in the rho-independent transcription terminal segnal.

14. The leader has two unusual features which enables it to play a regulatory role. First a portion of trp leader sequence is translated forming a leader peptide of 14 amino acid long within the mRNA sequence, coding for this peptide are two adjacent codon for amino acid tryptophan Second, the trp leader mRNA also contains four segments or sub-regions whose nucleotide can base pair with each other to form the severel distinctive hairpin loop structures. The region comprising region 3 and 4 plus an adjacent string of U6-8 is called the attenuator.
Which of the following mutation would lead to an increase in expression of trp operon.
a) Changing the two tryptophan codon
b) A mutation in sequence 3 that decreases pairing with sequence 4 without affecting 2:3 pairing
c) A mutation in sequence 2 without affecting 3:4 pairing
d) A mutation in rho gene.

15. The chromatin structure represses gene expression. For a gene to be transcribed, transcription factors, activators and RNA polymerases must bind to DNA. Before transcription, chromatin, structure changes and DNA become more accessible to transcription machinery. Chromatin structure change may involve histone modification and chromatin remodeling. Histone modification comprises the histone modification and the histone acetylation, methylation, phosphorylation, ubiqutinilation and sumoylation.
The following statements are related with chromatin modification
(A) The most common histone modification is acetylation. Acetyl group destablizes the nucleosome structure.
(B) The most common histone modification is histone phorphorylation and phosphate group is abundant in cells due to presence of ATP.
(C) Chromatin remodelling complexes bind directly to particular sites on DNA and reposition the nucleosomes allowing transcription factors to bind to promoters and initiate transcription

(D) Chromatin remodelling involves covalent modification or covalent alteration to histone molecules.

Which of the following combination is correct?

a) A, C and D b) B, C and D
c) A and C d) Only A

16. Eukaryotic gene may be controlled by RNA interference also known as RNA silencing. It appears to wide spread existing in fungi, plants and animals. RNA interference is triggered by double stranded RNA molecule which may arise in several ways; by transcription of inverted repeat into an RNA molecules that then base pairs with itself to form double stranded RNA, and by the simultaneous transcription of two different RNA molecules that are complementry to one another and that pairs forming double stranded RNA.

The following statements are related with RNA interference

(A) There is a strict requirement for si RNA to have 51 phosphorylated end to enter into RISC

(B) Target mRNA by si RNA pathway is cleaved at single site in the centre of the duplex region.

(C) Interferon triggers the degradation of mRNA by inducing 21-51 oligo adenylate synthase by si RNA mediated pathway.

(D) si RNA is processed once by RNAse III

Which of the following combinations is correct?

a) A, B, C and D b) B and D
c) A, B and C d) B, C and D

17. Three experiments were carried out with tryptophan operon: The leader sequence is deleted in one experiments, The represser gene sequence is deleted from the bacteria is second experiment, in third both sequences were deleted from the operon. These three experiments were carried out to check the importance of these regions in tryptophan biosynthesis.

Which of the following is correct?

a) No transcription and translation in case of experiment first and second
b) Transcription occurs only in case of second experiment
c) Transcription occurs in case of both first and second experiment
d) Transcription occur only in case of third experiment

18. When the lactose is absent from the growth medium. There is little nead of lactose processing enzymes and the structural genes specifying these protein are transcribed only in small amount. Transcription of these genes is regulated by regulatory gene, operator gene and promoter gene. Lactose operon is also regulated by the presence or absence of glucose in the medium.

	Glucose	Lactose	cAMP
A.	High	Low	Low
B.	High	High	Low
C.	Low	Low	High
D.	Low	High	Low

In which of following case lac operon is induced.

a) None
b) OnlyD
c) Only B
d) B and D

19. Match the following :

	Group I	Group II
A.	Shine-Dalgarno sequence	1. Aminoacylation of tRNA.
B.	Leucine zipper	2. Gene selencing
C.	Aminoacyl tRNA synthetase	3. Transcription factor
D.	RNAi	4. Ribosome binding and facilitation of translation initiation

a) A-4, B-3, C-1, D-2 b) A-4, B-3, C-2, D-1
c) A-2, B-3, C-1, D-4 d) A-3, B-2, C-4, D-1

20. A student of molecular biology isolated and purified RNA polymerase from prokaryotic and eukaryotic sample. But by mistake the samples were mixed. How would you experimently determine wheather a purified preparation of an RNA polymerase is from prokaryotic or eukaryotic source. Some of the possible explanations are given

(A) Treatment of α-amanitin: all forms of eukaryotic RNA polymerases are inhibited by the αamanitin but prokaryotic RNA polymerase is not.
(B) Treatment of α-amanitin : prokaryotic RNA polymerases is inhibited by α-amanitin but eukaryotic RNA polymerase are not.
(C) Treatment of rifampicin: prokaryotic RNA polymerase is inhibited by rifampicin but eukaryotic polymerases are not sensitive to this.
(D) Treatment of rifampicin: eukaryotic RNA polymerases are inhibited by rifampicin but prokaryotic RNA polymerase is not.

Which one of the following is most appropriate?

a) A and C b) B and D
c) A and D d) B and C

21. You are working with two strains of *E.coli*, one contains a wild type β-galactosidase gene and an I^- mutation. The other contains a temperature sensitive β-galactosidase gene and an O^c mutation. After mating these strains, you assay for the production of β-galactosidase at both permissive and nonpermissive temperatures, in the absence of lactose you expect to find

(A) Wild type gene would be regulated normally.
(B) Temperature sensitive gene will be expressed constitutively
(C) β-galactosidase will be produced at permissive temperature.
(D) β-galactosidase will be produced at non permissive temperature.
Which of the following combination is true?
a) A, B and D b) B, C and D
c) A, B and C d) B and C

22. The basic function of cell cycle is to duplicate DNA accurately and then distribute the copies of DNA precisely to daughter cells. But there are gaps between 'S' phase and 'M' phase. Some of the following statements could possibly explain this observation
(A) G2 check point prevents the initiation of mitosis until DNA replication is completed.
(B) G2 check points senses DNA damage, such as that resulting from irradiation.
(C) During G2 phase cell growth is continuous.
(D) During G2 proteins are synthesized in the preparation for mitosis.
Which of the following combination of statements is most appropriate?
a) A, B, C and D b) A and D
c) A, B and D d) A, C and D

23. Sigma factors direct bacterial RNA polymerase to promoters. Each sigma factor has a preferred promoter sequence to which it binds. If the sequences of promoter that are recognized by sigma factors are mutated then what would not be the possible outcome?
a) RNA polymerases can randomly transcribe any gene.
b) Efficiency of RNA polymerases decreases.
c) Bacterial cells cannot respond properly to a particular stimulus.
d) Two component signaling system becomes overactive.

24. RNA polymerase I and III do not have CTD domain that is present in RNA polymerase II. If CTD domain is incorporated in RNA polymerase I and III then which of the following would be a peculiar feature of RNAs that are synthesized by these modified RNA polymerases?
a) Transcription of RNAs by modified RNA polymerases will be fast.
b) RNAs will be capped and polyadenylated.
c) Translation of the transcripts is faster.
d) RNAs remain in the nucleus.

25. In, bacterium *E. coli* Mut S, Mut L and Mut H proteins are involved in mismatch DNA repair. Here, Mut S recognizes and binds mismatched base pairs, Mut H is an endonuclease that specifically nicks the newly synthesized

daughter strand, targeting repair to this strand, and Mut L recruits helicase II that displaces the nicked strand from the duplex. The bacterium is grown in culture medium containing mutagens. Mutations, which of the following protein is the primary requirement to induce mismatch replication?

a) Mut S
b) Mut L
c) Mut H
d) Helicase II

26. Glucose depletion in bacteria leads to increased synthesis of cAMP, which binds to the dimeric CAP and increases its affinity for DNA. The CAP dimer binds to specific DNA sites in or near target promoters and enhances the ability of the RNA polymerase holoenzyme to bind to its promoter and initiate transcription. If glucose levels are high and lactose is present in relatively less amount then

a) cAMP-CAP complex is formed to utilize glucose.
b) CAP does not bind DNA but cAMP-CAP complex is formed and lac operon does not switch on.
c) CAP does not bind DNA and the lac genes are transcribed at a much lower level.
d) CAP does not bind DNA and the lac genes are not transcribed.

27. The synthesis of proteins destined to leave the cell or become embedded in the plasma membrane begins on a free ribosome but, shortly after synthesis begins, it is halted until the ribosome is directed to the cytoplasmic site of the endoplasmic reticulum. The translocation consists of four components: the signal sequence, the signal recognition particle (SRP), the SRP receptor (SR), and the translocon. Following are some of the statements regarding translocation:

(A) SRP sequence is usually near the amino terminus of the nascent polypeptide chain.
(B) Some signal sequences are maintained in the mature protein, whereas others are cleaved by a signal peptidase from most proteins.
(C) SRP is a ribonucleoprotein consisting of 7S RNA and six different proteins. SRP54 is one of the six proteins of SRP which has GTPase activity.
(D) SRP can bind only to ribosomes that display the signal sequence.

Which one of the following combinations of above statements is true?

a) A and B
b) A and C
c) A, B, and C
d) A, B, C, and D

28. Genes required for galactose utilization in yeast are activated by a transcription factor called GAL4, which recognizes DNA binding sites with two 5'-CGG-3' sequences on complementary strands separated by 11 base pairs. Approximately 4000 potential GAL4 binding sites of the form 5'-

CGG(N)11CCG-3' are present in the yeast genome, but only 10 of them regulate genes necessary for galactose metabolism. Following reasons are suggested:

(A) Chromatin structure shields a large number of the potential binding sites in eukaryotic cells. GAL4 is thereby prevented from binding to sites that are unimportant in galactose metabolism.
(B) Chromatin structure is altered in active genes.
(C) This transcription factor is not crucial for RNA polymerase to bind promoter.
(D) Most of the binding sites for GAL4 possess mutated sequences while only a few are functional.

Which of the following combinations of above statements is true?

a) A and B
b) A and C
c) A and D
d) B and D

29. Some genes are transcribed frequently- as often as every 2 seconds in *E. coli.* The promoters for these genes are referred to as strong promoters. In contrast, other genes are transcribed much less frequently, about once in 10 minutes; the promoters for these genes are weak promoters. Some of the following statements could possibly explain this observation.

(A) The -10 and -35 regions of most strong promoters have sequences that correspond closely to the consensus sequences; where as weak promoters tend to have multiple substitutions at these sites.
(B) The distance between -10 and -35 regions is more in strong promoters than weak promoters.
(C) Strong promoters have U P element that is bound by the a subunit of RNA polymerase.
(D) σ factors have low affinity for weak promoters.

Which of the above statements are correct?

a) A and B
b) B and D
c) A and D
d) A and C

30. Eukaryotes have three different kinds of promoters in their RNA polymerase III transcription units, called types 1 to 3. Following statements relate to some characteristic features of these promoters.

(A) Type 1 promoter contains three short elements, the A box, the intermediate element (IE) and a C-box. It is present in 5S rRNA transcription unit and is upstream from the transcription initiation site.
(B) Type 2 promoter is present in most tRNA transcription units. It is divided into the A box and the B box. It is downstream from the transcription initiation site.
(C) Type 3 promoter controls U6 snRNA transcription units and is entirely upstream from the transcription initiation site.

(D) Type 3 promoters have TATA box and BRE element.
Which of the following combinations is correct?
(1) A and B (2) Only D
(3) B and C (4) Only A

31. A bacterial strain is growing in a natural habitat. When it is exposed to ultraviolet irradiation some of it operons are switched on which usually remain switched off in normal environmental conditions. It is also observed that the level of few proteins like RecA and LexA changes dramatically. Some of the following statements could possibly explain this observation.
(A) Ultraviolet irradiations cause DNA damage and SOS response is induced.
(B) RecA protein inhibits SOS response therefore its amount is decreased in the cell.
(C) LexA protein positively regulates genes that synthesize DNA repairing enzymes.
(D) RecA protein is activated when the DNA is exposed to UV light. Active RecA causes proteolytic cleavage of LexA.
Which one of the following combinations of the above statements is true?
a) A and B b) C and D
c) B and C d) A and D

32. Eukaryotes have multiple origins of replication along the chromosomes and the regulation of initiation is critically important. Each origin must fire once-and only once-in each cell cycle. If unregulated replication occurred, some region along the chromosome might be copied more than once and others not at all. The following possibilities are suggested to regulate origin sites.
(A) The pre-replicative complex can be activated only once in G1 phase.
(B) Cdc6 is a key licensing factor. It is highly unstable and is degraded during S phase. As a result it is not available to support reloading of MCM proteins onto the origin site.
(C) Cdt1 is a main component of pre-replication complex and it can work only once after it synthesis because it's DNA binding domain is inactivated by S phase Cdk.
(D) Replication origin sites can be recognized by origin recognition complex (ORC) for second cycle only when whole chromosome is replicated.
Which of the following is correct?
a) A and C b) Only B
c) B and D d) Only D

33. siRNAs and miRNAs are used for achieving gene silencing. Although, major steps are similar there are distinct differences in the key players of the two processing pathways. Following statements relate to some characteristic features of gene silencing.

A. Both siRNAs and miRNAs are processed by cytoplasmic endonuclease Dicer.
B. 'Drosha' is needed for processing miRNAs and precursor siRNAs.
C. Both siRNAs and miRNAs show association with Argonaute protein.
D. Both the processing pathways involve RISC complex.

Which of the following combinations is NOT correct?

a) A and C b) C and D
c) A and B d) D and A

[CSIR (NET/JRF) Exam. June 2011]

34. Genetic studies demonstrated that TBP mutant cell extracts are deficient in transcription of genes from all three promoters viz. class I, II and III. Following statements describe characteristic features of TBP.

A. TBP is considered as an universal basal transcription factor.
B. TBP is not required for transcription of archaeal genes.
C. TBP is involved in recognizing TATA box.
D. TBP operates at all promoters regardless of their TATA content.

Which of the following combination is correct?

a) A and D b) C and D
c) B and D d) A and C

[CSIR (NET/JRF) Exam. June 2011]

35. Presence of circular mRNAs for a specific protein in an eukaryotic cell reflects a rapid rate of synthesis of that protein. Following mechanisms are suggested:

A. eIF-4G and PABP promote this process through 5'-3' interaction of mRNA.
B. ribosomes are less active in recognizing circular mRNA.
C. PABP and eIF-4A promote this process.
D. ribosomes can reinitiate translation without being disassembled.

Which of the following is correct?

a) A and D b) B and D
c) A and C d) B and C

[CSIR (NET/JRF) Exam. June 2011]

36. It has been observed that in 5-10% of the eukaryotic mRNAs with multiple AUGs, the first AUG is not the initiation site. In such cases, the ribosome skips over one or more AUGs before encountering the favourable one and initiating translation. This is postulated to be due to the presence of the following consensus sequence (s):

A. CCA CC AUG G B. CCG CC AUG G
C. CCG CC AUG C D. AAC GG AUG A

Which of the following sequence sets related to the above postulations is correct?

a) A and B b) A and C
c) C and D d) B and D

[CSIR (NET/JRF) Exam. June 2011]

37. In eukaryotic chromatin, 30nm fiber (solenoid) can open up to give rise to two kinds of chromatin. In one type (A), the promoter of a gene within the open chromatin is occupied by a nucleosome whereas in the other (B), the promoter is occupied by histone H1.
The following possibilities are suggested.
A. The gene in (A) is repressed.
B. The gene in (B) is repressed.
C. The gene is (A) is active.
D. The gene in (B) is active.
Which of the following sets is correct?
a) A and D b) A and B
c) B and D d) C and D

[CSIR (NET/JRF) Exam. June 2011]

38. Lac repressor inhibits expression of genes in lac-operon whereas purine biosynthesis is repressed by the Pur repressor. The two proteins have 31% identical sequences and have similar three-dimensional structures. The gene regulatory properties of these proteins differ in relation to
A. binding of small molecules to the repressor.
B. presence of recognition sites on the genome.
C. oligomeric nature of the repressor.
D. DNA binding property.
The correct statements are
a) A and B b) A, B and C
c) A and C d) B, C and D

[CSIR (NET/JRF) Exam. June 2011]

39. During mitogenic stimulation, cells proliferate at a higher rate and it is primarily determined by an enhanced rate of protein synthesis. Among other mechanisms, MAP kinase pathway of signal transduction is involved in this. Global protein synthesis may be regulated by many mechanisms involving various steps of protein synthesis, namely, initiation, elongation and termination. Thus, many protein factors may be involved in the same. In the above process (mitogenic stimulation) the following factors are the portable targets.
A. elF -2 B. eEF-1
C. S6 kinase D. elF-4E BP
The correct answer is

a) A+B b) C+D

c) D+A d) B+D **[CSIR Model Paper 2011]**

40. DNA repair, synthesis and recombination are intimately connected and inter dependent. An apparent commonality between processes of DNA replication and repair in the enzymatically catalyzed synthesis of DNA polynucleotide segments, which can be assembled with preexisting polynucleotides, leading to repair or replication. Synthesis of these polynucleotide segments is catalyzed by a group of enzymes DNA-dependant DNA polymerases. In the case of E.coli, DNA polymerase has been isolated in three distinct forms whereas five main types of polymerase have been isolated from mammalian cells. All the polymerases synthesize polynucleotides only in the 5' 3' direction. If polynucleotide chains could be elongated in 3' 5' direction, the hypothetical growing 5' terminus, rather than the incoming nucleotide, would carry a triposphate that is unsuitable for further elongation. The 3' 5? exonuclease activity is not associated with all the polymerases and only present in

(A) All E. coli DNA polymerases but not all mammalian polymerases.

(B) Pol I, Pol II, Pol III, Pol α , Pol. β

(C) Pol I, Pol II, Pol δ , Pol, Pol γ

(D) Pol I, Pol II, Pol α, Pol. ε

The correct statements are

a) (A) and (B). b) (A), (B) and (C).

c) (A) and (C). d) (A), (C) and (D).

[CSIR Model Paper 2011]

41. Rho factor is involved in termination of transcription in prokaryotes. Genetic manipulations indicate that Rho-dependent termination requires the presence of a specific recognition sequence on the newly synthesized RNA upstream of the termination site. The recognition sequence must be on the nascent RNA rather than the DNA, as demonstrated by Rho?s inability to terminate transcription in the presence of pancreatic RNAse. The essential features of this termination site have not been fully elucidated. Construction of synthetic termination sites indicates that it consists of 80 to 100 nts that lack a stable secondary structure and contain multiple regions that are rich in C and poor in G. Which of the following is/ are suggested by the above observation?

a) Rho factor attaches to nascent RNA at its recognition sequence and then migrates along the RNA in the 51 31 direction until it encounters an RNAP paused at the termination site.

b) Rho unwinds the RNA-DNA duplex forming the transcription bubble, thereby releasing the RNA transcript.

c) Rho factor attaches to the RNA at its recognition sequence while

RNA is in the RNA-DNA hybrid condition.

d) There may be other factors and hence Rho factor does not need to unwind the RNA-DNA hybrid to release the transcript.

[CSIR Model Paper 2011]

42. During development and differentiation, there is a dynamic programme of differential expression of sets of genes. In bacteria, phage infections are among the simplest examples of developmental process. Typically, only a subset of the phage genome, often referred to as immediate early genes, are expressed in the host immediately after phage infection. As time passes, early genes start to be expressed, and the immediate early genes and bacterial genes are turned off. In the final stage of phage infection, the early genes give way to late genes. One of the simplest way it is achieved is through
(A) expression of cascade of σ factors
(B) expression of new RNA polymerases
(C) expression of different holoenzymes
(D) expression of different transcription factors
The correct reasons are
a) (A), (D) b) (A), (C), (D)
c) (A), (B), (D) d) (A), (B), (C)

[CSIR Model Paper 2011]

43. Conversion of proto-oncogene to oncogene may involve the following processes:
A mutation in coding sequence
B gene amplification
C chromosome rearrangement
D mutation in non-coding sequence
Which one is appropriate?
a) A, B and C b) B, C and D
c) A, C and D d) All **[CSIR Model Paper 2011]**

44. Transcription elongation is intrinsically discontinuous and is interrupted by frequent pausing, stalling and arrest. Paused RNA polymerases (RNAPs) have a tendency to move in a retrograde direction along the DNA template *in vivo* and *in vitro*. During this “backtracking”, the RNA 3’ end is extruded from the RNAP through the pore and RNA polymerisation cannot occur. RNAPs can over come this impediment by cleaving the transcript internally, releasing short (3 to 18 nucleotides) RNA 3’- cleavage products and creating a new 3’- OH on the RNA that is aligned in the active site and conducive to catalysis. Following statements are regarding transcription elongation by paused RNAPs.
(A) The endonucleolytic cleavage activity of RNAP is stimulated by tran-

script cleavage factor Gre B in archaea.

(B) In eukaryotes transcription elongation factor TFIIS stimulates transcript cleavage.

(C) Bacterial TFS stimulates transcript cleavage and helps in resumption of transcription elongation by paused RNAP.

(D) The mechanism of action of the Gre B proteins and TFIIS involves absolutely conserved Asp and Glu side-chains at tips of domains that intrude into the catalytic centre and co-ordinate Mg^{++} for catalysis of hydrolytic cleavage near the RNA 3' end.

Which one of the following combination of above statements is true?

a) A and B b) B and C
c) A and D d) B and D

45. Translation initiation and the identification of the proper start codon is regulated most extensively during the translation process. Following statements are regarding translation initiation control in eukaryotes.

(A) eIF3 and eIF 5 are required for the assembly of the translation initiation complex and scanning of the ribosome and also for the regulation of start codon selection.

(B) eIF6 is a translation initiation factor that interacts with the 60S subunit and prevents binding of the two subunits.

(C) eIF4E-BPs undergo phosphorylation and de-phosphorylation cycles leading to hypo- or hyper-phosphorylated eIF4E-BPs. In their hypo-phosphorylated form, eIF4E-BPs interact with eIF4E and thereby blocking eIF4E binding to eIF4G. This leads to a block of translation initiation.

(D) Phosphorylation of the elongation factor eEF2 slows down translation when a eukaryotic cell enters mitosis. Therefore, translation is strongly reduced during mitosis and eEF2 dephosphorylation allows for rapid protein synthesis when cells exit the mitotic phase.

Which one of the following combination of above statements is correct?

a) A and C b) A, B and C
c) B, C and D d) A and D

46. Nonsense-Mediated mRNA Decay (NMD) is the predominant and best studied mRNA quality control system in the cytoplasm of eukaryotic cells. Following statements are regarding NMD.

(A) The NMD pathyway targets mRNAs that contain a premature terination codon (PTC).

(B) Intron-less mRNAs efficiently undergo NMD.

(C) UPF1 is essential for rapid and efficient degradation of a PTC-containing mRNA.

Which one of the following combination of above statements is true?

a) A and B b) Only A
c) Only B d) A and C

47. MicroRNAs (miRNAs) are small non-coding RNAs which are involved in post transcriptional gene regulation. Following are some statements regarding miRNA.
   (A) Mirtrons are miRNA genes with precursors spanning and defining entire introns and require the action of the Drosha complex for biogenesis.
   (B) Most plant miRNAs function as siRNA.
   (C) Ago proteins that are bound by miRNAs, interact with a member of the GW protein family and induces deadenylation of the target mRNAs.

   Which one of the following combination of above statements is true?

   a) A and B b) B and C
   c) Only A d) Only B

Answer Sheet

Part – B

1.	a	2.	a	3.	a	4.	a	5.	d	6.	c
7.	d	8.	c	9.	d	10.	c	11.	b	12.	a
13.	a	14.	a	15.	b	16.	a	17.	a	18.	b
19.	c	20.	d	21.	d	22.	a	23.	c	24.	c
25.	c	26.	d	27.	a	28.	b	29.	b	30.	c
31.	b	32.	a	33.	c	34.	a	35.	c	36.	b
37.	b	38.	d	39.	c	40.	d	41.	d	42.	d
43.	b	44.	d	45.	c	46.	b	47.	c	48.	d
49.	b	50.	d	51.	a	52.	b	53.	c	54.	b
55.	b	56.	b	57.	c	58.	c	59.	b	60.	a
61.	c	62.	a	63.	c	64.	c	65.	b	66.	b
67.	b	68.	c	69.	a	70.	d	71.	d	72.	b
73.	a	74.	c	75.	b	76.	a	77.	b	78.	c
79.	c	80.	c	81.	d	82.	c	83.	d	84.	c
85.	c	86.	b	87.	c	88.	c	89.	c	90.	a
91.	c	92.	c	93.	b	94.	b	95.	b	96.	a
97.	c	98.	d	99.	c	100.	a	101.	b	102.	c
103.	a	104.	b	105.	a	106.	b	107.	d	108.	b
109.	b	110.	b	111.	b	112.	d	113.	b	114.	c
115.	d	116.	a	117.	d	118.	d	119.	b	120.	d
121.	d	122.	d	123.	d	124.	c	125.	a	126.	d
127.	d	128.	b	129.	c	130.	d	131.	d	132.	a
133.	d	134.	b	135.	b	136.	b	137.	d	138.	d
139.	d	140.	d	141.	d	142.	c	143.	d	144.	c
145.	c	146.	c	147.	d	148.	d	149.	c	150.	b
151.	c	152.	d	153.	b	154.	b	155.	a	156.	a
157.	d	158.	c	159.	c	160.	b	161.	a	162.	d
163.	b	164.	c	165.	a	166.	c	167.	b	168.	b
169.	b	170.	b	171.	b	172.	a	173.	b	174.	b
175.	c	176.	a	177.	a	178.	c	179.	a	180.	b
181.	b	182.	b	183.	d	184.	a	185.	a	186.	b
187.	d	188.	a	189.	b	190.	c	191.	a	192.	a
193.	c	194.	b	195.	a	196.	b	197.	b	198.	b
199.	b	200.	b	201.	d	202.	b	203.	c	204.	b
205.	b	206.	a	207.	c	208.	b	209.	c	210.	b

211.	b	212.	a	213.	c	214.	d	215.	a	216.	c
217.	d	218.	b	219.	d	220.	c	221.	c	222.	c
223.	d	224.	b								

Part – C

1.	a	2.	c	3.	d	4.	b	5.	c	6.	a
7.	d	8.	a	9.	b	10.	a	11.	b	12.	c
13.	c	14.	b	15.	c	16.	a	17.	c	18.	b
19.	a	20.	a	21.	c	22.	a	23.	a	24.	b
25.	a	26.	d	27.	d	28.	a	29.	d	30.	c
31.	d	32.	b	33.	a	34.	b	35.	c	36.	a
37.	b	38.	d	39.	b	40.	c	41.	d	42.	a
43.	a	44.	d	45.	c	46.	d	47.	b		

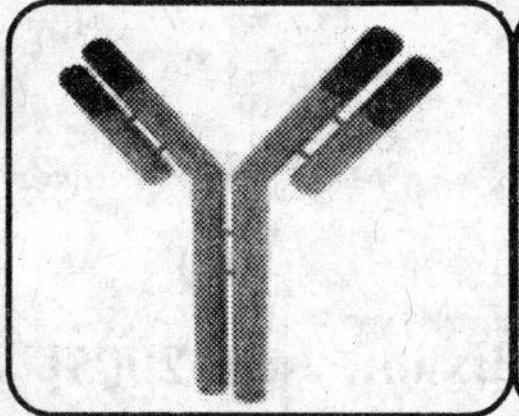

Chapter 4
Immunology

Part B

1. CD 4 receptors are specialized for
   a) MHC II
   b) MHC I
   c) Phagocytes
   d) Ig G

2. Toll-like receptors play a central role in the signaling process which results in
   a) Innate immunity
   b) Humoral immunity
   c) Cell-mediated immunity
   d) Artificial passive immunity

3. Which of the following immunoglobulin is pentameric?
   a) IgG
   b) IgM
   c) IgA
   d) IgE

4. Which of the following is not a component of complement system
   a) C3 convertase
   b) Mannose binding lectin
   c) MASP-2
   d) Adjuvants

5. Which of the following statement is correct?
   a) Super antigens are processed by endogenous pathway
   b) Super antigens are processed by exogenous pathway
   c) Super antigens are never processed
   d) Super antigens can be processed either by endogenous or exogenous pathway

6. A genetic region found in all humans whose products are primarily responsible for the rejection of grafts between individuals, is called
   a) Epitope
   b) Antigen
   c) Fc
   d) Major histocompatibility Complex

7. A secondary antibody response differs from a primary antibody response in
   a) Reaching lower maximal levels
   b) Being mounted faster
   c) Having a different effector function
   d) Being dependent on immune complexes

[CSIR (NET/JRF) Exam. Dec 2001]

8. Allergy response is caused by
   a) IgG b) IgM
   c) IgE d) IgD

[CSIR (NET/JRF) Exam. June 2005]

9. Immunoglobulins are antibodies synthesized by
   a) Both T-cell and B-cell b) Helper T-cell
   c) B-cell d) Antigen presenting cell

10. In case of humans, passive immunity observed in new-born child is due to the passage of the following immunoglobulin from the mother of the child through placenta
    a) IgD b) IgE
    c) IgG d) IgM

11. MHC II is
    a) CD 8 restricted b) CD 4 restricted
    c) Interleukines restricted d) Interferon restricted

12. Opsonization is an event which occurs in
    a) Cell-mediated immune response
    b) Humoral immune response
    c) Innate immunity
    d) All of the above

13. Systemic Lupus erythrmatosus is
    a) Infectious disease b) Autoimmune disease
    c) Metabolic disorder d) Immune deficiency disease

[CSIR (NET/JRF) Exam. Dec. 2005]

14. T and B-cells are activated by
    a) Cytotoxic cell b) T Helper cell
    c) B-cells d) Antibodies

15. T.B. Vaccine has
    a) Killed bacteria b) Extract of cell wall of bacteria
    c) Bacterial toxin d) Attenuated bacteria

[CSIR (NET/JRF) Exam. June 2001]

16. The immunoglobulin that results in histamine release is
    a) IgG b) IgM
    c) IgE d) IgD

17. The most immunogenic of all the macromolecular antigens of an infectious organism is
    a) Polysaccharide b) Nucleic acid
    c) Protein d) Glycolipid

[CSIR (NET/JRF) Exam. Dec 2001]

18. The prime target of HIV is helper T-cells of immune system because
    a) HIV has receptor only for CD 4
    b) Helper cells are very important part of immune system
    c) HIV can survive only in helper cells because they can replicate only in these cells
    d) None of the above

19. The recognition of target cell by CD 8 cytotoxic cells is
    a) MHC restricted
    b) MHC-I restricted
    c) MHC-II restricted
    d) MHC-III restricted

[CSIR (NET/JRF) Exam. Dec 2001]

20. The relative level of specific IgM antibodies can be of diagnostic significance because
    a) IgM is easier to detect than the other isotypes
    b) Viral infection often results in very high IgM response
    c) IgM antibodies are more often protective against reinfections than are the other isotypes.
    d) Relative high levels of IgM often correlate with a first recent exposure to the inducing agent

21. The T-cell receptor can bind to antigenic peptides
    a) Only in the free form
    b) Only when loaded on to MHC molecules
    c) Only when complexed to hapten
    d) Only when bound by antibody

22. Which of the following cell types does HIV preferentially infect?
    a) Cytotoxic T-cells
    b) Natural killer cells
    c) Helper T-cells
    d) Memory cells

[CSIR (NET/JRF) Exam. Dec 2003]

23. Which one of the following statements is true with regard to tissue macrophages?
    a) Have short life spans because they self-destruct after engulfing foreign invaders.
    b) Originate from monocytes that leave the circulation and enter the tissues
    c) Are most effective against parasites
    d) Do not attack microorganisms directly, instead, they destroy virus-infected body cells.

24. Which of the following surface marker distinguish helper T-cell lymphocyte from cytoxic T cell?
    a) CD 4
    b) CD 8
    c) CD 16
    d) CD 64

[CSIR (NET/JRF) Exam. Dec. 2005]

25. Which of the following vaccine consists of living microorganisms?
    a) Poliomyelitis
    b) Diphtheria
    c) Tetanus
    d) Small pox

[CSIR (NET/JRF) Exam. June 2001]

26. Which one of the following antibody is found attached to mast cells?
    a) Ig G
    b) Ig D
    c) Ig E
    d) Ig A

27. TH17 cells stimulate
    a) Macrophages
    b) Lymphocytes
    c) Neutrophiles
    d) Basophiles

28. Protein kinase - R inhibits
    a) Replication of tumour cells.
    b) Replication of bacterial cells.
    c) Replication of virus.
    d) Cell movement

29. α defensin a potent antibacterial and anti fungal is secreted from
    a) Paneth cells
    b) Kuffer cells
    c) Macrophage cells
    d) B cells

30. When any Tc cell binds to APC to antigen recognition by MHC I and TCR and CD 28 and B7. These two bindings produce two signals which release the cytokine known as IL-2 which has?
    a) An autocrine effect
    b) Paracrine effect
    c) Endocrine effect
    d) Juxtacrine effect

31. Toll like receptors are very important part of innate immunity. There are 10 TLR in humans are studied which functions for a special types of pathogen associated molecular pattern. Which of the following TLR is responsible against the G-rich oligonucleotide?
    a) TLR 8
    b) TLR 7
    c) TLR 6
    d) TLR 1 and 2

32. In compliment activation pathway by classical method C1q, C1r and C1s plays an important role for initation of autocatalysis. C1r is a protease and cleaves to C1s which cleaves to C4 and C2, if C1q gene is mutated then what would be the effect on activation of pathway?

a) No effect
b) Pathways would not initiated
c) C3 convertase will form but C5 convertase will not
d) Rate of reaftion during autocatalysis would be decreased.

33. Blood transfusion reaction is an example of
a) Type I hypersensitivity b) Type II hypersensitivity
c) Type III hypersensitivity d) Type IV hypersensitivity

34. The secondary structure of antibody is made up mostly of
a) α-helix b) β sheets
c) Left handed α-helix only d) α-helix and β-sheets both

35. Rabies virus enters the cell through
a) Nerve growth factor receptor
b) Nicotine-acetylcholine receptor
c) Cell-cell adhesion receptor
d) All of the above

36. Interleukin binding receptors on lymphocytes are example of
a) Receptor tyrosine kinases b) Tyrosine kinase associated receptors
c) GPCR d) Receptor serine/threonine kinases

37. Influenza virus binds with
a) N-acetylgalactosamine b) N-acetylglucosamine
c) N-acetylmuramic acid d) N-acetylneuraminic acid

38. Which of the following statement is incorrect?
a) Poliovirus and adenovirus infect cell by pore formation in the endosome.
b) Poliovirus is an enveloped virus.
c) Adenovirus is a nonenveloped virus.
d) Poliovirus enters the cell by receptor mediated endocytosis.

39. Which of the following statement is incorrect?
a) NK cells always kills the cells which have altered MHC I glycoprotein.
b) Macrophages digest exogenous antigens.
c) TNF-a is secreted by macrophage.
d) TAP is a P type ATPase transporter present in the ER membrane.

40. Which of the following molecular chaperon is present in the rough ER
a) Calnexin b) Calreticulin
c) Tapasin d) All of the above

41. Antigen binding with MHC II molecule is mediated by
a) Cathepsin-S b) CLIP
c) HLA-DM d) Peptidyltransferase

42. First made antibody by new born baby is
    a) IgM b) IgG
    c) IgA d) IgD

43. Delayed type hypersensitivity is
    a) Type I hypersensitivity b) Type II hypersensitivity
    c) Type III hypersensitivity d) Type IV hypersensitivity

44. Why don't we become immune to influenza viruses?
    a) Because they attack only the helper T cells there by suppressing the immune system.
    b) Because they alter their surface proteins and thus avoid recognition.
    c) Because they don't actually. generate an immune response.
    d) Because they are too small to serve as antigens.

45. If you want to design an artificial cell that could safely carry drugs inside the body. Which of the following molecule would need to mimic to deter the immune system?
    a) MHC I b) Interleukin I
    c) Antigen d) Complement

46. Which of the following disease is not caused by bacteria?
    a) Peptic ulcers b) The flu
    c) Tuberculosis d) Dental carries

47. Rabies virus replicates in
    a) RBCs b) WBCs
    c) Nerve cells d) Muscle cells

48. Poliovirus encodes a protease which proteolytically cleave
    a) Transmembrane protein b) TATA binding factor of TFIID
    c) p53 gene product d) Lysosomal enzymes

49. Antigen shifting is a process where
    a) Pathogen may defeat the immune system by changing its surface marker
    b) Pathogen moves from one host to another host
    c) Infection is caused by infected materials
    d) All of the above

50. Ig G mediated hypersensitivity response is
    a) Type-I b) Type-II
    c) Type-III d) Both (b) and (c)

51. What is critical to finding novel antigens for vaccine development?
    a) The growth of live infectious agents to create whole vaccines
    b) The engineering of genes to attenuate infectious agents

c) The identification of proteins that elicit an immune response
d) The identification of the immune system components unique to specific infectious agents

52. How are the variants of antibodies produced?
a) Each variant is encoded on one gene
b) By post-translational modification of the antibodies
c) By shuffling a small number of gene segments around
d) By splicing the transcript into various configurations

53. Graft rejection does not involve
a) erythrocytes
b) T cells
c) macrophages
d) polymorphonuclear leukocytes **[CSIR (NET-JRF) Exam. Dec. 2011]**

54. Toxic shock is caused by
a) toxins produced by some bacteria.
b) excessive stimulation of a large proportion of T cells by bacterial superantigens
c) abnormal cytokine production by B cells
d) excessive production of immuno-globulins

[CSIR (NET-JRF) Exam. Dec. 2011]

55. Indirect immunofluorescence involves fluorescently labelled
a) immunoglobulin-specific antibodies
b) antigen-specific antibodies
c) hapten-specific antibodies
d) carrier-specific antibodies **[CSIR (NET-JRF) Exam. Dec. 2011]**

56. To keep them in a totipotent state, embryonic stem cells need to be maintained in a medium supplemented with
a) growth hormone b) leukemia inhibiting factor
c) nestin d) insulin

[CSIR (NET-JRF) Exam. Dec. 2011]

57. Rapid but non- antigen specific immune response are produced by.
a) Adaptive immune response b) Innate immune response
c) Leukocytes d) Lymphatic system

58. The major component of pus is?
a) Dead or dying neutrophills b) Dead or dying eosinophills
c) Dead or dying leucocytes d) Dead or dying lymphocytes

59. C1q, C1r and C1s are the components of classical pathway of complement activation. In an experiment C1s coding gene is mutated.

    What would be the effect of this mutation on compliment activation pathway?
    a) No compliment activation takes place
    b) Compliment activation takes place but C3 convertage will not form.
    c) C3 convertage will form but C5 is not formed
    d) C1q can not bind to pathogen surface

60. Immunoglobulin G was fractionated by size exclusion chromatography and it was observed to have a molecular mass of 150 kDa. SDS-PAGE analysis under reducing condition revealed two bands of size 50 kDa and 25 kDa. The oligomeric status of the protein consists of.
    a) 3 polypeptide chains of molecular mass of 50 kDa
    b) 6 polypeptide chains of molecular mass of 25 kDa
    c) One polypeptide chain of 50 kDa and 4 polypepted of mass 25 kDa.
    d) Two of 50 kDa and two of 25 kDa

61. Anthrax vaccine has
    a) Inactivated virus
    b) Inactivated bacteria
    c) Extract of attenuated bacteria
    d) Extract of attenuated virus

62. Th2 response is generated and maintained mainly by which of the following pair of cytokines?
    a) IL-4 and IL-10.   b) IL-12 and IFN- .
    c) IFN- and TNF-   d) IL-2 and IL-12.

    [CSIR (NET/JRF) Exam. June 2011]

63. Which class of immunoglobulins will increase in case of a chronic infection?
    a) IgA   b) IgG
    c) IgM   d) IgE

    [CSIR Model Paper 2011]

Part C

1. Survival of intracellular pathogens depends on the levels of pro-inflammatory and anti-inflammatory cytokines in macrophages. In an experimental condition, Mycobacteria infected macrophages were treated with IL-6 or IL-12 for 4 hours at 370C. Untreated cells were used as control. Cells were lysed and number of bacteria in each experimental set was counted by measuring colony forming unit (CFU). Which of the following observations true?
   a) IL-12 treated cells contain more intracellular bacteria than control
   b) IL-12 treated cells contain less intracellular bacteria than control
   c) IL-6 treated cells contain more intracellular bacteria than control
   d) IL-6 treated cells contain less intracellular bacteria than control

   [CSIR (NET/JRF) Exam. Dec. 2011]

2. In order to prevent tetanus in neonates, one of the following treatments can be adopted.
   A. Treatment of the infant with anti-toxin and the toxoid.
   B. Immunize the mother with the toxoid.

   In case of A, the treatment can be given
   a. immediately after birth
   b. after the onset of the condition.

   In case of B, the immunization has to be done
   c. before pregnancy.
   d. late in the pregnancy.

   The correct combination is
   a) A/a b) A/b
   c) B/c d) B/d

   [CSIR (NET/JRF) Exam. Dec. 2011]

3. Many of the bacteria that cause infectious diseases in humans multiply in the extracellular spaces of the body, and most intracellular pathogens spread by moving from cell to cell through the extracellular fluids. The extracellular spaces are protected by the humaral immune response, in which antibodies are produced by B cells and result in the destruction of microorganism. The following statements are related with the humoral immune response
   (A) Stimulation of B cells by helper T cells
   (B) Secretion of antibodies that specifically recognize foreign molecules
   (C) Presentation of an antigen-antibody complex to cytotoxic T cells
   (D) Destruction of antigen-antibody by macrophages

Which of the following is correct about humoral immunity.

a) A, B, C and D b) A, B and D
c) B, C and D d) A and B

4. The internal epithelia are known as mucosal epithelia because they secrete a viscous fluid called mucus. Which contain many glycoproteins called mucins.Microorganisms coated in mucus may be prevented from adhering to epithilium such as that of respiratory tract microorganisms can be expelled in the flow of mucus driven by beating of cilia.

Read the following?

(A) Epithial surface also produce chemical substances that are microbicidal or that inhibit microbial growth
(B) The antibacterial enzymes, lysozymes and phospholipase A are secreted in saliva
(C) Saliva contains various histatins which are cystine rich peptides with anti- microbial properties
(D) -defensins are made by respiratory and urino-genital epithelium

Which of the following is corret?

a) A, B, C and D b) A, B and D
c) B, C and D d) A, B and C

5. Microorganisms typically bear repeating patterns of molecular structure on their surface. The cell walls of gram positive and gram negative bacteria are composed of matrix of carbohydrates, proteins and lipids in a repetitive array. These repeatitive structures are known as generally "pathogen associated molecular patterns" (PAMPs) and the receptors that recognize it, pattern recognition receptors. (PRR).

The following statements are associated with PAMPs and PRRs interaction

(A) Scavanger receptors, recognize various anionic polymers and acetylated low density lipoproteins.
(B) Some scavanger receptors recognize structures that are sheilded by sialic acid on normal host cells.
(C) Mannose binding lectin responsible for complement activation in lectin pathway is a kind of PRR.
(D) Macrophage mannose receptors are C type lectin.

a) A, B, C, D b) A, C, D
c) B, C, D d) A and D

6. There are 10 expressed TLR genes is mice and humans, and each of the 10 protiens they produced is devoted to recognize a distinct set of molecular patterns that are characteristic components of pathogenic microorganisms at one or other stage of infection.

The following statements are associated with TLRs
(A) TLR -1, TLR 2 and TLR 2 and TLR 6 work as heterodimer and are activated by peptidoglycan and lipoproteins etc.
(B) TLR- 9 are exclusively activated by unmethylated CpG DNA
(C) TLR - 4 functions as a dimer with MD-2 and CD-14 and are exclusively activated by gram positive bacteria
(C) Toll like receptor 8 is activated by 'G' rich oligonucleotides
Which of the following combination is correct?

(a) A, B, C and D (b) B and D
(c) A and C (d) A, B and D

7. Complement activation pathways depand on the different molecules for their initiation, but they converge to generate the same set of effector complement proteins.
Follwing informations were collected
(A) Lectin patway of complement activation can be activated by ficolin which bind to carbohydrate on pathogen surface
(B) C3b is a part of C3 convertage which binds to complement receptor on phagocytes
(C) C3a and C5a are peptide mediators of inflamation phagocyte recruitment.
(D) C5b, C6, C7, C8 and C9 are important in lysis of certain pathogens and cells
Which one of the following combination is correct?

a) A, B, C and D b) B and C
c) B, C and D d) A and D

8. There are two classes of MHC molecules. MHCI and MHC II which differ in both their structure and function and expression pattern on the tissues of the body. MHC I and class II molecules are closely related in overall structure but differ in their subunit composition.
The following statements are associated with MHC molecules
(A) chain of MHC I is coded by chromosome 6
(B) In class I and form the antigen binding cleft
(C) In class II and form the antigen binding cleft
(D) MHC II is also encoded by chromosome 6
Which one of the following combination is correct?

a) A, B, C and D b) A, B and C
c) B, C and D d) B and C

9. A group of 10 humans was tested for the penicillin. Penicillin was injected in all the individuals in equal amount but in 3 invividuals penicillin caused allergic reaction and in 7 individiuals it did not activate immune system and did not show any allergic reaction. On the basis of above information penicillin is a

a) Hapten
b) Antigen
c) Adjuvant
d) Both hapten and antigen

10. The major histocompatibility complex referred to as the HLA complex in human and the H-2 complex in mice. Although the arrangement of genes is somewhat different in both cases, the MHC genes are organized into regions encoding three classes of molecules. On the basis of this information these results were observed:-

(A) Class II MHC genes encode various secretory proteins that have not any immune function

(B) A monoclonal antibody specific for B2 microglobulin can be used to detect both class I and classII molecules on cell surface.

(C) Class II MHC molecules typically binds to longer peptides than class I.

(D) The majority of peptides displayed by class I and class II MHC molecules on the cell surface are derived from self protein.

Which of the following combination is not correct:

a) Only A
b) A and B
c) B and D
d) A and D

11. Antigen presenting cells have been shown to present lysozyme peptide with class II MHC. When CD4+TH cells are incubated with APC and native lysozyme peptide, TH cells activation occurs. If the chloroquine is added to the incubation mixure, presentation of antigen is inhibited but the peptide continues to induce the TH cell activation. Explain why this occurs?

a) Chloroquine increases the pH of medium
b) Chloroquine degrades the antigenic peptide
c) Chloroquine inhibits the MHC synthesis
d) Chloroquine inhibits endocytons.

12. Cyclosporin is powerful immunosuppressive drug given to transplant recipient. This drugs prevents the formation of a complex between calcineurin and Ca+2/calmodulin. Explain how this compound supress T-cell mediated aspects of transplant rejection?

A. Cyclosporin blocks production of NFAT. one of the transcription factor necessory for proliferation of antigen activated cells.

B. Cyclorporin blocks this complex which results into activation of phosphatase calcineurin

C. Cyclosporin activate the production of NFAT and results in the suppression of immune system

D. Cyclosporin inhibits the activation of calcineurin.

Which of the following is correct?

a) A, C and D
b) B, C and D
c) A and D
d) Only A

13. Graft rejection reactions have various time courses depending upon the type of the tissue or organ grafted and the immune response involved. Hyperacute rejection reaction occurs within the first 24 hours after transplantation accute rejection reaction usually begin in the first few weeks after transplantation and chronic rejection reaction can occur from month to year after transplantation.
The following statements are related with tissue / organ rejection.
(A) Acute rejection is mediated by pre existing host antibodies specific for antigen on the grafted tissue.
(B) Cytokines produced by host TH cells activated in response to alloantigens play a major role in graft rejection.
(C) Passenger leukocytes are host dendritic cells that migrate into grafted tissue and act as antigen presenting cells
(D) All allograft between individual with identical HLA haplotype will be accepted
Which of the following is not true?
a) A,B, C and D b) A, C and D
c) B, C and D d) A, B and D

14. Intracellular pathogens like *Mycobacteria*, *Salmonella*, *Leishmania* and *Listeria* survive in macrophages by modulating host cellular machinery. In order to study the fate of these intracellular pathogens in macrophages, cells were labelled with lysotracker Red and infected with GFP-labelled organisms. After 2 hours at 370C, cells were fixed, stained with anti-transferrin receptor antibody and probed with secondary antibody conjugated-blue dyes. Cells were viewed under confocal microscope.

Observation: GFP-labelled *Mycobateria*, *Salmonella* and *Listeria* were lacolized in the same compartment labelled with blue dyes, whereas GFP-Leishmania colocalize with red labelled compartment. Which of the following statement is true based on these observations?
a) *Mycobacteria*, *Salmonella* and *Listeria* reside in the lysosomes.
b) *Leishmania* reside in lysosome like compartment
c) *Leishmania* reside in a compartment which bears characteristics of early endocytic compartment.
d) *Mycobacteria*, *Salmonella* and *Listeria* lyse the phagosomal membrane and reside in cytosol. **[CSIR (NET/JRF) Exam. June 2011]**

15. Toll-like receptor 4 is associated with responsiveness to LPS, an endotoxin that causes lethal endotoxic shock. The mice deficient in Toll-like receptor 4 and BALB/c mice were injected with *Escherichia coli*. In addition, some BALB/b mice were also injected with the same bacteria alone or with anti-interleukin-10 (IL-10) antibody. The mice resistant to the lethal effect of the bacteria were:

a) BALB/b mice receiving the bacteria.
b) BALB/b mice receiving the bacteria and the anti-IL-10 antibody.
c) Mice deficient in Toll-like receptor
d) BALB/c mice receiving the bacteria.

[CSIR (NET/JRF) Exam. June 2011]

16. A patient undergoes liver transplantation and during the course of post-operative treatment, becomes susceptible to infection. The patient can be treated in two different modes and can have alternative outcomes. Which of the following statements is correct?
    a) Treatment with immunostimulatory drugs reducing the infection but rejecting the transplant.
    b) Treatment with immunostimulatory drugs reducing the infection and retaining the transplant.
    c) Treatment with antibiotics reducing the infection but retaining the transplant.
    d) Treatment with antibiotics reducing the infection but rejecting the transplant. **[CSIR (NET/JRF) Exam. June 2011]**

17. Monoclonal antibodies (mAb) can be potentially used as therapeutic agents. The major advantage is that they can specifically target aberrant cells. However, there is a practical difficulty. Monoclonals are raised in mouse and therefore it is expected that an immune reaction will develop if these are injected into humans. It is therefore necessary to 'humanize' monoclonal antibody by
    a) expressing the genes for the mAb in cultured human cells and isolating the mAb from these cells
    b) replacing the Fv region of a mAb with one derived from a human IgG
    c) replacing CL and CH regions of the Mab with that obtained from a human IgG.
    d) taking a human IgG and replacing the CDRs by those derived from the mouse mAb. **[CSIR (NET/JRF) Exam. June 2011]**

18. Polyclonal antibodies are raised against bovine serum albumin in rabbit. Subsequently IgG in the antiserum is purified and digested with either pepsin or papain. Out of the following possibilities, which one is correct?
    a) Pepsin-digested antibodies cannot precipitate the antigen
    b) Papain-digested antibodies cannot precipitate the antigen
    c) Pepsin digestion will produce two Fab molecules
    d) Pepsin-digested antibodies will lose all interchain disulfide bonds

[CSIR Model Paper 2011]

Answer Sheet

Part – B

1.	a	2.	a	3.	b	4.	d	5.	c	6.	d
7.	b	8.	c	9.	c	10.	c	11.	b	12.	b
13.	b	14.	b	15.	d	16.	c	17.	c	18.	a
19.	b	20.	d	21.	b	22.	c	23.	b	24.	a
25.	d	26.	c	27.	c	28.	c	29.	a	30.	a
31.	b	32.	b	33.	b	34.	b	35.	a	36.	b
37.	d	38.	b	39.	d	40.	d	41.	c	42.	a
43.	d	44.	b	45.	a	46.	b	47.	c	48.	b
49.	a	50.	d	51.	c	52.	c	53.	a	54.	b
55.	a	56.	b	57.	b	58.	a	59.	a	60.	d
61.	a	62.	a	63.	b						

Part – C

1.	b	2.	d	3.	b	4.	b	5.	a	6.	a
7.	a	8.	a	9.	a	10.	c	11.	d	12.	c
13.	b	14.	b	15.	b	16.	c	17.	d	18.	b

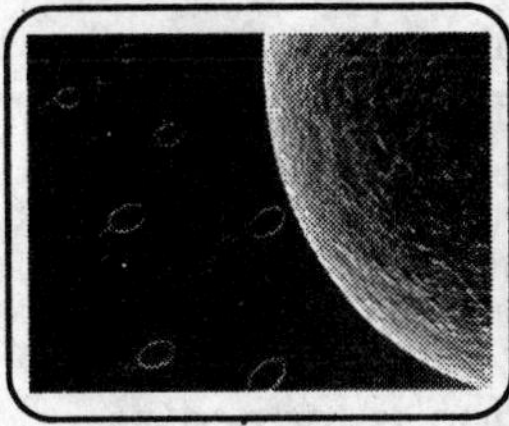

Chapter 5
Developmental Biology

Part B

1. Cell fusion is an essential phenomenon in development of
   a) Nerve　　b) Muscle
   c) Spleen　　d) Liver

   [CSIR (NET/JRF] Exam. Dec. 2006]

2. Gene amplification is common in
   a) Developing oocytes　　b) Senescing cells
   c) Differentiated cells　　d) Every dividing cell

3. Which of the following are the anterior determinants in Drosophila
   a) Hunchback RNA and nanos RNA
   b) Caudal RNA and bicoid RNA
   c) Hunchback RNA and caudal RNA
   d) Hunchback RNA and bicoid RNA

4. Dorsal mutant in *Drosophila* will result in
   a) Dorsalization of ventral side
   b) Ventralization of dorsal side
   c) There would be no effect
   d) Anterior-posterior pattern formation will be effected

5. Sxl gene of *Drosophila* regulates expression at
   a) Transcription level　　b) Post transcription level
   c) Translation level　　d) Post translation level

6. Mosaic developmental pattern is always
   a) Autonomous　　b) Non autonomous
   c) Conditional　　d) Regulative

7. In an early embryonic transplantation experiment prospective skin cells were transferred near future muscle cell but they still differentiate into skin cell. The cell would be termed as
   a) Determined　　b) Committed
   c) Totipotent　　d) Differentiated

8. The emergence of polarity of an embryo is the result of
   a) Positive and negative charges interacting in early development.
   b) Cytoplasmic differences between cells.
   c) Cytoplasmic determinants within cells.
   d) All of the above.

9. Rolling of sheet of cell over other cells during gastrulation is termed as
   a) Epiboly b) Ingression
   c) Involulation d) Delamination

10. Factor responsible for formation of early embryonic axis during early developmental pathway of plants is
    a) Auxin gradient b) Morphogens
    c) Orientation of embryo sac d) Plane of cell division

11. During germination of seeds, after imbibition of water first step would be
    a) Mobilization of reserve food
    b) Transcription of specific genes
    c) Cell division
    d) Embryo differentiation

12. In ABCE model of flower development genes A, B, C and E regulates the development of flower in Arabidopsis. If a loss-of-function mutation occurs in the E-type genes, what will be the composition of the flower whorls?
    a) Sepals-petals-stamens-carpels
    b) Sepals-sepals-sepals-sepals
    c) Petals-stamens-carpels-carpels
    d) Sepals-sepals-petals-petals

13. Which statement is correct for capacitation?
    a) Is the maturation of mammalian spermatozoa after entering into oviduct of female.
    b) Meiotic division in egg after penetration of sperm
    c) Maturation of egg in oviduct after fertilization
    d) Maturation of spermatozoa in male body

14. Morphallaxis can be defined as
    a) Production of lost organ by division in remaining cell
    b) Reinitiation of cell division in existing cell, followed by repatterning of those cells
    c) Production of complete organism by single cell
    d) Movement of organism toward stimulus

15. During development homing of cells is mediated by
   a) Integrin b) Laminin
   c) Cadherin d) Selectin

16. In regulative development, the prospective potency of cells
   a) Equal to prospective fate
   b) More than prospective fate
   c) Lesser than prospective fate
   d) Not determined

17. Anterior-posterior polarity in *Drosophila* is determined by
   a) Zygotic genes b) Maternal effect genes
   c) Paternal effect genes d) Both (b) and (C)

18. What would happen if "bicoid" gene is injected in the center of bicoid - deficient embryo?
   a) Develops normal anterior - posterior polarity.
   b) Middle region of the embryo become head.
   c) Two heads emerged one at either end.
   d) No effect on the development of embryo.

19. The major function of cortical granules in cytoplasm of egg is
   a) Early block to polyspermy
   b) Late Block to polyspermy
   c) Allowing meiosis to complete
   d) Helping in reorganization of sperm

20. The development of identical twins is an example of
   a) Mosaic development b) Conditional specification
   c) Syncytial specification d) Morphallaxis

21. In C. elegans anterior - posterior axis formation is governed by
   a) PAR proteins b) P - granules
   c) SKN - 1 protein d) PIE-1 protein

22. In Drosophila if Dorsal protein does not translocate from cytoplasm to the nuclei of any embryonic cell
   a) All the cells an dorsalized
   b) All the cells an ventralized
   c) Dorsalized and ventralized cells are formed equally
   d) Embryo does not survive

23. In tissue culture experiment to initiate shoots from undifferentiated mass of cell, the medium must contain
   a) Low auxin and high cytokinin b) High auxin and high cytokinin
   c) High auxin and low cytokinin d) Low auxin and low cytokinin

24. In *Drosophila* the protein product encoded by "bicoid" and "nanos" are critical for establishing the
    a) Anterior - posterior polarity of embryo.
    b) Dorsal - ventral polarity of embryo.
    c) Latero-posterior axis of the embryo.
    d) All of the above

25. Which of the following represent the gametophyte generation in plants
    a) Ovule
    b) Megaspore
    c) Embryo sac
    c) Egg

26. First cell to be differentiated in developing embryo is
    a) Epidermal cells
    b) Bods
    c) RBC
    c) Nerve cells

27. Homeotic genes are responsible for
    a) Maintaining gaps in segments
    b) Provide gradient in developing embryo
    c) Codes morphogens
    d) Mutation results in formation of organ at unusual locations

28. Induction of parthenocarpic fruit development is mediated by
    a) Auxin
    b) Ethylene
    c) ABA
    d) Cytokinin

29. Which of the following group contains organisms that represent early stages in the evolution of the eukaryotic cell?
    a) Archaea
    b) Fungi
    b) Protista
    d) Animalia

30. During oogenesis of mammals, the second meiotic division occurs
    a) In the formation of the primary oocyte
    b) In the formation of the secondary oocyte
    c) Before ovulation
    d) After fertilization

31. In frog morula is
    a) 16 celled stage
    b) 32 celled stage
    c) 64 celled stage
    d) 128 celled stage

32. In frog an enzyme is produced from acrosome which dissolve vitteline membrane is
    a) Hyalurinidase
    b) Spermlysin
    c) Amphibilinidase
    d) Tigrinase

33. Which of the following are the gap genes
    a) kruppel and giant b) kruppel and hairy
    c) wingless and hedgehog d) wingless and giant

34. During the development of *Drosophilla* which of the following specification takes place?
    a) Autonomous b) Conditional
    c) Non autonomous d) Syncytial

35. Energids are formed in the development of
    a) *Drosophilla* b) *C. elegans*
    c) *Arabidopsis* d) Frogs

36. Pipe protein coding gene is found on both plates, that is, dorsal and ventral. But by a special experiment pipe gene is mutated only in the ventral plate. What would be the effect of this mutation?
    a) Dorsolization of ventral side.
    b) Ventralization of dorsal side.
    c) Normal development.
    d) A mass of cells will form.

37. In mosaic development the prospective potency of cell is
    a) Equal to prospective fate.
    b) Is greater than prospective fate
    c) Is less than prospective fate.
    d) Fates are unrelated.

38. In *Drosophila*, bicoid and hunchback genes define
    a) Anterior axis only b) Posterior axis only
    c) Dorso-ventral part d) Both (a) and (b)

39. Why are embryonic stem cells important?
    a) They can be passed from one generation to the next
    b) These cells carry retroviral genes
    c) They can develop into any tissue in the body, including the germ line
    d) The cells are differentiated and can therefore be manipulated

40. Merozygotes are formed in
    a) *Drosophila* b) *Neurospora*
    c) Yeast d) Bacteria

41. If a bud is able to flower when given the appropriate developmental signal, it is called.
    a) Determined b) Competent
    c) Expressed d) Phase transition

42. When a cell or tissue is capable to differentiate autonomously even when placed into another region of the embryo, it is called
a) Specification b) Determination
c) Differentiation d) Epiboly

43. When cells achieve their respective fates by interacting with other cells, it is called
a) Autonomous specification b) Conditional specification
c) Syncytial specification d) Competence

44. The product of which of the following gene is responsible for generating dorsal-ventral pattern in *Drosophila*?
a) bicoid gene b) hunchback gene
c) dorsal gene d) gap genes

45. In plants vernalization causes deacetylation of histone protein which
a) Suppress the gene FLOWERING LOCUS T (FLT)
b) Suppress the gene FLOWERING LOCUS C (FLC)
c) Activates FLT
d) Activates FLC

46. Which of the following phytohormone seems to play a role in establishing apical-basal polarity in the embryo?
a) Cytokinin b) ABA
c) Auxin d) Gibberellins

47. Which of the following is NOT involved in animal development?
a) Wnt signaling b) Notch receptors
c) GPCRs d) Hedgehog receptors

48. "Copia element" is a retrotransposon. It is present in
a) Yeast b) *Arabidopsis thaliana*
c) *Drosophila* d) Human

49. In the early development in *Drosophila* karyokinesis occurs without cytokinesis and the rapid rate of division is accomplished by eliminating the gap (G) stages of the cell cycle resulting in the formation of a syncytium. During 10th cleavage cycle nuclei reach the periphery of the egg and form
a) Pole cells b) Syncytial blastoderm
c) Energids d) Germ band

50. In *Drosophila* Smaug protein controls maternal-to-zygote transition. If this protein is artificially added to the anterior of an early Drosophila embryo what would not be a result
a) Cleavage cell cycle delay b) Cellularization
c) Gastrulation delay d) Zygotic gene expression

51. Which of the following cadherin type is found predominantly on the placenta in vertebrate embryos?
a) E-cadherin b) P-cadherin
c) N-cadherin d) D-cadherin

52. When a cell has already been specified for initiating a new gene expression and needs only an environment that allows the expression, it is called
a) Instructive interaction b) Permissive interaction
c) Determined d) Competent

53. During early embryonic development embryos develop like a mosaic of individually laid tiles-with each receiving its instructions independently. It is called
a) Conditional specification b) Autonomous development
c) Permissive interaction d) Determination

54. In which of the following oocytes are developed in egg chamber?
a) *Xenopus* b) *Drosophila*
c) *Dictyostelium* d) *C. elegans*

55. In Drosophila dorsal-ventral patterning in the oocyte is governed by
a) Gurken protein b) Dorsal protein
c) Bicoid protein d) Cactus protein

56. When concentration of dorsal protein is increased in cells of developing embryo of Drosophila it instruct the cells to become
a) Lateral ectoderm b) Amnioserosa
c) Dorsal ectoderm d) Mesoderm

57. Morphogen gradient provides a very important mechanism for
a) Mosaic embryos b) Regulative embryos
c) Gastrulation d) Formation of blastema

58. In embryonic development when the fate of cells depends on the cell's neighbors rather than some cytoplasmic factors, is called
a) Conditional specification b) Autonomous specification
c) Instructive interaction d) Syncytial specification

59. Bindin is an insoluble protein which mediates species-specific sperm-egg recognition. The receptors for this protein are found on
a) Sperm membrane b) Egg membrane
c) Vitelline envelop d) Jelly coat

60. If *nanos* mRNA is absent in the *Drosophila* embryo which of the following body part is not formed?
a) Head b) Thorax
c) Abdomen d) Telson

61. Maskin inhibits translation of mRNA in unfertilized eggs of
    a) Birds
    b) Amphibians
    c) Drosophila
    d) C. elegans

62. Which of the following pair of protein-protein interaction represent sperm-egg fusion in mammals?
    a) CD9-bindin
    b) Izomo-CD9
    c) Resact-RGC
    d) ZP3-acrosome

63. In gastrulation the migration of individual cells from the surface layer into the interior of the embryo is called
    a) Invagination
    b) Involution
    c) Ingression
    d) Epiboly

64. In an experiment some genes of *Drosophila* are knocked out and it results in defects in every segment of the body. These genes fail to encode
    a) Torso-like protein
    b) Hedgehog protein
    c) Hunchback protein
    d) Caudal protein

65. In *Drosophila* the unsegmented anterior and posterior extremities are regulated by the activation of
    a) Torso protein
    b) Cactus protein
    c) Oskar protein
    d) Pelle kinase

66. In mammals which of the following represent totipotent cells?
    a) Zygote
    b) Blastocyst
    c) Embryo
    d) Hematopoietic stem cells

67. When differentiated cells re-divide but maintain their differentiated functions, the phenomenon is called
    a) Epimorphosis
    b) Morphallaxis
    c) Compensatory regeneration
    d) Stem cell mediated regeneration

68. Stem cell niches provide microenvironment that regulate stem cell renewal, survival and differentiation. The niches retain the cells in an uncommitted state. Once the cells leave the niche they begin differentiating. The stem cell niches regulate stem cell proliferation and differentiation usually by
    a) Autocrine factors
    b) Juxtacrine factors
    c) Paracrine factors
    d) Endocrine factors

69. The induction of lens and optic placodes from the head epidermis of vertebrate neurulae is an example of
    a) Instructive induction
    b) Appositional induction
    c) Permissive induction
    d) Lateral inhibition

70. Which of the following appears to be the active agent of the zone of polarizing activity (ZPA)?
    a) Fgf 10
    b) Wnt 3
    c) Shh
    d) nAG
71. The creation of the amphibian regeneration blastema depends, in part, on the maintenance of ion currents driven through the stump. In Xenopus which of the following proton pump is activated after tail amputation, changing the membrane voltage and establishing flow of protons through the blastema?
    a) P type ATPases
    b) V type ATPases
    c) ABC transporters
    d) H^+/Na^+ antiporters
72. In a mutant analysis study of developing plant embryo it was found that FACKEL (FK) gene was mutated. Which of the following would be a result of this mutation in Arabidopsis embryogenesis?
    a) Cotlydons and shoot apical meristem are reduced or missing.
    b) Multiple shoot and root meristems developed.
    c) Polar distribution of PIN auxin carrier is defective.
    d) Auxin response factor is not found.
73. Since the A, B and C genes were identified, another class, the D genes, has been discovered. If D activity is specified by the SEPALLATA (SEP1-3), by expressing D class genes in combination with A and B genes, which of the following is a possibility?
    a) Conversion of leaves into petals.
    b) Conversion of petals into sepals.
    c) Conversion of leaves into stamen.
    d) Conversion of leaves into sepals.
74. Quadruple-mutant *Arabidopsis* plant (*ap1*, *ap2*, *ap*3, and *ag*) produce floral stems that develop as
    a) Sepal-sepal-petal-petal
    b) Sepal-petal-stamen-carpel
    c) Pseudoflowers
    d) Flowers continue to form within flowers
75. In mammalian females meiosis begins in the embryonic gonads while in males meiosis is not initiated until puberty. This critical difference in timing is due to
    a) Production of retinoic acid (RA) by the mesonephric kidneys in females which stimulates the germ cells to undergo meiosis.
    b) Secretion of RA-degrading enzyme Cyp26b1 which promotes meiosis in females but not in males.
    c) High production of FSH during embroyonic stage of mammalian females.

d) Secretion of gonadotropin releasing hormone starts in early embryonic stage in females but not in males.

76. Amphibian primary oocytes can remain in the diplotene stage of meiotic prophage for years and resumption of meiosis in the amphibian oocyte is thought to require progesterone. The mediator of the progesterone signal is
   a) c-mos protein that activates cdc2 of MPF
   b) Cytostatic factor (CSF)
   c) Calmodulin
   d) MAP kinase

77. What would happen if the functions of SHOOTMERISTEMLESS (STM) and MONOPTERUS (MP) are reversed?
   a) The embryo suspensor axis would be reversed.
   b) Embryo suspensor axis would be duplicated.
   c) Root-shoot axis would be reversed.
   d) Root-shoot axis would be duplicated.

78. The most obvious difference between plant embryonic development and animal embryonic development is that
   a) A plant develops from unfertilized eggs while animal develops from fertilized eggs.
   b) Plant morphogenesis is entirely growth dependent while animal morphogenesis involves movement of cells within the embryo.
   c) Plant embryos have an available source of nutrients while animal embryos needs feeding.
   d) None of the above.

79. In an experiment the Veg T transcripts of *Xenopus* oocytes are destroyed using antisence oligonucleotides. What would be the fate of the embryo?
   a) The entire embryo becomes mesoderm.
   b) The entire embryo becomes endoderm.
   c) The entire embryo becomes epidermis.
   d) The embryo cannot survive.

80. Which of the following serves as master regulator gene for the initiation of floral development?
   a) SOC1
   b) LFY
   c) AP1
   d) FLT

81. Which of the following statement is not correct?
   a) CONSTANS gene expression is involved in flowering in long day plants
   b) FLOWERING LOCUS T(FLT) protein is the phloem mobile signal that stimulates flower evocation in the meristem

c) Phytochrome is the primary photo- receptor in photoperiodism
d) FLT is a chromoprotein

82. Loss of type C activity in ABC flowering model results in the formation of
a) Petals instead of stamens b) Carpels instead of stamens
c) Sepals instead of stamens d) Stamens instead of carpels

83. Which of the following statement is not correct for ABC model?
a) AP1 alone specifies sepals
b) AG alone specifies the carpels
c) In the ag mutant, stamens and carpel are not formed and all four whorls are filled with sepals or petals
d) AP1 in combination with AG specifies petals

84. Which germ layer is involved in development of heart
a) Ectoderm b) Mesoderm
c) Endoderm d) Both (b) and (c)

85. Neural crest develops from
a) Mesoderm b) Endoderm
c) Ectoderm d) Archenteron

86. Holoblastic cleavage is found in
a) Reptiles b) Birds
c) Mammals d) Both (a) and (b)

87. Which of the following RNA can regulate the developmental timing in some organisms?
a) piRNA b) stRNA
c) miRNA d) siRNA

88. The blastopore region of amphibian embryo that secretes BMP inhibitors and dorsalizes the surrounding tissue is known as
a) Brachet's cleft b) Nieuwkoop center
c) Spemann's organizer d) Hensen's node

[CSIR (NET/JRF) Exam. Dec. 2011]

89. Which of the floral whorls is affected in agamous (ag) mutants?
a) Sepals and petals b) Petals and stamens
c) Stamens and carpels d) Sepals and carpels

[CSIR (NET/JRF) Exam. Dec. 2011]

90. Which of the following maternal effect gene products regulate production of anterior structures in *Drosophila* embryo?
a) Bicoid and Nanos b) Bicoid and Hunchback
c) Bicoid and Caudal d) Nanos and Caudal

[CSIR (NET/JRF) Exam. Dec. 2011]

91. The first division of zygote in a flowering plant is asymmetric and generates cells with two different fates. One daughter cell is small and the other larger daughter cell. If you could use microlaser to destroy the larger cell in a two cell plant embryo, how would it likely affect embryonic development?
    (a) The embryo would develop normally except it would not become anchored in seed wall.
    (b) The embryo would develop normally except it would have multiple cotyledons.
    (c) The embryo would fail to develop, but a fully functionally suspensor would form.
    (d) The embryo would immedeatly be aborted and the seed would not form.

92. How would plant development changes if the functions of SHOOT MERISTEMLESS (STM) and MONOPTERUS (MP) were reversed?
    (a) The embryo suspensor axis would be reversed.
    (b) Embryo suspensor axis would be duplicated.
    (c) Root-shoot axis would be reversed.
    (d) Root-shoot axis would be duplicated.

93. Which of the following is not evident from looking at a plant embryo?
    (a) plant is a monocot or dicot (b) where shoot will form
    (c) where root will form (d) when seed will germinate.

94. The longest period of time that a seed can remain dormant is?
    (a) Days (b) Months
    (c) Weeks (d) Years

95. Fruits are complex organs that are specialized for dispersal of seeds. Which of the following plant tissue does not contribute to mature fruit?
    (a) Sporophytic tissue from the previous generation
    (b) Gametophytic tissue from previous generation
    (c) Sporophytic tissue from the next generation
    (d) Gametophytic tissue from the next generation

96. If you want to ensure that seed is failed to germinate. Which of the following strategy would be most effective?
    (a) Prevent imbibition (b) Prevent desiccation
    (c) Prevent fertilization (d) Prevent dispersal

97. How would a loss of function mutation in α-amylase gene affect seed germination?
    (a) Seed could not imbibe water
    (b) Embryo would starved
    (c) Seed coat would not rupture
    (d) Seed would germinate prematurely

98. Apomixis is a type of reproduction in plants in which?
    (a) Fertilization does not take place
    (b) Male nucleus take part in fertilization
    (c) Pollen fusion take place
    (d) Generative nucleus takes part in fertilization

99. Embryonic stem cells are derived from.
    a) Fertilized embryo b) Sperm
    c) Unfertilized Embryo d) Kidney

100. Developmental processes of *Drosophila* are governed by many maternal genes like bicoid, nanos, hunckback, caudal, bithorax, dorsal, antennapedia and others. Suppose that during a mutagenesis screen to isolate mutation in Drosophila, you came across a fly with legs growing out of its head. Which gene cluster is likely to be affected?
    (a) Bicoid (b) Hunchback
    (c) Bithorax (d) Antennapedia

101. In ABC model for flowering, class A and B genes together specify
    a) Sepals only b) Petals only
    c) Sepals and petals only d) Petals and stamens only

102. Capacitation is a developmental transition of sperms of
    a) Amphibians b) Birds
    c) Reptiles d) Mammals

[CSIR (NET/JRF) Exam. Dec 2004]

103. The vulva is the epidermal structure that is formed in larval life around the mid-ventral opening of the gonad in *Caenorhabditis elegans.* Its formation is controlled by EGF-liked signal from an internal cell called
    a) The anchor cell b) Equivalence group cells
    c) P_2 cells d) AB_p cells

104. In amphibian oocyte, the germplasm which gets segregated during cleavage to give rise to primordial germ cells (PGC's) is normally
    a) distributed evenly throughout the oocyte.
    b) localized at animal pole.
    c) localized at vegetal pole.
    d) aggregated in central part of oocyte.

[CSIR (NET/JRF) Exam. June 2011]

105. In mature *Arabidopsis* embryo, root apical meristem consists of cells derived from
    a) embryo and apical suspensor cell.
    b) embryo only.

c) suspensor only.
d) hypophysis only. **[CSIR (NET/JRF) Exam. June 2011]**

106. Cytoplasmic determinants coding for anterior structure of *Drosophila* embryo, if injected elsewhere in the recipient embryo, would lead to
a) normal development.
b) formation of additional ectopic head.
c) degeneration
d) a phenotype with two heads and two tails.

[CSIR (NET/JRF) Exam. June 2011]

107. When prospective neuroectoderm from an early amphibian gastrula is transplanted in the prospective epidermal region of a recipient (early gastrula) embryo, the donor tissue will give rise to
a) neural tube.
b) epidermis.
c) neural tube and notochord.
d) neural tube and epidermis. **[CSIR Model Paper 2011]**

108. Amphibian oocytes remain for years in the diplotene stage of meiotic prophase. Resumption of meiosis is initiated by
a) gonodatropic hormone. b) growth hormone.
c) oestrogen. d) progesterone.

[CSIR Model Paper 2011]

109. A group of six cells called 'equivalence group cells' divide to form the vulval structure in *Caenorhabditis elegans.* They are called so because
a) they have similar fates during development of vulva.
b) all the six cells are competent to form vulva and can replace each other under various experimental conditions.
c) they are all under the influence of the anchor cell, signals from which initiate vulval development.
d) they interact with each other to form the vulval structure.

[CSIR Model Paper 2011]

Part C

1. In an experiment a large amount of *bicoid* mRNA was injected into the posterior end of a wild type embryo of *Drosophila*. The following statements correlate with this experiment?
   A. Anterior-posterior polarity does not developed.
   B. Posterior end becomes anterior without head.
   C. Head emerges at posterior end and anterior end becomes posterior.
   D. Two heads emerged, one at either end.
   Which of the following combination is correct?
   a) A and D b) C and D
   c) Only B d) Only D

2. Which of the following statement is NOT correct for early embryonic development of C. elegans?
   a) CYK-4 protein from sperm is essential for anterior-posterior axis formation.
   b) ABp cell defines the future dorsal side of the embryo while the EMS cell marks the future ventral surface of the embryo.
   c) The specification of the AB blastomere is autonomous.
   d) When sperm enters the egg, the egg nucleus is undergoing meiosis.

3. In an experiment the researchers infected the pancreas of living 2-month-old mice whose normal ß cells were destroyed, with harmless viruses containing the genes for three transcription factors: Pdx1, Ngn3 and Mafa. After a time period it was observed that pancreatic endodermal cells were converted into insulin-secreting ß ells. The following statements explain the above observation.
   A. Transcription factors Pdx1, Ngn3 and Mafa induce transdifferentiation in pancreas.
   B. Pdx1 and Mafa signal for dedifferentiation in pancreas.
   C. Pluripotent pancreatic stem cells start differentiation after viral infection.
   D. Viral transcription factors promote formation of stem cells.
   Which of the following combination is correct?
   a) A and B b) Only A
   c) A, C and D d) Only D

4. Which of the following statement is NOT correct?
   a) In the early divisions of the *C. elegans* zygote, one daughter cell becomes a founder cell and the other becomes a stem cell.
   b) Blastomere identity in *C. elegans* is regulated by both autonomous and conditional specification.

c) Capaicited mammalian sperm must penetrate the cumulus and bind to the zona pellucida before undergoing the acrosome reaction.
d) Sperm and egg activation involve Na+ ions.

5. In an experiment the optic vesicle of one side from *Xenopus* embryo is removed at early stages of development. The following observations were made.
   A. Formation of functional pigmented retina will not take place if optic vesicle is removed from the embryo.
   B. Formation of retina will take place and eye will develop normally.
   C. Optic vesicles induce the formation of lens placod which then invaginates to forms the lens.
   D. Development of eye in *Xenopus* involves optic vesicle mediated induction of Sox transcription factors in lens formation.

   Which of the following combination is correct?
   a) A and D
   b) A and C
   c) Only B
   d) A, C and D

6. In an experiment the entire progress zone (PZ) from an early embryo was placed on the limb bud of a later-stage embryo, new proximal structures were produced beyond those already present. Conversely, when older progress zone were added to young limb buds, distal structures developed immediately, so that digits were seen to emerge from the humerus without an intervening ulna and radius. The following explanations are suggested for the above observation.
   A. The positional information for proximal-distal polarity resides in the mesenchyme.
   B. The AER provides the positional information for proximal-distal polarity.
   C. Older AERs combine with younger mesoderm and produce limb without deletion in the middle.
   D. Younger AERs combine with older mesenchyme and produce duplication of structures.

   Which of the above statement is true?
   a) Only A
   b) A and B
   c) B and C
   d) Only D

7. In an experiment the embryonic chick fibroblasts which normally would never synthesize Sonic hedgehog, were transfected with a viral vector containing the shh gene. Which of the following would be the possible outcome of this experiment?
   a) Mirror-image digit duplications formed.
   b) New proximal structures were produced.
   c) A new limb bud is formed.
   d) Only digit 1 is formed.

8. An inducing factor is an extracellular signal substance that can alter the developmental pathway of cells exposed to it. If the factor is simply necessary for continued development of the target cells it is said to be permissive. The following statements are related with the permissive induction.
   A. In permissive induction the signal is necessary for the successful self differentiation of the responding tissue but cannot influence the developmental pathway selected.
   B. Permissive interactions are very important in early development.
   C. In the absence of signal permissive induction simply fails to develop, and does not form any alternative tissue.
   D. Permissive inductions lead to a subdivision of the competent tissue.
   Which of the following combination is true?
   a) A and C b) A and B
   c) A and D d) B and C

9. In a developmental biology experiment when a region of prospective epidermal cells from an early gastrula of one species was transplanted into an area in an early gastrula of the other species and placed in a region where neural tissue normally formed, the transplanted gave rise to neural tissue. This indicates that
   a) Cells of the early newt gastrula exhibit regulative development.
   b) Cells of the newt gastrula develop autonomously.
   c) The prospective fate of early gastrula is determined.
   d) Development of neural tissue is inhibited by epidermal cells.

10. When gsk3 mRNA is injected into a normal amphibian embryos from outside their dorsal axis formation is inhibited. Conversely, injection of a dominant negative version of gsk3 can rescue the formation of a dorsal axis in UV embryos or induce a second axis in normal embryos. The following statements correlate the above observation
   A. Gsk3 protein phosphorylates, and thereby inhibits, β-catenin.
   B. Gsk3 protein combines with Tcf-3 transcription factor and activate genes that are needed to form dorsal structure.
   C. β-catenin is a key player in the formation of the dorsal tissues.
   D. Gsk3 protein activates expression of twin and siamois genes whose activity is critical for axis formation.
   Which of the following combination is true?
   a) A and B b) B and C
   c) A and C d) B and D

11. AP1 (APETLA 1) is one of the floral meristem identifying genes. In wild type Arabidopsis thaliana plants transformed with AP1 :: GUS, glucuronidase (GUS) activity is seen in floral meristem, only after the commitment to

flowering. Ectopic expression of AP1:: GUS in the EMBRYONIC FLOWER (emf) mutant background results in GUS activity throughout the shoots in four day old seedlings. These observations suggest that AP1 is:

a) not involved in flowering.
b) involved in repression of flowering.
c) involved in promoting flowering.
d) stimulation of flowering in the emf background.

[CSIR (NET-JRF) Exam. Dec. 2011]

12. The figure above represents a late zebrafish gastrula. The following concepts may be proposed during further development of the embryo.

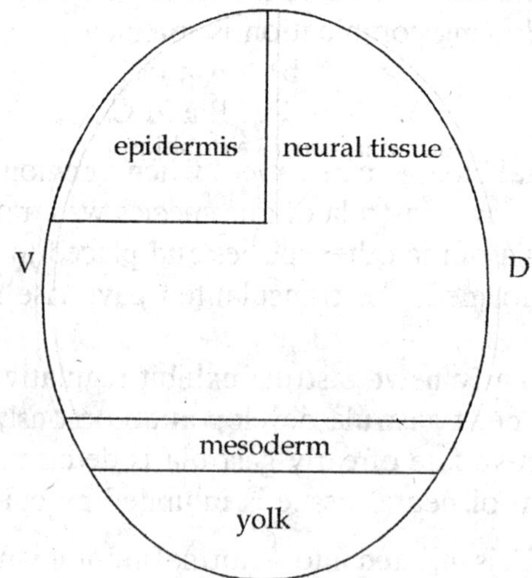

A. The concentration of FGF decreases from the yolk towards the epidermis, along with the increase of BMP activity from the dorsal to the ventral axis.
B. Increase in FGF activity in the epidermis with concomitant decrease in BMP activity towards the ventral axis.
C. Neural induction in Zebrafish is independent of the organizer and depends on activation of BMP signalling.
D. In comparison, both Xenopus and chick embryos require activation of FGF for neural induction to occur in addition to BMP inhibition.

Which of the above statements are true?

a) A and C b) B and C
c) A and D d) C and D

[CSIR (NET/JRF) Exam. Dec. 2011]

13. When the prospective neurons from an early gastrula of a frog were transplanted into the prospective epidermis region, the donor cells differentiated into epidermis. However, when a similar experiment was done

with the late gastrula of frog, the prospective neurons developed into neurons only. These observations could possibly be explained by the following phenomena.

A. The early gastrula show conditional development whereas the late gastrula shows autonomous development.
B. The early gastrula show autonomous development whereas the late gastrula shows conditional development.
C. The prospective neurons from the early gastrula are only specified whereas those from the late gastrula are determined.
D. The prospective neurons from the early gastrula are determined whereas those from the late gastrula are specified.

Which of the conclusions drawn above are correct?

a) A and B b) A and C
c) A and D d) B and C

[CSIR (NET-JRF) Exam. Dec. 2011]

14. In case of morphallactic regeneration:
  a) there is repatterning of the existing tissues with little new growth
  b) there is repatterning of the existing tissues after the stem cell division has taken place
  c) there is cell division of the differentiated cells which maintain their differentiated state to finally form a complete organism.
  d) there is dedifferentiation of the cells at the cut surface which become undifferentiated. These undifferentiated cells then divide to redifferentiate to form the complete structure. **[CSIR (NET-JRF) Exam. Dec. 2011]**

15. The decision to become either a trophoblast or inner cell mass blastomere is one of the first decisions taken by any mammalian embryo. Below is a diagrammatic representation of the different cells formed during development from the morula with the help of different molecules. Identify the molecules 1-4, sequentially.

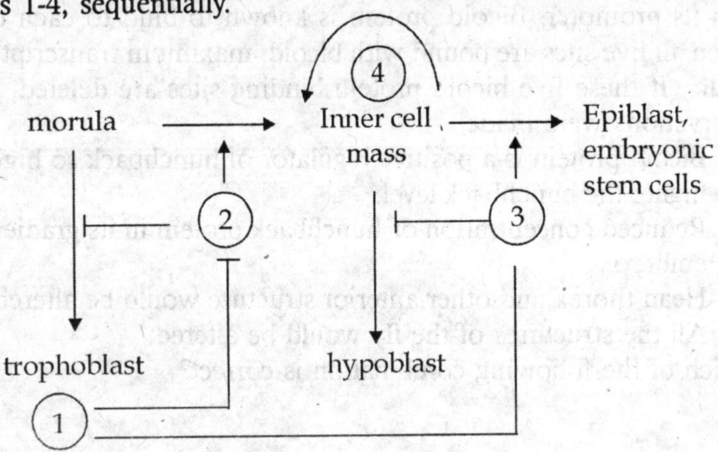

a) cdx 2, Oct 4, Nanog, Stat 3   b) cdx 2, Nanog, Stat 3, Oct 4
c) cdx 2, Nanog, Oct 4, Stat 3   d) cdx 2, Oct 4, Stat 3, Nanog

[CSIR (NET-JRF) Exam. Dec. 2011]

16. Loss of function mutations in the suspensor gene in *Arabidopsis* lead to development at two embryos in a seed. After analysing the expression of this gene in early embryo you find high level of suspensor mRNA in the developing suspensor cells. What is the likely function of the suspensor protein?
    (a) Suspensor protein likely stimulates development of the embryonic tissue
    (b) Suspensor protein likely stimulates development of the suspensor tissue
    (c) Suspensor protein likely inhibits embryonic development in suspensor.
    (d) Suspensor protein likely inhibits suspensor development in the embryo.

17. The arrival of viable pollen grains on a receptive stigma does not guarantee fertilization. Interspecific incompatibility refers to failure of pollen from one species to germinate or grow on the stigma of another species. Intraspecific incompatibility occurs within species
    The following statements are related with self-incompatibility
    (A) Self incompatibility blocks fertilization between two genetically similar gametes.
    (B) Gametophytic self incompatibelity occurs when S allele of pollen grain matches either of S allele of stigma.
    (C) Sporophytic self incompatibility occurs when one of the two S alleles of pollen producing sporophyte matches one of the S allele of stigma.
    (D) The S locus consists of several physically linked gene that regulate recognition and rejection of pollen.
    Which of the following combination is correct?
    (a) A, B, C and D   (b) A, B and C
    (c) B, C and D   (d) A, B and D

18. The *Drosophila* gene hunchback contains five repeats of 5'-TCTAATCCCC-3' in its promoter. Bicoid protein is known to bind to each of these sites. When all five sites are bound with bicoid, maximum transcription activation occurs. If these five bicoid protein binding sites are deleted, the following observations were made
    (A) Bicoid protein is a positive regulator of hunchback so higher the bicoid higher the hunchback level.
    (B) Reduced concentration of hunchback protein in its gradient throughout embryo.
    (C) Head thorex and other anterior structure would be altered.
    (D) All the structures of the fly would be altered.
    Which of the following combination is correct?

(a) A, B and D (b) B, C and D
(c) A, B and C (d) A and C

19. There are two very important processes in the development of embryo, that is, cell specification and determination. What would be a result of transplantation experiment in a chick embryo in which cells determined to become a forelimb were replaced by cells determined to become hindlimb?
(a) A hindlimb would form in the region where the forelimbs should be.
(b) A forelimbs would form in the region where hindlimbs should be.
(c) Nothing : the forelimbs would form normally.
(d) Neither a forelimb nor a hindlimb would form because cell were already determined.

20. The invertebrate *Drosophila* is the best understood in terms of the events of early pattering, a hierarchy of gene control development of Drosophila. The anterior- posterior axis formation is completely depend on signaling process. The following statements are related with the anterior-posterior axis formation in Dorsophila
(A) The anterior-posterior axis is formed based on a gradient of bicoid protein.
(B) Oskar is a posterior determining protein
(C) Dynein appears to be necessary for the localization of bicoid.
(D) Action of bicoid protein is to control the expression of gap genes.
Which one of the following combination is correct?
(a) A and B (b) A and D
(c) B and C (d) A, B, C and D

21. The dorsal-ventral axis in *Drosophila* is controlled by a different mechanism that does not involve localized cytoplasmic determinants like bicoid. Instead an accumulation of message on one side of the nucleus activates a transcription factor that results in directional translation and the surface of oocyte. The following statements are related with the dorsal-ventral axis formation in Drosophila:
(A) The gurken mRNA accumulates on one surface of the nucleus, that would be the future dorsal side of embryo.
(B) Transcription factor Dorsal plays an important role in the formation of ventral side.
(C) Gurken is a maternally expressed gene
(D) Dorsal is negatively regulated by cactus protein.
Which of the following combination of statements is true?
(a) A, C and D (b) A, B and D
(c) B, C and D (d) A, B, C and D

22. Figure (A) Below represents the distribution of mRNA of different genes involved in Drosophila development. Figure (B) represents the distribution of their protiens in early cleavage embryo.

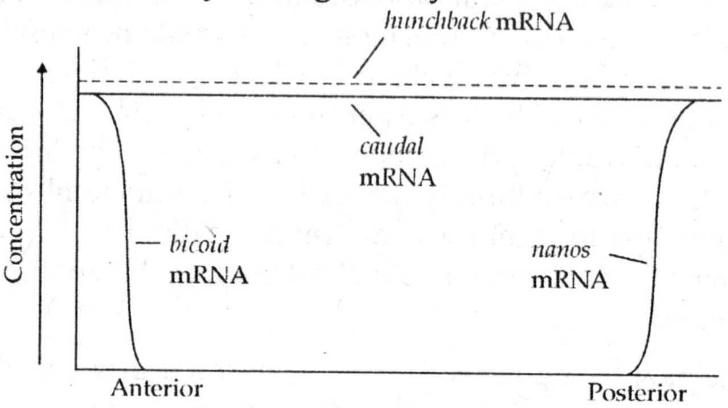

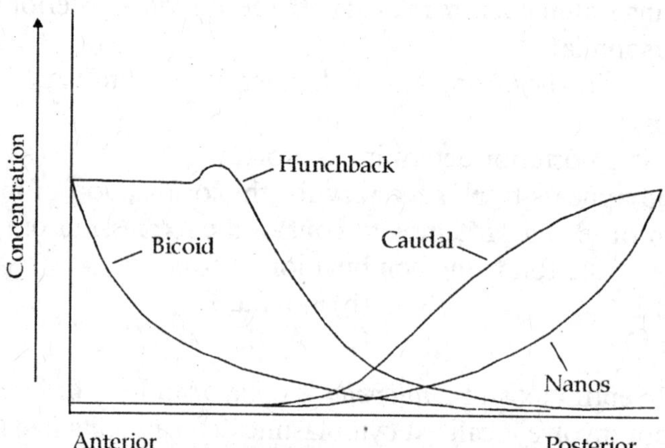

On the basis of above figure following results were made:

(A) The oocyte mRNA are transcribed in nurse cells of embryo.

(B) Hunchback and bicoid are responsible for anterior and nanos and caudal are responsible for posterior axis determination.

(C) Bicoid is an activator of hunchback where as nanos plays a role as an inhibitor for hunchback.

(D) The concentration of hunchback and caudal protein is equal in whole occyte.

Which of the following combination is correct?

(a) A, B and C (b) A, B, C and D

(c) B, C and D (d) A, C and D

23. Three classes of organ identity genes, A, B and C are involved in specifying the four whorls of a flower. Sepals (Se) are determined by the action of 'A'

class of genes, petals (Pe) are determined by both 'A' and 'B', and Stamens (St) by 'B' and 'C' while carpels (Ca) are detemined by 'C' alone. Mutation in these genes lead to homeotic transformation. Given below is the phenotype of floral whorls observed in wild type and mutants of floral identity genes

Whorl	1	2	3	4
Wild type	Se	Pe	St	Ca
Apetala-2	Ca	St	St	Ca
Pistillata	Se	Se	Ca	Ca
agamous	Se	Pe	Pe	Se

To which class (A, B or C) do the genes apetata 2, pistilla and agamous belong?

(a) Apetala 2 - class A
Pistillata - class B
Agamous - class C

(b) Apetala 2 - class A
Pistillata - class A
Agamous - class C

(c) Apetala 2 - class B
Pistillata - class B
Agamous - class C

(d) Apetala 2 - class B
Pistillata - class A
Agamous - class C

24. The following table shows the results obtained from a tissue transplantation experiment during early and late gastrula stages in newt.

Donar region	Host region	Differentiation of donar tissue
EARLY GASTRULA Propective neuron	Prospective epidermis	Epidermis
LATE GASTRULA Prospective Neuron	Prospective epidermis	Neurons

On the basis of above informations following explanations were made.

(A) The cells of early gastrula are specified to form prospective neurons.
(B) The cells of late gastrula are determined to form prospective neurons.
(C) Due to conditional specification prospective neurons convert their fate to epidermis.
(D) Due to autonomous specification cells of prospective neurons did not modulate their fate and formed neurons.

Which one of the following combination is correct?

(a) A, B, C and D (b) A, C and D
(c) A, B and D (d) C and D

25. During early cleavage of *Caenorabditis elegans* embryos, each asymmetrical division produces one founder cell which produces differentiated descendants and one stem cell. The very first cell division produces one anterior founder cell, namely AB and one posterior stem cell, namely P1. When these blastomeres are experimentally separated and allowed to proceed further with development, one could get the following possible outcomes:
    a) P1 cell would develop autonomously while the AB would show conditional development.
    b) P1 cells would show conditional development while AB would show autonomous development.
    c) Both would show autonomous specification and result in mosaic development.
    d) Both would show conditional specification and result in regulative development. **[CSIR (NET/JRF) Exam. June 2011]**

26. cAMP signalling plays a very important role in the development and differentiation of *Dictyostelium discoideum*. This morphogen is synthesized by different adenyl cyclases expressed at different stages of its life cycle. The following statements (A-D) refer to the effect of mutations in different adenyl cyclase genes:
    A. aca deficient cells can be allowed to aggregate by exposing them to pulses of cAMP.
    B. acb deficient cells would form normal fruiting bodies and the spores can germinate when exposed to favourable conditions.
    C. acg deficient cells develop normally and the spores germinate in the spore head itself.
    D. spores formed from the acg deficient cells will germinate irrespective of the osmotic conditions.

    Which of the above statements are correct?
    a) A and D　　b) A only
    c) A and B　　d) C and D

    [CSIR (NET/JRF) Exam. June 2011]

27. Mutations in CONSTANS (CO) of *Arabidopsis thaliana* results in late flowering phenotype. Transcript levels of CO were determined in long day and short day seedlings. Which of the following would likely represent the transcript profile of CO?

	Long-day seedling	Short-day seedlings
a)	**—**	—
b)	—	**—**
c)	—	—
d)	**—**	**—**

[CSIR (NET/JRF) Exam. June 2011]

28. When a wrist blastema from a recently cut Axolotl forelimb is placed on a host hind limb cut at the mid thigh level, it will generate only a wrist. The host (whose own hind limb was removed) will fill the gap and regenerate the limb upto the wrist. However, if the donor blastema is treated with retinoic acid on grafting, the wrist blastema will regenerate a complete limb and will not allow the host to fill the gap. This happens because retinoic acid:
   a) helps in the proximalization of the blastema and activates the Hox genes differentially across the blastema.
   b) helps in the distalization of the blastema and activates the Hox genes differentially across the blastema.
   c) helps block the receptors of FGF essential for limb development.
   d) helps vigorous proliferation of the cells at the cut surface.

[CSIR (NET/JRF) Exam. June 2011]

29. Injection of *noggin* mRNA into a 1-cell, UV-irradiated embryos of frog completely rescues dorsal development and allows the formation of a complete embryo. Some of the following statements (A-D) could possibly explain this observation.
   A. *Noggin* is a secreted protein which induces dorsal ectoderm to form neural tissue and it dorsalizes the mesoderm cells which would otherwise contribute to ventral mesoderm.
   B. Noggin binds directly to BMP4 and BMP2 thus preventing complex formation with their receptors.
   C. Noggin along with other molecules prevent BMP from binding to and inducing ectoderm and mesoderm cells near the organizer.
   D. Noggin is a secreted protein which induces the dorsal ectoderm to form the epidermis and it ventralizes the mesoderm cells which would otherwise contribute to dorsal mesoderm.

   Which of the above statements are correct?
   a) A, B and C. b) A and B.
   c) B and C. d) A and D.

[CSIR (NET/JRF) Exam. June 2011]

30. In case of sea urchin, which of the following is the correct sequence of events taking place during the interaction of sperm and egg?
   a) Chemoattraction of sperm to the egg by soluble molecules secreted by the egg → exocytosis of the sperm acrosomal vesicle to release its enzymes → binding of the sperm to the extracellular matrix of the egg → passage of sperm through this extracellular matrix → fusion of egg and sperm cell membranes.
   b) Chemoattraction of sperm to the egg by soluble molecules secreted by the egg → binding of the sperm to the extracellular matrix of the egg

→ exocytosis of the sperm acrosomal vesicle to release its enzymes → passage of sperm through this extracellular matrix → fusion of egg and sperm cell membranes.

c) Chemoattraction of sperm to the egg by soluble molecules secreted by the egg → binding of the sperm to the extracellular matrix of the egg → passage of sperm through this extracellular matix → exocytosis of the sperm acrosomal vesicle to release its enzymes → fusion of egg and sperm cell membranes.

d) Chemoattraction of sperm to the egg by soluble molecules secreted by the egg → passage of sperm through this extracellular matrix → binding of the sperm to the extracellular matrix of the egg → exocytosis of the sperm acrosomal vesicle to release its enzymes fusion of egg and sperm cell membranes. **[CSIR (NET/JRF) Exam. June 2011]**

31. Fill in the blanks (a, b, c and d) in the following statements with a proper combination of m, n, o and p.

Wherein m represents - longer
n represents - shorter
o represents - prevents
p represents - induces

Short day (SD) plants flower when night lengths are___a___than a critical dark period. Interruption of the dark period by a brief light treatment ___b___flowering in SD plants. Long day (LD) plants flower when night length is___c___than a critical period. Shortening of the night with a brief light treatment___d___flowering in LD plants.

	a	b	c	d
a)	m	o	n	p
b)	n	p	m	o
c)	n	o	m	p
d)	m	p	n	o

[CSIR (NET/JRF) Exam. June 2011]

32. During vertebrate limb development, a specialised ectodermal structure, called Apical Ectodermal Ridge (AER), forms at the dorso-ventral ectodermal boundary at the distal tip of the developing limb bud.
The following experimental facts about the AER is available:
(A) FGF 2, 4, and 8 are expressed in the AER (B) Removal of the AER causes cessation of limb growth
(C) Removal of AER along with implantation of beads soaked in FGF 8 or
(D) FGF 4 or FGF 2 protein rescues the AER removal phenotype and gives rise to normal limb

Which of the following statements cannot be made based on the above facts?
a) FGF 2, 4, and 8 are secreted proteins.
b) FGF 2, 4, and 8 are necessary and sufficient for AER function
c) FGF 2, 4, and 8 are sufficient for AER function
d) FGF 2, 4, and 8 have largely redundant functions

[CSIR Model Paper 2011]

33. During fertilization in amphibians, the fusion of egg and sperm plasma is preceeded by
(A) release of enzymatic contents from the acrosomal vesile through exocytosis
(B) binding and interaction of the sperm to vitelline membrane
(C) chemoattraction of the sperm to the egg by soluble factors secreted by egg
(D) passage of sperm through extracellular envelope
Which of the following is the correct sequence?
a) (A) → (B) → (C) → (D)
b) (B) → (A) → (C) → (D)
c) (C) → (A) → (B) → (D)
d) (C) → (B) → (A) → (D) **[CSIR Model Paper 2011]**

34. In many different contexts of cell differentiation, two distinct cell populations emerge from a uniform cell population. This process is referred to as lateral inhibition. Which one of the following must not be true about lateral inhibition?
(A) lateral inhibition results from morphogen action
(B) lateral inhibition requires direct cell cell contacts
(C) lateral inhibition requires reciprocal signalling between two neighbouring cells
(D) lateral inhibition is preceded by stochastic changes in gene expression in two neighbouring cells
a) (D) b) (A) and (D)
c) (B) and (C) d) (A) **[CSIR Model Paper 2011]**

35. Which of the following statements is true about dorso-ventral patterning of drosophila embryo?
(A) This is dictated by the location of the nurse cells
(B) dorsal is the default fate
(C) The whole process is regulated by preventing the entry of a transcription factor to the nucleus of dorsal cells
(D) Homeobox containing genes play a critical role in this process.
a) (A), (B) and (C) b) (A),(B), (C) and (D)
c) (A) and (D) d) (B) and (C)

[CSIR Model Paper 2011]

36. Which of the following is true about amphibian limb regeneration?
    (A) It requires a minimum number of functional nerves.
    (B) The blastema of an amputated limb, if transplanted in the trunk region between two existing limbs in a host, will still give rise to a limb.
    (C) The size of the regenerated limb is often grossly different from the original limb.
    a) (A)
    b) (B) and (C)
    c) (A) and (C)
    d) (A), (B) and (C)

    [CSIR Model Paper 2011]

37. In agamous mutant (flower within flower phenotype) which of the following statements is valid?
    a) Class A genes are expressed in the first two whorls, Class B genes are expressed in the second and third whorls and Class C genes are expressed in the third and fourth whorls.
    b) Class A genes are not expressed. Class B and C genes are expressed in all the whorls.
    c) Class A genes are not expressed. Class B genes are expressed in the second and the third whorls and Class C genes are expressed in all the whorls.
    d) Class A genes are expressed in all the whorls. Class B genes are expressed in the second and the third whorls. **[CSIR Model Paper 2011]**

38. Following are the different ways of obtaining human stem cells-
    (A) Cells from morula are dispersed and cultured to give rise pluripotent stem cells.
    (B) Isolated inner cell mass of a blastocyst are cultured and they become pluripotent stem cells.
    (C) The primordial germ cells from a fetus are collected and cultured, which grow into pluripotent stem cells.
    (D) Stem cells are collected from adult tissues and grown in specific manner to develop into pluripotent stem cells.

    Which of the above cell type(s) is extensively used for somatic cell gene therapy in human?
    a) (A) and (B)
    b) (B) only
    c) (B) and (D)
    d) (D) only **[CSIR Model Paper 2011]**

Answer Sheet

Part – B

1.	b	2.	a	3.	d	4.	a	5.	b	6.	a
7.	a	8.	c	9.	a	10.	a	11.	b	12.	b
13.	a	14.	b	15.	c	16.	a	17.	b	18.	b
19.	b	20.	b	21.	a	22.	a	23.	a	24.	a
25.	c	26.	c	27.	d	28.	a	29.	a	30.	d
31.	b	32.	b	33.	a	34.	d	35.	a	36.	a
37.	a	38.	a	39.	c	40.	d	41.	b	42.	b
43.	b	44.	c	45.	b	46.	c	47.	c	48.	c
49.	b	50.	c	51.	b	52.	b	53.	b	54.	b
55.	a	56.	d	57.	b	58.	a	59.	c	60.	c
61.	b	62.	b	63.	c	64.	b	65.	a	66.	a
67.	c	68.	c	69.	b	70.	c	71.	b	72.	b
73.	a	74.	c	75.	a	76.	a	77.	c	78.	b
79.	c	80.	b	81.	d	82.	a	83.	d	84.	a
85.	c	86.	c	87.	b	88.	b	89.	c	90.	b
91.	a	92.	c	93.	d	94.	d	95.	b	96.	a
97.	b	98.	a	99.	a	100.	d	101.	b	102.	d
103.	a	104.	b	105.	d	106.	b	107.	b	108.	d
109.	b										

Part – C

1.	d	2.	c	3.	b	4.	d	5.	a	6.	a
7.	a	8.	a	9.	a	10.	c	11.	c	12.	a
13.	b	14.	a	15.	a	16.	d	17.	d	18.	c
19.	a	20.	d	21.	d	22.	a	23.	a	24.	a
25.	a	26.	d	27.	a	28.	a	29.	b	30.	b
31.	a	32.	d	33.	d	34.	b	35.	b	36.	a
37.	d	38.	b								

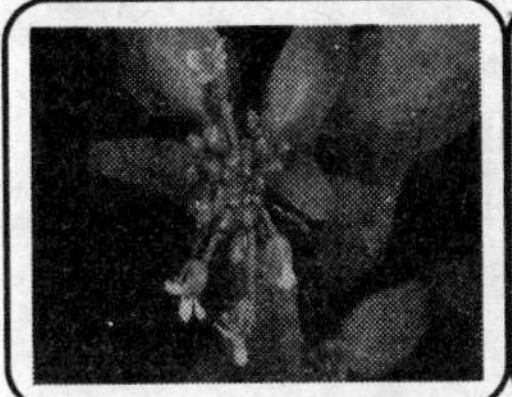

Chapter 6
Plant Physiology

Part B

1. 'Dicamba' is a synthetic analog of
   a) ABA b) GA
   c) Auxin d) Cytokinin

2. A central region of the root apical meristem (RAM) characterized by low mitotic activity is known as
   a) Root cap b) Elongation zone
   c) Quiescent centre d) Maturation zone

3. A common symptom of molybdenum deficiency in plants is the accumulation of nitrate in the cytosol which results from
   a) Reduced nitrite reductase activity
   b) Reduced nitrate reductase activity
   c) Reduced transport of nitrate into the vacuoles
   d) Reduced transport of the nitrate into the chloroplasts

4. A feature of the plant citric acid cycle that is absent in many other organisms is the activity of
   a) NAD+ malic enzyme b) NADP+ malic enzyme
   c) PCK d) PFK

5. A group of chemicals that have been implicated in attraction of rhizobia during nodule formation is
   a) Nod factors b) Flavonoids
   c) Lipo-chito oligosaccharides d) Lectins

6. A plant hormone responsible for producing α-amylase is
   a) Cytokinin b) GA
   c) IAA d) Ethylene

   [CSIR (NET/JRF) Exam. Dec 2001]

7. α- amylase production by aleurone layers is induced by
   a) Cytokinins b) Auxins
   c) ABA d) Gibberellin

   [CSIR (NET/JRF) Exam. Dec 2009]

8. Which of the following statement is correct?
   a) In oxidative phosphorylation movement of electrons is downhill
   b) In oxidative phosphorylation movement of electrons is uphill
   c) In photophosphorylation movement of electrons is downhill
   d) Oxygen is released in oxidative phosphorylation

9. Alkaloid production in plants is regulated by a change in the endogenous pool of
   a) Gibberellins   b) Jasmonates
   c) Brassinosteroids   d) ABA

10. All of the following are the intermediates of reductive pentose phosphate pathway except
   a) DHAP   b) Glyceraldehyde-3-phosphate
   c) Erythrose-4-phosphate   d) 6-phosphogluconate

11. Alternate oxidase of plant mitochondria is inhibited by
   a) Azide   b) Cyanide
   c) SHAM   d) DCMU

[CSIR (NET/JRF] Exam. Dec. 2005]

12. Z
   CoQ -------> cytochrome b. Here Z indicates
   a) Amytal   b) Rotenone
   c) Antimycin A   d) Azide

13. Among the following which chemical does not inhibit the mitochondrial ETS?
   a) Streptomycin   b) Amytol
   c) Antimycin A   d) Azide

14. Antimycin inhibits
   a) Complex-I of respiratory chain
   b) Complex-II of respiratory chain
   c) Complex-III of respiratory chain
   d) Complex-IV of respiratory chain

15. At permanent wilting point, plants can not regain turgor pressure even if transpiration stops because
   a) Water potential of soil is less than or equal to osmotic potential of the plant
   b) Water potential is higher than osmotic potential
   c) Water potential and osmotic potential are unaltered
   d) Osmotic potential remains unaltered

16. At which step of glycolysis substrate level phosphorylation occurs?
a) G-3-P ----------> 1,3-BPG b) 1,3-BPG ----------> 3-PG
c) 2-PG ----------> PEP d) 3-PG ----------> 2-PG

17. ATP and NADPH are consumed in the
a) Oxidative pentose phosphate pathway
b) Reductive pentose phosphate pathway
c) Fermentation
d) Photosynthetic carbon oxidation pathway

18. Azide can block electron flow from
a) NADH to ubiquinone b) Ubiquinone to cytochrome b
c) FADH2 to ubiquinone d) Cytochromes a/a3 to oxygen

[CSIR (NET/JRF) Exam. Dec 2004]

19. Base modification of tRNA nucleotide leads to formation of
a) Auxins b) Cytokinin moities
c) GA d) ABA

20. Blue light- dependent phototropism of the hypocotyls is mediated by
a) Phytochrome b) Cryptochrome
c) Phototropin d) Zeaxanthin

21. Blue light response is involved in
a) Photomorphogenesis b) Stomatal movement
c) Photophosphorylation d) Protoplasmic streaming

22. C4 cycle is common in
a) Temperate plants b) Tropical plants
c) Xerophytic plants d) Aquatic plants

23. Carbon monooxide inhibits
a) Complex I b) Complex II
c) Complex IV d) ATP synthase

24. Cardiolipin is an important component of
a) Thylakoid membrane of chloroplast
b) Inner membrane of mitochondria.
c) Outer membrane of mitochondria
d) Bacterial cell membrane

25. Chlorosis in leaves is generally due to deficiency of
a) Mg^{++} b) Ca^{++}
c) Na^{+} d) Mn^{++}

[CSIR (NET/JRF) Exam. Dec 2005]

26. Chlorosis occurs due to deficiency of
    a) N b) P
    c) K d) C

27. Circadian rhythmic phenomena in higher plants does not inlcude
    a) Stomatal opening b) Sleep movements
    c) Stem Growth d) Fruit ripening

28. Circadian rhythm in plants is mediated by
    a) Phototropin b) Turgorin
    c) Phytochrome d) Cryptochrome

[CSIR (NET/JRF) Exam. Dec 2008]

29. Cold stress can not cause
    a) Ice crystal formation within cell
    b) Water deficit
    c) Desaturation of fatty acids of membrane
    d) Saturation of fatty acids of membrane

30. Compatible substances are accumulated within the cell during
    a) Physical water deficit b) Physiological water deficit
    c) Both (a) and (b) d) Heat stress

31. Cyclic electron transport in chloroplast can be inhibited by
    a) Antimycin A b) Chloramphenicol
    c) DCMU d) Streptomycin

32. Cytochrome P_{450} is a component of
    a) Electron transport system of mitochondria
    b) Electron transport system of thylakoid membrane
    c) Drug detoxification system
    d) Defence system of oxidative stress

33. Direct oxidation of peroxide in plants is carried out by
    a) SOD b) Catalase
    c) Peroxidase d) Glutathione

34. During aerobic respiration, the substrate level phosphorylation takes place in
    a) Cytoplasm only
    b) Mitochondria only
    c) Cytoplasm and mitochondria
    d) Cytoplasm and Golgi complex

35. During photorespiration serine is formed in
    a) Chloroplast b) Mitochondria
    c) Peroxisome d) None of these

36. During photorespiration which organelle is involved in conversion of glycolate into glyoxylate?
   a) Mitochondria b) Peroxisome
   c) Chloroplast d) Nucleus

37. During saline stress compatible solutes in plant cells-
   a) Decrease solute potential b) Increase solute potential
   c) Decrease pressure potential d) Increase water potential

38. Electron flow in cytochrome oxidase in the respiratory chain can be blocked by-
   a) Rotenone b) Cyanide
   c) Amytol d) Cycloheximide

39. Electrons removed from substrate in the citric acid cycle are ultimately passed to
   a) NAD^+ b) FAD
   c) Oxygen d) NAD^+ and FAD

[CSIR (NET/JRF) Exam. June 2009]

40. Energy overflow hypothesis explains
   a) Photorespiration
   b) C4 syndrome
   c) Cyanide resistant respiration
   d) Energy transduction in thylakoid

41. Fixation of one molecule of $^{14}CO_2$ by photosynthesis will yield
   a) One molecule of ^{14}C-phosphoglyceric acid
   b) Two molecules of ^{14}C-phosphoglyceric acid
   c) Three molecules of ^{14}C-acetate
   d) One molecule of ^{14}C-glucose

42. Flooding and submergence of plants leads to anoxic condition, usually flood tolerant species alter their developmental programme, resulting in
   a) Increased activity at the apical meristem
   b) Growth retardation of foliage
   c) Elongation growth of their stems
   d) Increased proliferation of root system

43. Formation of glucose from acetyl CoA is called
   a) Glycogenesis b) Gluconeogenesis
   c) TCA cycle d) Glycolysis

44. Fruit set is triggered by
   a) Auxin b) Gibberellin
   c) ABA d) Cytokinin

45. Genetic dwarfs are often deficient in
   a) Auxin b) Gibberellins
   c) ABA d) Cytokinin

46. Gluconeogenesis can not occur in
   a) Liver b) Kidney
   c) Small intestine d) Brain

47. Glucose synthesis from amino acids is called
   a) Glucogenolysis b) Glucogenesis
   c) Gluconeogenesis d) Transamination

48. Glycolysis is inhibited by iodoacetate. This compound inhibits glycolysis specifically by inhibition of?
   a) Hexokinase
   b) Phophofructokinase
   c) Pyruvate Kinase
   d) Glyceraldehyde-3-phosphate dehydrogenase

49. Glycolysis usually occurs in cytosol but in some lower eukaryotes its some steps are restricted in a specific structure. This structure is
   a) Acidocalcisome b) Apicoplast
   c) Glycosome d) Hydrogenosome

50. In animals the glycolysis is primarily controlled by
   a) PFK - I b) Pyruvate kinase
   c) Hexokinase d) Phosphoglycerate kinase

51. In C_4 plants NO_3^- assimilation occurs in-
   a) Bundle sheath cells b) Mesophyll cells
   c) Phloem parenchyma cells d) Xylem vessels

52. In eukaryotes β-oxidation occurs in
   a) Mitochondaria b) Peroxisomes
   c) Endoplasmic reticulum d) Both (a) and (b)

53. In glycolysis ATP is synthesized by
   a) Fructose-1, 6-bisphosphate
   b) 6-phosphofructo kinase
   c) Glyceraldehyde 3-phosphate dehydrogenase
   d) Phosphoglycerate kinase

54. In plant seed storage tissue β-oxidation occurs in
   a) Mitochondria b) Glyoxysome
   c) Peroxisome d) Chloroplast

55. In plants IAA causes cell elongation due to
   a) Increase in pH of apoplast
   b) Increase in pH of cytoplasm
   c) Decrease in pH of apoplast
   d) Decrease in pH of cytoplasm **[CSIR (NET/JRF) Exam. June 2005]**

56. In plants systemic acquired resistance (SAR) is induced by an endogenous signal. This signal is likely to be
   a) Jasmonic acid b) Systemin
   c) Salicylic acid d) Flavonoids

57. In storage chambers fruits and flowers are kept under
   a) Low oxygen concentration and high temperature
   b) High oxygen concentration and low temperature
   c) High ethylene concentration and high pressure
   d) Low oxygen concentration and low temperature

58. In TCA cycle malonate is competitive inhibitor. It is structurally similar to
   a) Succinate b) Fumarate
   c) Oxaloacetate d) α-ketoglutarate

59. In which of the following phases of Calvin cycle ATP is not comsumed?
   a) Carboxylation phase b) Reduction phase
   c) Regeneration phase d) None of these

60. Inhibition of photosynthesis by oxygen is called
   a) Emerson effect b) Warburg effect
   c) Pasteur effect d) Red drop phenomenon

61. Keton bodies are formed in
   a) Liver b) Kidney
   c) brain d) Heart

62. Ketone bodies are formed during catabolism of
   a) Glucose b) Amino acids
   c) Lipids d) Nucleotides

63. LEA proteins are synthesized late in embryogenesis and during dehydration stress. The synthesis of these polypeptides is induced by
   a) Auxins c) Cytokinins
   b) Gibberellins d) ABA

64. Leaf senescene can be delayed by
   a) Ethylene b) ABA
   c) Cytokinin d) Salicylic acid

65. Mitochondria are associated with all of the following except
    a) ATP synthesis
    b) DNA synthesis
    c) Apoptosis
    d) Hydrolysis of various macromolecules at low pH

66. Most heat sensitive part of photosynthetic machinery is
    a) PS I complex b) PS II complex
    c) Carbon metabolism d) Chloroplast integrity

67. NAD+ are regenerated in
    a) Glycolysis
    b) Citric acid cycle
    c) Pentose phosphate pathway
    d) Anaerobic fermentations **[CSIR (NET/JRF) Exam. Dec 2007]**

68. Osmotic adjustment cannot be achieved by
    a) Proline b) Glycine betaine
    c) Pinitol d) Glycine

69. Oxidative pentose phosphate pathway occurs in
    a) Mitochondria and cytosol b) Cytosol and plastids
    c) Cytosol and peroxisome d) Mitochondria and plastids

70. Oxygen evolving complex of PS II does not possess
    a) Ca^{2+} b) Cl^{-}
    c) Mn d) Tyrosine

71. Paraquate inhibits light reaction. It acts at
    a) PS I b) PS II
    c) cyt b\f complex d) Q cycle

72. Photopigment that removes reactive oxygen species formed during light reaction is
    a) Phycobilin b) Phytochrome
    c) Carotenoid d) Cryptochrome

73. Photoperiodic signal is perceived by
    a) Buds b) Stem
    c) Aptical meristem d) Leaves

74. Photoperiodic stimulus from leaves to shoot apical meristem/floral meristem is transported through
    a) Xylem b) Phloem
    c) Plasmodesmata d) Apoplast

75. Photophosphorylation in chloroplast requires movement of
   a) Electrons across the membrane
   b) Ions across the membrane
   c) Protons across the membrane
   d) Electrons and protons across the membrane

76. Photosynthetically-active radiation lies in the wavelength range of
   a) > 700 nm b) < 400 nm
   c) 400-700 nm d) 200-300 nm

77. Phototropism is regulated by the photoreceptor phototropin. It is a
   a) Nucleoprotein b) Flavoprotein
   c) Heatshock protein d) DNA binding protein

78. Phycobillin proteins are found in
   a) Higher plants
   b) Green algae
   c) Cyanobacteria and red algae
   d) Diatoms **[CSIR (NET/JRF) Exam. Dec 2005]**

79. Pitcher plant *Nepenthes clato* would be expected to have
   a) NO_3^- specific ion channel b) H^+ - NO_3^- symporters
   c) Peptide transporters d) ATP powered pumps for NO3-

80. Plant mitochondrial electron transport chain differs from that of animals in having
   a) ATP synthase b) Cytochrome oxidase
   c) Alternate oxidase d) Cytochrome C

81. Plants growing in cold environments generally have
   a) High cholesterol
   b) High saturated fatty acids
   c) High unsaturated fatty acids
   d) Short chain fatty acids

82. Plants uptake nitrate through
   a) Ca^{2+}/NO_3^- symporter b) H^+/NO_3^- antiporter
   c) H^+/NO_3^- symporter d) Ca^{2+}/NO_3^- antiporter

83. Polymer trap model explains
   a) Transport of amino acids b) Phloem loading
   c) Phloem unloading d) Starch synthesis

84. Precious germination and vivipary can be inhibited by
   a) Auxin b) Gibberellin
   c) ABA d) Ethylene

85. Primary acceptor of CO_2 in photosynthesis is
a) Ribose
b) Ribulose-5-P
c) Ribulose1,5-bisphosphate
d) Phosphoglycerate

86. Production of ethylene increases during
a) Drought
b) Cold
c) Flood
d) Heat

87. Proline and glycine betain are accumulated in plant cells during
a) Heat stress
b) Cold stress
c) Water stress
d) Oxidative stress

88. Proline can function as compatible substance in plant cells during
a) Water stress
b) Salt stress
c) Both (a) and (b)
d) Heat stress

89. Pyruvate ferredoxin oxidoreductase (PFO) is an enzyme which convert pyruvate into CO2 and acetyl co-enzyme. This enzyme is exclusively reported from
a) Mitochondria
b) Glycosome
c) Hydrogenosome
d) Glyoxysome

90. Respiratory crisis is related to the
a) Anaerobic respiration
b) Photo respiration
c) Superoxide formation
d) Cyanide resistance respiration

91. Ribulose-5-phosphate is formed in
a) Oxidative phosphorylation
b) Pentose phosphate pathway
c) Kerb's cycle
d) Glycolysis

[CSIR (NET/JRF) Exam. Dec 2007]

92. Rubisco is the most abundant protein on Earth because
a) It is involved in CO_2 fixation
b) Its Km value is very low
c) Its Km value is very high
d) It has oxygenase activity

93. RUBP carboxylase is estimated to be the most prevalent enzyme on the planet. This makes sense because the enzyme is involved in
a) ATP synthesis
b) Autotrophic CO_2 fixation
c) Nitrogen fixation
d) Biodegradation

94. Salt exclusion is mechanism necessary for
a) Halophytes
b) Xerophytes
c) Plants in cold habitat
d) Hydrophytes

[CSIR (NET/JRF) Exam. June 2005]

95. Salt glands help plant to overcome
   a) Drought stress   b) Heat stress
   c) Water stress   d) Saline stress

96. Stem elongation is caused by?
   a) IAA   b) Gibberellins
   c) Ethylene   d) Cytokinins

97. Substrate level phosphorylation occurs in
   a) Cytosol   b) Mitochondria
   c) Hydrogenosome   d) All of these

98. Symbiotic nitrogen fixing bacteria provide plants nitrogen in the form of
   a) NH_4^+ b) NO_3^-
   c) NO_2^- d) Ureids

99. Systemic acquired resistance in plants is mediated by
   a) Jasmonic acids   b) Salicylic acid
   c) Systemin   d) ABA

100. The alternative pathway of respiration can be inhibited by
   a) Cyanide   b) Arachodoic acid
   c) Ampicilin   d) SHAM

[CSIR (NET/JRF) Exam. Dec 2005]

101. The blue light -stimulated stomatal opening is completely inhibited by DTT because
   a) It blocks PS I in guard cells
   b) It blocks PS II in guard cells
   c) Zeaxanthin formation is blocked by DTT.
   d) It inhibits cryptochrome synthesis.

102. The carriers of mitochondrial electron transport chains are present in the
   a) Mitochondrial matrix   b) Inner mitochondrial membrane
   c) Cristae   d) Outer membrane

103. The characteristic softening of fruit during ripening is due to breaking down of
   a) Primary cell wall   b) Plasma membrane
   c) Middle lamella   d) Both (a) and (b)

104. The endogenous signal which is likely to be involved in systemic acquired resistance (SAR) is
   a) Benzoic acid   b) Salicylic acid
   c) Flavonoids   d) Anthocyanin

105. The enzyme responsible for conversion of superoxide to H_2O_2 is
a) Catalase
b) Ascorbate
c) Peroxidase
d) SOD

106. The enzyme cytochrome oxidase is found in
a) Mitochondrial matrix
b) Mitochondrial inner membrane
c) Mitochondrial outer membrane
d) Intermembranous space of Mitochondria

107. The first acceptor of electron in photosystem II is
a) Phytocyanin
b) Phycoerythrin
c) Ferredoxin
d) Pheophytin

108. The floral stimulus is transported in
a) Phloem
b) Xylem
c) Apoplast
d) Symplast

109. The lack of the enzyme superoxide dismutase may explain why certain bacteria are
a) Unable to produce oxygen radicals when exposed to oxygen
b) Killed by exposure to O_2
c) Unable to use O_2 in metabolism
d) Able to grow in the absence of O_2

110. The major difference in PS I and PS II found in chloroplast is
a) Position on lamellae
b) Chlorophyll a
c) Position of electron carriers
d) Energy harvesting

[CSIR (NET/JRF) Exam. Dec 2004]

111. The mitochondrial membrane contains a transporter for
a) NADH
b) Acetyl Co-A
c) GTP
d) ATP

112. The out growth of the axillary bud is inhibited by
a) Cytokinin
b) ABA
c) Auxin
d) Ethylene

113. The phytohormone which provides desiccation resistance to embryo in germinating seed is
a) Gibberellic acid
b) Ethylene
c) ABA
d) cytokinin

114. The pigment that plays a key role in photomorphogenesis is
a) Chlorophyll
b) Phytochrome
c) Cryptochrome
d) Anthocyanine

115. The polymer-trapping model explains
   a) Symplastic phloem loading b) Apoplastic phloem loading
   c) Short distance transport d) Mass flow

116. The region of visible light which is most useful for photomorphogenesis is
   a) Blue, red b) Blue, red and far-red
   c) Green, Blue d) Blue, green

117. The repeating structure common in haemoglobin, chlorophyll and cytochrome is
   a) Pentose b) Phenol
   c) Benzene d) Porphyrin

118. The repetition of local configuration in protein is found in
   a) Primary structure b) Secondary structure
   c) Tertiary structure d) Quaternary structure

119. The *Rht* mutation in wheat that were pivotal for "green revolution" cause reduction in plant height due to impairment in
   a) Gibberellic acid biosynthesis pathway
   b) Gibberellic acid signaling pathway
   c) Auxin biosynthetic pathway
   d) Auxin response pathway

120. The role of carrier proteins in light is
   a) To transfer energetic electrons from PS II to PS I
   b) Pumping of protons
   c) Formation of ATP
   d) Transferring of high energy electrons from PS I to PS II

121. The secondary metabolites which may protect plants against damage by ultraviolet light are
   a) Alkaloids b) Flavonoids
   c) Anthocyanin d) Lignin

122. The site of action of the herbicide DCMU is
   a) cyt b/f ------------> PC b) Q_A ------------> Q_B
   c) PS I ------------>Fd d) Fd ------------> $NADP^+$

123. The site of synthesis and degradation of H2O2 in a plant cell is
   a) lysosome b) Sphaerosome
   c) Peroxisome d) Microsome

124. The site of oxygen evolution and photophosphorylation in chloroplast is
   a) Grana stacks b) Matrix
   c) Inner wall of chloroplast d) Surface of chloroplast

125. The structure of the reaction centre of PSII corresponds to that of the reaction centre of?
   a) Green bacteria
   b) Purple bacteria
   c) Halobacteria
   d) Cyanobacteria

126. The symptoms of potassium deficiency in plants appear initially on the more mature leaves towards the base of the plant because
   a) It is macroessential element
   b) It is immobile
   c) It delays leaf senescence
   d) It is mobile

127. There is net gain of energy in the form of ATP, if glucose which has converted into acetyl CoA enters
   a) TCA cycle
   b) Glycolysis
   c) β-oxidation
   d) Pentose phosphate pathway

128. Water potential decreases when
   a) Solute concentration increases
   b) Osmotic pressure increases
   c) Solute concentration decreases
   d) None of the above

129. Water shortage and high salt content of the soil causes accumulation of .... in plant cells
   a) Compatible substances
   b) Secondary metabolites
   c) Heavy metals
   d) None of these

130. Which element is present in oxygen evolving complex of PSII?
   a) Mn2+
   b) Mg2+
   c) Fe2+
   d) Cu2+

[CSIR (NET/JRF) Exam. Dec 2005]

131. Which hormone induces formation of Late Embryogenesis Abundant (LEA) protein during seed maturation?
   a) Ethylene
   b) Cytokinin
   c) Gibberellic acid
   d) ABA

[CSIR (NET/JRF) Exam. June 2007]

132. Which ion gradient is formed across the thylakoid membrane if light is incident on isolated thylakoid?
   a) Na^+
   b) Cl^-
   c) H^+
   d) Both Na^+ and H^+

133. Which is not true about TCA cycle?
   a) It takes place in mitochondrial matrix
   b) It is single largest source of ATP
   c) It is linked to glycolysis via pyruvate
   d) There is formation of NADH and $FADH_2$

[CSIR (NET/JRF) Exam. June 2007]

134. Which mineral ion plays an important role in functioning of photosystem II
   a) Magnesium b) Iron
   c) Manganese d) Molybdenum

135. Which of the following phytohormones plays no role in overcoming water stress?
   a) Gibberellin b) ABA
   c) Ethylene d) Auxin

136. Which of the following are required for the growth of pollen tube?
   a) Cytokinins b) Brassinosteroids
   c) ABA d) Gibberellins

137. Which of the following are the photoreceptor for photoperiodism?
   a) Phytochrome and phototropin
   b) Phototropin and carotenoids
   c) Cryptochrome and phototropin
   d) Phytochrome and cryptochrome

138. Which of the following can inhibit complex IV of ETS?
   a) Rotenone b) Azide
   c) Amytal d) Antimycin

139. Which of the following compatible substance can scavenge hydroxyl radicals?
   a) Proline b) Sucrose
   c) Trehalose d) Glycine betaine

140. Which of the following electron carrier in photosynthesis is a form of chlorophyll *a* in which the magnesium ion has been replaced by two hydrogens?
   a) Pheophytin b) Oxygen evolving complex
   c) Quinones d) Reaction centre chlorophyll

141. Which of the following enzyme of Krebs cycle has iron-sulphur cluster as prosthetic group
   a) Succinyl Co-A synthetase b) Malate dehydrogenase
   c) Fumarase d) Aconitase

142. Which of the following enzymes of the glycolytic pathway is not obligatory for bacteria?
a) PFK I
b) Hexokinase
c) Pyruvate kinase
d) Triose phosphate isomerase

143. Which of the following forms reaction centers of light reaction?
a) Chlorophyll a
b) Chlorophyll b
c) Chlorophyll a+b
d) Chlorophyll a, b and accessory pigments

144. Which of the following involves epigenetic changes?
a) Floral induction
b) Stem elongation
c) Fruit ripening
d) Vernalization

145. Which of the following ion plays a vital role in stomatal physiology?
a) H^+
b) K^+
c) Na^+
d) Mg^{++}

[CSIR (NET/JRF) Exam. June 2007]

146. Which of the following is a proteinaceous phytohormone?
a) Auxin.
b) Cytokinin
c) Systemin
d) Jasmonate

147. Which of the following is a regulatory enzyme of cholesterol biosynthesis?
a) HMG-CoA reductase
b) HMG-CoA synthase
c) Phosphomevalonate kinase
d) Acetoacetyl CoA thiolase

148. Which of the following is a water soluble copper containing electron carrier of chloroplast electron transport chain?
a) Pheophytin
b) Plastoquinone
c) Plastocyanin
d) Ferredoxin

149. Which of the following is free-living and aerobic nitrogen fixing bacteria?
a) *Azotobacter*
b) *Rhizobium*
c) *Rhodospirillum*
d) *Clostridium*

150. Which of the following is known as pacemaker enzyme of glycolytic pathway?
a) Hexokinase
b) Phosphofructokinase
c) Pyruvate kinase
d) Triose phosphate isomerase

151. Which of the following is not a compatible substance
a) Proline
b) Pinitol
c) Glycine betaine
d) PEG

152. Which of the following is not a component of pyruvate dehyrogenase complex?
a) Lipoamide b) Coenzyme A
c) FMN d) NAD^+

153. Which of the following is not a mobile mineral nutrient?
a) N b) K
c) Fe d) P

154. Which of the following is not a part of any of the four complexes of ETS?
a) Cytochrome-c b) Cytochrome-b
c) Cytochrome-c_1 d) Fe-S proteins

155. Which of the following is not an electron carrier in cyclic photoposphorylation?
a) Cytochrome-b b) Plastoquinone
c) Pheophytin d) Cytochrome-f

156. Which of the following is not formed in photosynthetic carbon oxidation cycle?
a) Glycolate b) NH_3
c) NADH d) Serine

157. Which of the following is not involved in checking oxidative stress?
a) Carotenoids b) Glutathione
c) Ascorbate d) Glycine betaine

158. Which of the following is often called as facultative pathway?
a) C_3 pathway b) C_4 pathway
c) CAM pathway d) C_2 pathway

159. Which of the following is the primary photoreceptor in photoperiodism?
a) Cryptochrome b) Phototropin
c) Zeaxanthin d) Phytochrome

160. Which of the following light dependent movement of ion regulates Calvin cycle enzymes?
a) Ca^{2+} b) Cl^-
c) Mg^{2+} d) H^+

161. Which of the following mineral nutrient activates many enzymes involved in photosynthesis and respiration?
a) K^+ and Mg^{2+} b) Mn^{2+} and Mg^{2+}
c) Zn^{2+} and Mn^{2+} d) K^+ and Ca^{2+}

162. Which of the following monochromatic lights are more suitable for growth and development of plants.
   a) Red/far red
   b) Red/green
   c) Red/blue/far red
   d) Blue/far red
163. Which of the following photopigment is similar to photolyase and mediate photomorphogenic responses?
   a) Phytochromes
   b) Phototropins
   c) Cryptochromes
   d) Carotenoids
164. Which of the following photosynthetic pigment absorb light energy in the green region of the visible spectrum?
   a) Chlorophyll a
   b) Chlorophyll b
   c) Phycoerythrin
   d) Bacteriochlorophyll
165. Which one of the following is not a ketone body?
   a) Acetoacetate
   b) Acetone
   c) 3-hydorxybutyrate
   d) Acetoacetyl-CoA
166. Which of the following phytochrome controlled response displays red/far red reversibility?
   a) Very low- fluence responses
   b) Low- fluence responses
   c) High- irradiance responses
   d) Very high -irradiance responses
167. Which of the following phytochrome has been implicated in clock entrainment?
   a) Phytochrome C
   b) Phytochrome B
   c) Phytochrome A
   d) Phytochrome E
168. Which of the following phytohormone can be an alternative of cold treatment?
   a) ABA
   b) Gibberellins
   c) Cytokinins
   d) Ethylene
169. Which of the following phytohormone can check drought stress?
   a) Auxin
   b) Gibberellin
   c) ABA
   d) Cytokinin
170. Which of the following phytohormone helped greatly in the spreading of green revolution?
   a) Auxin
   b) Cytokinin
   c) Gibbberellin
   d) Ethylene
171. Which of the following phytohormone induces vascular differentiation?
   a) Auxin
   b) Gibberellin
   c) Cytokinin
   d) ABA

172. Which of the following phytohormone is synthesized in roots?
   a) Auxins b) Ethylene
   c) ABA d) Cytokinines

173. Which of the following phytohormone is used to break seed dormancy?
   a) ABA b) Ethylene
   c) Auxin d) Gibberellin

174. Which of the following phytohormone play a significant role in plants to overcome water stress (flooding)?
   a) ABA b) Gibberellins
   c) Auxins d) Ethylene

175. Which of the following phytohormone promote chloroplast development?
   a) Gibberellin b) Ethylene
   c) ABA d) Cytokinin

176. Which of the following phytohormone regulates vivipary?
   a) Auxin b) ABA
   c) Brassinoids d) Gibberellins

177. Which of the following phytohormone stimulate mobilization of nutrient reserves during germination of cereal grains?
   a) Ethylene b) Cytokinins
   c) Jasmonates d) Gibberellins

178. Which of the following phytohormone stimulates abscission
   a) ABA b) Auxin
   c) Ethylene d) Cytokinin

179. Which of the following process can not be prevented by glycine betaine?
   a) Inactivation of Rubisco
   b) Sucrose synthesis
   c) Inactivation of Rubisco and destabilization of PS-II
   d) Scavenging of hydroxy radicals **[CSIR (NET/JRF) Exam. June 2001]**

180. Which of the following provides seed maturation and antistress signal?
   a) Ethylene b) Cytokinin
   c) Salicylic acid d) ABA

181. Which of the following statement is not true?
   a) In hot, dry climates, the C_4 cycle reduces photorespiration and water loss
   b) C_4 cycle has higher energy demand than the Calvin cycle
   c) Light regulates the activity of key C_4 enzymes
   d) The C_4 cycle concentrates CO_2 in the chloroplast of mesophyll cells.

182. Which of the following statement is not correct about blue light response?
   a) Blue light rapidly inhibits stem elongation.
   b) Blue light stimulates stomata opening.
   c) Blue light regulates osmotic relations of guard cells.
   d) Blue light inhibits a proton pump at the guard cell plasma membrane.

183. Which of the following statement is not correct?
   a) C_4 plants are adapted to high temperature and drought
   b) Phloem translocation occurs by mass transfer
   c) Phloem unloading may occur symplastically or apoplastically
   d) Companion cells are the principal cellular constituents of the phloem

184. Which of the following statement is not correct?
   a) Gibberellins enhance the transcription of α-amylase mRNA
   b) Gibberellins promote seed development and germination
   c) Auxin delays the onset of leaf abscission
   d) ABA promotes precocious germination and vivipary

185. Which of the following statement is not correct?
   a) Nitrogen fixation requires anaerobic environment
   b) *Frankia* fixes nitrogen in alder trees.
   c) Nodule formation involves brassinosteroids.
   d) Amides and ureids are the transported forms of nitrogen.

186. Which of the following statement is not correct?
   a) Osmotic adjustment of cells helps maintain water balance.
   b) CAM plants consume more water
   c) LEA proteins accumulate in vegetative tissue in plants during heat stress.
   d) Ion exclusion and compartmentalization reduce salinity stress.

187. Which of the following statement is not correct?
   a) The C_4 cycle has higher energy demand than the Calvin cycle
   b) Malate and aspartate are carboxylation products of the C_4 cycle
   c) The C_4 cycle concentrates CO_2 in the chloroplasts of mesophyll cells
   d) Two different types of cells participate in the C_4 cycle

188. Which of the following statement is not correct?
   a) The phytochromes are serine/threonine kinases
   b) Phytochromes are imported into the nucleus in the active Pfr form
   c) Photoreversibility is the hallmark of phytochrome action
   d) Phytochrome structure is similar to DNA repair enzymes

189. Which of the following statement is not correct?
   a) Water moves the soil along a water potential gradient
   b) Water moves through the soil by bulk flow

c) Increased solute concentration within a cell increases water potential
d) Aquaporins are specific channel for water uptake.

190. Which one of the following enzyme of krebs cycle closely resembles the PDC in both structure and function?
a) Aconitase
b) Isocitrate dehydrogenase
c) Succinyl Co-A sythetase
d) α-Ketoglutarate dehydrogenase

191. The most common route by which plants absorb minerals and nutrients into their roots is
a) Along cell walls
b) Through root cells
c) Passively, by diffusion from the soil
d) Directly into the phloem

192. In terms of plant structure, what we call the wood of a tree consists of
a) Cork cambium
b) Layers of secondary xylem
c) Layers of secondary phloem
d) All of the above

193. Roots and shoots lengthen through activity at
a) Apical meristems
b) Vascular cambium
c) Lateral meristems
d) Cork cambium

194. ABA is a plant stress hormone, it is
a) Monoterpene
b) Diterpene
c) Triterpene
d) Sesquiterpene

195. Which of the following is the only plant growth hormone that has been clearly shown to be transported polarly?
a) Auxin
b) Gibberellin
c) Cytokinin
d) ABA

196. *Arabidopsis thaliana* is a
a) Long day plant
b) Short day plant
c) Day neutral plant
d) Dual-day length plant

197. Which of the following second messenger does not induces stomatal physiology?
a) cAMP
b) ROS
c) IP3
d) cADPR

198. Which of the following phytohormone is also found in humans?
a) Auxin
b) Gibberellin
c) ABA
d) Brassinosteroids

199. Which of the following statement is not correct?
   a) Osmotic adjustment of cells helps maintain water balance.
   b) CAM plants consume more water
   c) LEA proteins accumulate in vegetative tissue in plants during heat stress
   d) Ion exclusion and compartmentalization reduce salinity stress.

200. Monocots lack
   a) Phytochorme A and B
   b) Phytochrome B and C
   c) Phytochrome A and C
   d) Phytochorme D and E

201. Which of the following is an example of "chemical chaperon"?
   a) HSPs b) Proline
   c) Glucose d) ABA

202. The sucrose-H+ symporter of companion cells of tomato is reffered as
   a) SUC2 b) SUT1
   c) SLAC1 d) SOS1

203. Phenolic compounds in plants are derived from
   a) Tyrosine b) Isoleucine
   c) Phehylalanine d) Tryptophan

204. Which of the following statement is not correct?
   a) DELLA proteins are nuclear-localized
   b) Light inhibits hypocotyl elongation in a DELLA-dependent manner
   c) *Rht* mutants are dwarf because GA receptor is not formed and thus GA signaling is halted
   d) Pfr facilitates degradation of PIFs

205. Which of following phytohormone can be used to induce the formation of embryos from somatic cells?
   a) ABA b) GA
   c) Cytokinin d) Auxin

206. Bacterial phytochromes are light dependent
   a) Serine/threonine kinases b) Histidine kinases
   c) Tyrosine kinases d) Histidine/threonine kinases

207. PIN transporters are involved in
   a) Auxin efflux from the cell b) Auxin influx from the cell
   c) ABA transport d) Ethylene perception

208. In tomato never-ripe mutants are formed when
   a) Ethylene receptors are mutated and it cannot release bound ethylene

b) Mutated ethylene receptors cannot bind ethylene
c) CTR 1 kinases becomes more active
d) None of the above

209. CHLH knockout mutant does not fail to
a) Embryo maturation
b) Vivipary
c) Producing inviable seeds that lack storage reserves and LEA proteins
d) Stomatal and seed dormancy regulation.

21. Brassinosteriod biosynthesis takes place in
a) Plastids
b) Endoplasmic reticulum
c) Peroxisome
d) Cytosol

211. If a plant is growing near the equator where the day length is constant throughout the year, the flowering in this plant is regulated by
a) Photoperiod
b) Internal developmental control that is autonomous
c) Environmental conditions
d) Temperature

212. When plants grow in saline soil influx of Na^+ occurs through nonselective voltage insensitive gated channels that passively transport cytotoxic cations into cells. Closure of these channels is caused by
a) Physiological levels of Ca^{++}
b) Physiological levels of K^+
c) High concentration of Mg^{++}
d) High concentration of H^+

213. Jasmonic acid is synthesized from
a) Linolenic acid
b) Linoleic acid
c) Arachidonic acid
d) Sialic acid

214. Which of the following is not involved in stomatal opening and closing?
a) K^+
b) Cl^-
c) Malate
d) Mg^{++}

215. The herbicide triazine inhibits light reaction in thylakoid membrane. It binds to
a) QB binding site of the D1 protein
b) QA binding site of the D2 protein
c) Cytochrome b6/f complex
d) NADP+ oxidoreductase

216. Phytoalexines are
   a) Falvonoids
   b) Alkaloids
   c) Terpenes
   d) Fatty acids

217. Sulphur deficiency will not influence the synthesis of
   a) Biotin
   b) Thiamine
   c) Coenzyme A
   d) PLP

218. Physiologically active form of phytochrome is maintained by
   a) Red light
   b) Blue light
   c) Far-red light
   d) UV-light

219. Which of the following entrain circadian clock in *Arabidopsis*?
   a) Phytochrome
   b) Cryptochrome
   c) Carotenoids
   d) Both (a) and (b)

220. A decrease in solute potential (Ψs) would
   a) Lower water potential (Ψw)
   b) High water potential
   c) Lower matric potential (Ψm)
   d) All of the above

221. When water stress increases, in C_3 plants the leaf carbon isotope ratio
   a) Increases
   b) Decreases
   c) Remain constant
   d) First increases and then decreases

222. Which of the following enzyme is inhibited by mercury in glycolysis?
   a) Hexokinase
   b) Phosphofructokinase 1
   c) Pyruvate kinase
   d) Glyceraldehydes-3-phosphate dehydrogenase

223. Glucose reabsorption from the lumen is mediated by
   a) Glucose permease
   b) Na^+ - glucose symporter
   c) H^+ - glucose symporter
   d) H^+ - glucose antiporter

224. Amytol inhibits
   a) Complex-I
   b) Complex-II
   c) Complex-III
   d) Complex-IV

225. Which of the following hormone promotes root growth and inhibit shoot growth at low water potential
   a) Gibberelin
   b) Cytokinin
   c) Auxin
   d) ABA

226. The final electron acceptor in lactic acid fermentation is
   a) Pyruvate b) NAD+
   c) Lactic acid d) Oxygen

227. Wounding in a leaf leads to the production of
   a) Jasmonic acid b) Salicylic acid
   c) Systemin d) None of the above

228. Glutamate glyoxylate aminotransferase enzyme is involved in the photorespiration which is located in
   a) Chloroplast b) Mitochondria
   c) Peroxisome d) Both (b) and (c)

229. Which of the following statement is not correct
   a) Photorespiration becomes important only under condition when CO_2 levels are very low
   b) Erythrose-4-phosphate is a precursor of aromatic amino acid
   c) C_4 plants show special temporal separation while CAM plants show spacial separation
   d) C_4 plants can grown in nitrogen deficient soil

230. Which of the following is not the characteristic of guard cell
   a) The primary function of guard cell chloroplast is sensory transduction.
   b) They lack rubisco and $NADP^+$- linked triose phosphate dehydrogenase enzyme.
   c) Guard cell chloroplasts are rich in PSI.
   d) Guard cells function as multisensory hydraulic valves.

231. Acidification of chloroplast lumen causes
   a) Zeaxanthin formation
   b) Violaxanthin formation
   c) Inactivation of the serine-threonine kinase
   d) All of the above

232. Seed germination and formation of leaf primordia are mediated by
   a) Cryptochrome b) Phytochrome
   c) Phototropin d) Phytochrome and phototropin

233. Which of the following statement is incorrect?
   a) Phytochrome is a serine-threonine kinase.
   b) Phototropin is a serine-threonine kinase.
   c) Cryptochrome response is activated by blue light.
   d) Circadian rhythm in animal is mediated by phototropin.

234. In apoplastic phloem loading, sucrose transportation in the transfer cells is mediated by
a) H^+-sucrose symporter b) H^+-sucrose antiporter
c) Na^+-sucrose symporter d) Facilitated diffusion

235. CO_2 formation in pyruvate dehydrogenase complex is mediated by
a) Pyruvate dehydrogenase
b) Pyruvate decorboxylase
c) Dihydrolipoamide transacetylase
d) Dihydrolipoamide dehydrogenase

236. Target site for the toxic action of fluroacetate is
a) Aconitase b) Isocitrate dehydrogenase
c) Succinate dehydrogenase d) Malate dehydrogenase

237. Salt induced inactivation of rubisco is prevented by
a) Glycine betaine b) Proline betaine
c) Alanine betaine d) 3-hydroxyproline betaine

238. HSP-90 is found in
a) Cytosol b) Chloroplast
c) Mitochondria d) All of the above

239. Pterin is component of
a) Nitrate reductase b) Nitrite reductase
c) Dinitrogenase d) GOGAT

240. Histidine amino acid is formed by
a) Pyruvate b) Erythrose-4-phosphate
c) Oxaloacetate d) Ribose-5-phosphate

241. Ureids are translocated in
a) Tropical origin plants b) Temperate origin plants
c) Mediterranian origin plants d) All of the above

242. Tannin is a derivative of
a) Flavonoids b) Phenols
c) Alkaloids d) Lignin

243. Which of the following is largely found in mitochondria?
a) HSP 70 b) HSP 90
c) HSP 60 d) smHSP

244. G-3-P is transported from chloroplast into cytosol through
a) Diffusion b) PO_4^--/triose symporters
c) PO_4^--/triose antiporters d) Triose uniporters

245. Which of the following is NOT a prosthetic group of nitrate reductase?
  a) FAD b) Heme
  c) Mo d) Pterin
[CSIR (NET/JRF) Exam. Dec. 2011]

246. Which of the following acts as a branch point for the biosynthesis of sesquiterpenes and triterpenes?
  a) Farnesyl pyrophosphate
  b) Geranyl pyrophosphate
  c) Isopentyl pyrophosphate
  d) Hydroxymethylglutaryl-CoA **[CSIR (NET/JRF) Exam. Dec. 2011]**

247. Which of the following set of cell organelles are involved in the biosynthesis of jasmonic acid through octadecanoid signaling pathway?
  a) Chloroplast and peroxisomes
  b) Chloroplast and mitochondria
  c) Mitochondria and peroxisomes
  d) Golgi bodies and mitochondria **[CSIR (NET/JRF) Exam. Dec. 2011]**

248. During development of embryos in plants, PIN proteins are involved in
  a) Establishment of auxin gradients
  b) Regulation of gene expression
  c) Induction of programmed cell death
  d) Induction of cell division **[CSIR (NET/JRF) Exam. Dec. 2011]**

249. Chloroplast distribution in a photosynthesizing cell is governed by blue light sensing phototropin 2 (PHOT2). When the cells are irradiated with high intensity blue light, the chloroplasts
  a) Move to the side walls
  b) Aggregate in the middle of the cell
  c) Are sparsely distributed
  d) Aggregate in small clusters **[CSIR (NET/JRF) Exam. Dec. 2011]**

250. Ethylene binding to its receptor, does NOT lead to
  a) Dimerization of the receptor
  b) Phosphorylation of the receptor
  c) Activation of CTR Raf kinase
  d) Endocytosis of ethylene-receptor complex
[CSIR (NET/JRF) Exam. Dec. 2011]

251. Which of the following features is NOT shown by glyphosate, a broad spectrum herbicide?
  a) Little residual soil activity
  b) Ready translocation in phloem

c) Inhibition of a chloroplast enzyme catalyzing the synthesis of aromatic amino acids

d) Inhibition of early steps in the bio-synthesis of branched chain amino acids **[CSIR (NET/JRF) Exam. Dec. 2011]**

252. The transition of flowering in plants requires

a) Growth of plants under long-day conditions.

b) Growth of plants under short-day conditions.

c) Reprogramming of the shoot apical meristem.

d) Synthesis of the flowering hormone florigen.

[CSIR (NET/JRF) Exam. June 2011]

253. Which of the following statements with respect to alternate oxidase activity in Cyanide-resistant respiration in plants, is not correct?

a) Alternate oxidase accepts electrons directly from cytochrome c.

b) Some plants exhibit thermogenesis during inflorescene development.

c) Transcription of alternate oxidase gene is often induced by various abiotic stresses.

d) When electrons pass to alternate oxidase, two sites of proton pumping are bypassed. **[CSIR (NET/JRF) Exam. June 2011]**

254. The dwarf pea mutant (le) used by Mendel was defective in which of the following enzyme involved in gibberellin biosynthesis?

a) ent-Kaurene synthase. b) GA 3 -hydroxylase.

c) GA 20-oxidase. d) ent-Kaurenoic acid hydroxylase.

[CSIR (NET/JRF) Exam. June 2011]

255. DCMU inhibits electron transport in chloroplast by preventing the reduction of

a) P 680. b) QA.

c) PQ. d) QB.

[CSIR Model Paper 2011]

256. In higher plant leaves, the reduction of nitrate to ammonium takes place by the combined action of nitrate reductase localized in cytosol and nitrite reductase localized in

a) Peroxisomes. b) Mitochondria.

c) Chloroplasts. d) Cytosol. **[CSIR Model Paper 2011]**

257. In higher plants, the red/far-red sensory photoreceptor, phytochrome, is a light-regulated kinase. Which of the following classes of kinases does it represent?

a) Two-component sensor regulator (histidine kinase).

b) Two-component sensor regulator (serine/threonine kinase).

c) Leucine rich repeat (LRR) receptor kinase.
d) Calcium-dependent protein kinase. **[CSIR Model Paper 2011]**

258. Vesicular-arbuscular mycorrhiza (VAM) represents a beneficial association between plant roots and fungus, where fungus assists plants in obtaining from the soil
a) Iron
b) Zinc
c) Sulphate
d) Phosphate **[CSIR Model Paper 2011]**

259. In the endodermis of higher plants, the role of Casperian strip is to control the water movement so that it flows
a) Between the cells.
b) Through the plasma membrane.
c) Through the cell wall.
d) Through the transfusion tissue. **[CSIR Model Paper 2011]**

Part C

1. During an experiment the leaf of a short-day plant exposed to short days is excised and grafted to a non induced plant maintained in long days, it causes flowering. This result indicates that
   a) photoperiodic induction depends on long days.
   b) floral stimulus is transported through phloem to flowering buds.
   c) photoperiodic induction depends on events that take place exclusively in the leaf.
   d) phloem is the prerequisite for flowering because grafting is not possible without phloem.

2. The seedlings of a plant having a single growing axis with few lateral branches are exposed to mutagens. The mutant seedlings tend to be bushy. Which of the following would be the possible reason?
   a) auxin biosynthesis is compromised in mutants.
   b) cytokinin production is halted.
   c) Gibberellin signaling is stopped.
   d) mutants are cytokinin-over producing.

3. Which of the following statement is not correct?
   a) Upon absorption of light, the Pr chromophore undergoes a cis-trans isomerization of the double bond between carbon 15 and 16 and rotation of the C14-C15 single bond
   b) Upon absorption of light, Pfr chromophore undergoes a cis-trans isomerization of the double bond between carbon 15 and 16 and rotation of the C14-C15 single bond
   c) The phytochromobilin attaches to the apoprotein through a thioether linkage to a cysteine residue
   d) Photolyases absorb blue light by the pterine and the excitation energy is then transferred to FAD

4. Following are some statements regarding plant growth hormones.
   A. Ethylene regulates abscission.
   B. Gibberlins do not play any role in flowering
   C. Auxin and cytokinin promote cell division
   D. Over expression of cytokinin oxidase would promote root growth.
   E. ABA inhibits root growth and promotes shoot growth at low water potential.
   F. ABA promotes leaf senescence independent of ethylene.

   Which one of the following combination of above statements is correct?

a) A, C and F b) B, C and D
c) D, E and F d) B, D and E

[CSIR (NET/JRF) Exam. Dec. 2011]

5. Following are some statements about low temperature stress in plants.
   A. Fatty acid composition of mitochondria isolated from chilling resistant and chilling sensitive plants differs significantly.
   B. Ratio of unsaturated fatty acids to saturated fatty acids is lower in chilling resistant species.
   C. The cellular water does not freeze even at -40°C, because of the presence of solutes and other antifreeze proteins.
   D. Heat shock proteins do not play any role during low temperature stress.

   Which one of the following combination of above statement is correct?
   a) A and B b) A and C
   c) B and C d) B and D

   [CSIR (NET/JRF) Exam. Dec. 2011]

6. Following are some of the statement regarding the effect of CO2 concentration on photosynthesis in plants.
   A. With elevated CO2 levels, C3 plants are much responsive than C4 plants under well watered conditions.
   B. In C3 plants, increasing intracellular CO2 partial pressure can stimulate photosynthesis only over a narrow range.
   C. In C4 plants, CO2 compensation point is nearly zero.

   Which one of the following combination of above statements is correct?
   a) A and B b) B and C
   c) A and C d) Only C

   [CSIR (NET/JRF) Exam. Dec. 2011]

7. The quantum yield of photosynthetic carbon fixation in a C3 plant and C4 plant is studied as a function of leaf temperature. Following are some statements based on this study.
   A. At lower temperature the quantum yield of C3 plant is lower than C4 plant.
   B. In C4 plant quantum yield does not show a temperature dependence.
   C. Since the photorespiration is low in C4 plants because of CO2 concentrating mechanism, quantum yield is not affected.
   D. At higher temperature the quantum yield of C3 plant is lower than C4 plant.

   Which one of the following combination of above statements is correct?
   a) A, B and D b) B, C and D
   c) A, B and C d) A, C and D

   [CSIR (NET/JRF) Exam. Dec. 2011]

8. Following are some statements for synthesis of jasmonic acid in plants
   A. 12-oxo-phytodienoic acid is produced in chloroplast and transported to peroxisome.
   B. Action of lipoxygenase, allene oxide synthase and allene oxide cyclase takes place in peroxisome.
   C. 12-oxo-phytodicnoic acid is first reduced and then converted to jasmonic acid by -oxidation.
   D. Final production of jasmonic acid takes place in chloroplast.
   E. Action of allene oxide synthase and allene oxide cyclase takes place in chloroplast.

   Which one of the following combination of above statements is correct?
   a) A, B and C   b) B, D and E
   c) C, D and E   d) A, C and E

   [CSIR (NET/JRF) Exam. Dec. 2011]

9. In the global nitrogen cycle, the following microbial organisms are involved in three important process-denitrification, nitrification and nitrogen fixation.
   A. Rhizobium   B. Nitrosomonas
   C. Nitrobacter   D. Pseudomonas
   E. Azotobacter.

   Which of the following is the correctly matched pair of process and its causative species?
   a) Denitrification - (b); nitrogen fixation - (c) and (e); nitrification - (d)
   b) Denitrification - (d); nitrogen fixation - (a) and (e); nitrification - (c)
   c) Denitrification - (e); nitrogen fixation - (a) and (d); nitrification - (d)
   d) Denitrification - (b); nitrogen fixation - (a) and (d); nitrification - (c)

   [CSIR (NET/JRF) Exam. Dec. 2011]

10. Osmolytes are low molecular weight organic compounds that are used by cells to maintain turgor pressure and cell volume, especially under stressed conditions. Under stress conditions, these compounds play an important role in maintaining the structural integrity of enzymes, membranes, hormones and other components. Some of the following statement could possibly explain this observation.
    (A) They stabilize proteins under stressed conditions by reducing the exposure of hydrophobic surface of the proteins.
    (B) They increase the stability of native proteins and assist in the proper refolding of unfolded polypeptides.
    (C) The accumulation of osmolytes in response to osmotic stress is ubiquitously present in diverse organisms from bacteria to plants and animals.
    (D) Osmo-protectants are species-specific

    Which of the following combinations of above statements is NOT true?
    a) A and B   b) B and C
    c) only B   d) only D

11. In an experiment sugar beet leaves are fed exogenous sucrose through the xylem. After few days it was noticed that there was decline in sucrose-H+ symporter in mRNA in companion cells of phloem. The following statements correlate the above observations:
 (A) Decreased sink demand leads to low sucrose levels in the vascular tissue.
 (B) High sucrose levels lead to down regulation of the symporter in the source.
 (C) Decreased loading results in increased sucrose concentration in the source.
 (D) High sucrose levels lead to up regulation of the symporter in the source.
 Which of the above statements are correct?
 a) A and C b) B and D
 c) A and D d) B and C

12. Sieve tubes of phloem conduct translocation of photoassimilate and other organic molecules. They are under very high internal turgor pressure and sieve elements in a sieve tube are connected through open sieve plate pores. When a sieve tube is cut or punctured the release of pressure causes the contents of the sieve elements to surge toward the cut end, from which the plant could loss much sugar-rich phloem sap if there were no sealing mechanisms. The following mechanisms are suggested:
 A) P-protein appears to function in sealing off damaged sieve elements by plugging up the sieve plate pores.
 B) P-proteins are found in sieve tube and they are involved in short-term sealing mechanism.
 C) Long-term mechanism for preventing sap loss entails closing sieve plate pores with callose.
 D) Callose is synthesized by an enzyme found in the cell wall and it plays a central role in short-term sealing mechanism
 Which of the following combinations is NOT correct?
 a) A and B b) Only D
 c) B and C d) Only A

13. Phytochromes are red/far-red light photoreceptors that play fundamental roles in photoperception of the light environment and the subsequent adaptation of plant growth and development. The following are some of the statements characterizing phytochromes:
 (A) They are soluble proteins and exist as tetramers.
 (B) Their N-terminal domain binds phytochromobilin in their NTE domain.
 (C) Their C-terminal domain harbors NLS.
 (D) They have three phosphorylation sites.
 Which one of the following combinations of the above statements is true?
 a) A and B b) C and D

c) B and C
d) A and D

14. CONSTANS (CO) plays acentral role in the induction of flowering by long days. The following statements correlate the CO functions:
(A) CO encodes a nuclear protein containing zinc fingers, and activates the transcription of floral regulators such as FLOWERING LOCUS T (FT) in the light.
(B) The mRNA level of CO is tightly controlled by the circadian clock and shows a striking temporal pattern of expression.
(C) Under SDs CO mRNA peaks before Dusk and stays high until the following dawn.
(D) Under LDs CO mRNA peaks during the night.
Which of the following combinations of above statements is true?
a) A and C
b) Only B
c) A and B
d) Only D

15. Atmospheric CO_2 contains the naturally occurring stable carbon isotopes ^{12}C and ^{13}C in the proportion of 98.9% and 1.1%, respectively. Following are some of the statements regarding CO_2 assimilation:
A. Both C_3 and C_4 plants assimilate less $^{13}CO_2$ than $^{12}CO_2$.
B. Both C_3 and C_4 plants assimilate less $^{12}CO_2$ than $^{13}CO_2$.
C. C_3 plants assimilate lesser $^{13}CO_2$ than $^{12}CO_2$ as compared to C_4 plants.
D. C_4 plants assimilate lesser $^{13}CO_2$ than $^{12}CO_2$ as compared to C_3 plants.
Which one of the following combinations of above statements is true?
a) A and B
b) A and C
c) C and D
d) A and D

[CSIR (NET/JRF) Exam. June 2011]

16. The dependence of the rate of sucrose uptake with respect to sucrose concentration in plant cell was studied and data are shown in the following graph. From the above data it can be inferred that

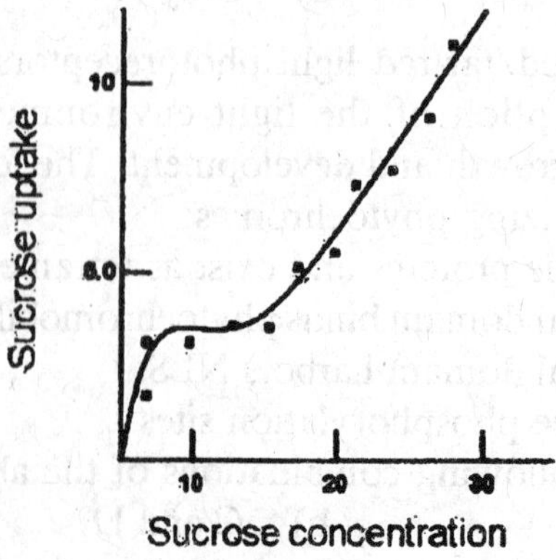

a) the sucrose uptake is energy independent and no special carrier is involved.
b) the sucrose uptake is energy dependent and a special carrier is involved.
c) at lower concentration of sucrose the uptake of sucrose is energy dependent and carrier mediated.
d) at higher concentration of sucrose the uptake is energy dependent and carrier mediated. **[CSIR (NET/JRF) Exam. June 2011]**

17. Following are some statements for synthesis of secondary metabolites in plants.
   A. Terpenes are synthesized by shikimic acid pathway and mevalonic acid pathway.
   B. Alkaloids are nitrogen containing compounds and are synthesized by shikimic acid pathway.
   C. Phenolic compounds are synthesized by shikimic acid pathway and mevalonic acid pathway.
   D. Both alkaloids and terpenes are synthesized by mevalonic acid pathway and MEP pathway.

   Which one of the following combinations of the above statement is true?
   a) A and D b) A and C
   c) B and C d) B and D

   [CSIR (NET/JRF) Exam. June 2011]

18. During episodes of anoxia in plants, pyruvate produced in glycolysis is initially fermented to lactate. During later stage, there is an increase in the fermentation to ethanol and decrease in the fermentation to lactate, a phenomena which helps plants survive anoxia. Which of the following statements is correct about this change of fermentation flux from lactate towards ethanol?
   a) The cytosolic pH increases, thus activating both lactaste dehydrogenase and pyruvate decarboxylase activity.
   b) The cytosolic pH increases, thus inhibiting lactate dehydrogenase activity and activating pyruvate decarboxylase activity.
   c) The cytosolic pH decreases, thus activating both lactate dehydrogenase and pyruvate decarboxylase activity.
   d) The cytosolic pH decreases, thus inhibiting lactate dehydrogenase and activating pyruvate decarboxylase activity.

   [CSIR (NET/JRF) Exam. June 2011]

19. Plants grown in greenhouse at 25°C when exposed first to 35°C for 6 hours and subsequently to 42°C for 12 hours adapt better to the high temperature (42°C) in comparison to those directly transferred to 42°C for the same duration. What is the phenomenon called and what is its main physiological

basis?

a) Acquired thermo-tolerance because of the induction of mutagens resulting into improved stability of all the proteins.
b) Induced thermo-tolerance because of the induction of heat shock proteins.
c) Induced thermo-tolerance because changes in RNA polymerase II resulting in efficient and improved transcription.
d) Acquired thermo-tolerance because of efficient post translational modification of proteins. **[CSIR Model Paper 2011]**

20. In which molecule would the radiolabel appear the earliest when wheat and sugar cane leaves are fed with $^{14}CO_2$?
   a) Wheat - malate, sugarcane - 3phosphoglycerate.
   b) Wheat - aspartate, sugarcane - malate.
   c) Wheat - 3phosphoglycerate, sugarcane - 3phosphoglycerate.
   d) Wheat - 3phosphyoglycerate, sugarcane - malate.

   [CSIR Model Paper 2011]

21. A young dicot seedling (e.g soyabean) is subjected to gravity stimulus by laying it horizontally on a surface the shoot bends upwards and root bends downward. Indicate the reason.
   a) Redistribution of auxin throughout the seedlings is responsible for stimulatory unequal growth in shoots and roots.
   b) Redistribution of auxin in shoots while cytokinine in roots is responsible for stimulatory unequal growth.
   c) Redistribution of auxin in roots while cytokinine in shoots is responsible for stimulatory unequal growth.
   d) Redistribution of cytokinine throughout the seedlings is responsible for stimulatory unequal growth in shoots and roots.

   [CSIR Model Paper 2011]

22. Which of the following statements are associated with the process of photorespiration in plants?
   (A) Photorespiration takes place in only C3 plants.
   (B) Photorespiration takes place in only C4 plants.
   (C) Photorespiration takes place in both C3 and C4 plants.
   (D) Glycolate is oxidized to glyoxylate in the peroxisome.
   (E) Glycolate is oxidized to glyoxylate in the mitochondira.
   a) (A) and (D) b) (C) and (D)
   c) (B) and (E) d) (C) and (E)

   [CSIR Model Paper 2011]

23. Aspartate kinase is a key enzyme in the lysine amino-acid biosynthesis in plants. With an objective of increasing the lysine content in maize seeds, maize plants were transformed with *E.coli* aspartate kinase with a strong seed specific plant promoter. Resulting transgenic plants were found to express the transgene; however, the content of lysine did not increase. Which of the following option best explain the possible reason?
   a) Bacterial proteins are not stable in plants.
   b) Bacterial proteins are not properly folded in plants.
   c) Proper post-translational modification did not take place in plants.
   d) Lysine causes feed back inhibition of aspartate kinase

[CSIR Model Paper 2011]

24. For C_3 plants, as many as 400 molecules of water are lost for every molecule of CO_2 fixed by photosynthesis, giving a transpiration ratio of 400. The large ratio of H_2O efflux to CO_2 influx results from three factors:
   (A) The concentration gradient driving water loss is about 50 times larger than that driving the influx of CO_2 because of the low CO_2 concentration in air and high concentration of water vapour within the leaf.
   (B) CO_2 diffuses about 16 times more slowly through air than water does.
   (C) CO_2 must cross the plasma membrane, the cytoplasm, and the chloroplast envelope before it is assimilated in the chloroplast.

   Which one of the following combination of above statements is correct?
   a) A and B b) B and C
   c) A and C d) Only C

25. In most algae and plants nonphotochemical quenching appears to be an essential part of the regulation of antenna systems. Following are some statements regarding nonphotochemical quenching
   (A) Nonphotochemical quenching is the quenching of chlorophyll fluorescence by photochemistry.
   (B) Nonphotochemical quenching is thought to be involved in protecting the photosynthetic machinery against over excitation and subsequent damage.
   (C) Nonphotochemical quenching appears to be preferentially associated with a peripheral antenne complex of photosystem I.
   (D) As a result of nonphotochemical quenching, a large fraction of the excitations in the antenne system caused by intense illumination are quenched by conversion into heat.

   Which one of the following combination of above statements is correct?
   a) A, B and C b) B, C and D
   c) B and D d) A and C

26. Arabidopsis mutants devoid of photorespiratory enzymes grow normally at high levels of CO_2 (2%), but they die rapidly when transferred to normal air (0.03% CO_2). The following explanation were proposed for this observation.
    (A) The C_2 oxidative photosynthetic cycle dissipates excess reducing equivalents, thereby preventing over-reduction of the photosynthetic electron chain.
    (B) H_2O_2 produced by photorespiration acts as a signaling molecule and regulates cellular redox homeostasis.
    (C) Oxygenation reaction becomes significant for regeneration of RUBP when levels of O_2 increased in the atmosphere.

    Which one of the following combination of above statements is correct?
    a) Only A b) A and C
    c) A and B d) A, B and C

27. Rubisco plays a critical role in the carbon cycle of the biosphere. CO_2 functions both as activator and as substrate in the reaction catalyzed by rubisco. As modulator, CO_2 reacts slowly with the amino group of a specific lysine within the active site of rubisco. The resulting carbamate derivative then rapidly binds Mg^{2+} to yield the activated enzyme. The tight binding of sugar phosphate-like molecules, such as ribulose 1,5 bisphosphate, to rubisco prevents carbamylation. However, the interaction of rubisco with rubisco activase brings about a structural change of rubisco that releases sugar phosphate-like molecules and prepares the enzyme for activation via carbamylation and metal binding. Following are some statements regarding rubisco activase.
    (A) Rubisco activase is a member of a protein family that exhibits ATPase activity associated with chaperon-like functions.
    (B) Before interaction with rubisco, 20 to 50 rubisco activase polypeptides oligomerise.
    (C) Arabidopsis mutants that lack rubisco activase exhibit severely impaired photosynthesis at atmospheric levels of CO_2.

    Which one of the following combination of above statements is correct?
    a) A and C b) B and C
    c) A, B and C d) A and B

28. Following are some of the statements regarding the effect of light on photosynthesis in plants
    (A) Increasing light above the light compensation point proportionally increases photosynthesis.
    (B) Light compensation points are lower for shade plants because respiration rates in shade plants are very high.

(C) Low respiratory rates allow shade plants to survive in light-limited environments through their ability to achieve positive CO_2 uptake rates at lower values of PAR than sun plants.

(D) Sun plants have low light compensation points and have high maximal photosynthetic rates than shade plants.

Which one of the following combination of above statements is true?

a) A and B b) C and D
c) A and C d) Only D

29. The polymer-trapping model explains symplastic loading in plants with intermediary cells. The following statements are about polymer-trapping model

(A) Sucrose should be more concentrated in the mesophyll than in the intermediary cells.

(B) The enzymes for raffinose and stachyose synthesis should be preferentially located in the mesophyl cells.

(C) The plasmodesmata linking the bundle sheath cells and the intermediary cells should exclude molecules larger than sucrose

Which of the above statements are true?

a) A and B b) B and C
c) A, B and C d) A and C

30. Following are some statements about secondary metabolites

(A) Terpenes are synthesized via malonic acid pathway

(B) Phenolic compounds are synthesized via mevalonic acid pathway.

(C) In higher plants, most phenolics are derived at least in part from tyrosine

(D) The malonic acid pathway is an important source of phenolic secondary products in fungi and bacteria.

Which one of the following combination of above statements is correct?

a) A, B and C b) C and D
c) Only B d) Only D

31. Phototropins are involved in auxin mediated phototropism. Following are some statements about phototropins

(A) They are chromoproteins and are the photoreceptors for the blue-light signaling pathway.

(B) Phototropins are autophosphorylating protein kinases which are normally found in plasma membrane.

(C) Phototropin 1 displays a lateral gradient in phosphorylation during exposure to low-fluence unilateral blue light.

(D) Their phosphorylation results in dissociation of the protein from the plasma membrane and subsequent interactions with auxin transporters, resulting in auxin transport inhibition.

Which one of the following is correct?

a) A and B
b) B and C
c) B and D
d) B, C and D

32. Following are some statements about phytohormones
   (A) Auxin delays the onset of leaf abscission.
   (B) Gibberellins promote pollen development and tube growth.
   (C) Cytokinin has been linked to the inhibition of a Cdc 25-like phosphatase.
   (D) ABA-insensitive mutants embryo accumulates high amount of LEA protein

   Which one of the following combination of above statements is correct?

   a) A and D
   b) B and C
   c) B, C and D
   d) A and B

33. Many plants have the capacity to acclimate to cold temperatures. The ability to tolerate freezing temperature under natural conditions varies greatly among tissues. Seed and other partially dehydrated tissues, as well as fungal spores, can be kept indefinitely at temperatures near absolute zero, indicating that these very low temperatures are not intrinsically harmful. The following are some statements about cold acclimation in plants
   (A) During cold acclimation, temperate woody species withdraw water from the xylem vessels, thereby preventing the stem from splitting in response to the expansion of water during subsequent freezing.
   (B) Cold acclimation involves Ca^{2+} influx to the cytosol from the apoplast, the endoplasmic reticulum, and vacuolar pools, resulting in cytosolic transients necessary for induction of some low temperature-responsive genes required for cold acclimation
   (C) Mutations of *Arabidopsis thaliana* that cause ABA-deficiency result in plants that are capable in serviving in extreme cold.

   Which are the following combination of above statement is correct?

   a) A and B
   b) B and C
   c) A, B and C
   d) A and C

34. Following are some statements describing unique feature of plant mitochondria
   (A) Plant mitochondrial electron transport chain has a proline dehydrogenase which oxidizes the amino acid proline accumulated during osmotic stress.
   (B) Plant mitochondrial matrix has malic enzyme which catalyzes the oxidative decarboxylation of malate.
   (C) Plant mitochondrial electron transport chain has an alternative oxidase which functions as a tetramer.

   Which one of the following combination of above statements is true?

a) Only C b) Only B
c) A and C d) A and B

35. The enzyme dinitrogenase is required for nitrogen fixing bacteria. Dinitrogenase synthesis is directed by a set of genes known as *nif* genes. Following are some statements about *nif* genes.
(A) The *nif* D and *nif* K genes encode the two different subunits of the MoFe protein.
(B) The Fe protein and ferredoxin are encoded by *nif*H and *nif* F, respectively.
(C) *nif* genes are involved in the synthesis and regulation of dinitrogenase in free-living forms as well as in symbiotic nitrogen fixers.
Which of the following combination is correct?
a) A and B b) B and C
c) A, B and C d) Only C

36. Following are some statements regarding oxidative pentose phosphate pathway
(A) Oxidative pentose phosphate pathway is present in both the chloroplast as well as the cytosol in plants
(B) The first step in the oxidative pentose phosphate pathway is the oxidation of glucose-6-phosophate to 6-phosphogluconate. This step is apparently the rate-determining step for the pathway.
(C) In animals, this pathyway, is extremely active in fatty tissues where NADPH is required for active fatty acid breakdown.
(D) Erythrose-4-phosphate is an intermediate of oxidative pentose phosphate pathway which is utilized in synthesis of alkaloids in plants.
Which one of the following combination of above statements is correct?
a) A and D b) B and C
c) B, C and D d) A and B

37. Following are some statements regarding phytohormones and their receptors
(A) The cytokinin receptor is a membrane based histidine kinase monomer. Binding with cytokinin induces dimerization and autophosphorylation of the receptor.
(B) The sensor domain of ethylene receptor contains a copper cofactor that is necessary for ethylene binding.
(C) DELLA proteins are gibberellin receptors.
(D) The receptor for brassinosteroids are plasma-membrane associated heterodimer. Which one of the following combination of above statements is correct?
a) A, B and D b) B, C and D
c) A and B d) A, B and C

38. Cryptochromes are blue-light receptors in plants and are involved in photomorphogenesis. Following are some statements regarding cryptochromes
    (A) They are permanently located in the nucleus.
    (B) In the nucleus cryptochrome interacts directly with the COP1 which is an E3 ubiquitin ligase.
    (C) After blue-light absorption, cryptochrome undergoes a conformational change which leads to the activation of COP1.
    (D) The phosphorylated form of cryptochrome is inactive.

    Which one of the following combination of above statements is correct?

    a) A, B and C   b) Only D
    c) Only B   d) A, B and D

39. Following are some statements regarding abiotic stress in plants.
    (A) UV-C radiation induces a high frequency of somatic homologous recombination in *Arabidopsis.* This trait is meiotically transmitted across generation through epigenetic processes.
    (B) ABA induces chromatin remodeling by histone H3 acetylation and methylation to regulate gene expression and abiotic stress-induced growth arrest.
    (C) *Arabidopsis* HOS15, a component of the chromatin repression complex involved in histone deacetylation, plays a key role in heat stress tolerance.
    (D) Submergence-stress induces the expression of alcohol dehydrogenase (ADH1) and pyruvate decarboxylase (PDC1) genes in rice through histone H3 trimethylation and acetylation.

    Which one of the following combination of above statements is true?

    a) A, B and C   b) B, C and D
    c) A, B and D   d) B and C

40. Stomata are turgor-responsive valves in the leaf epidermis in plants. Stomatal movements are due to the regulation of gurard cell turgor via the control of osmolyte concentrations in their cytosol. Following are some statements regarding stomatal physiology.
    (A) Several monovalent cations can affect guard cells osmotic potential but K^+ is the most relevant as it accumulates at high concentrations in gurar cells, which leads to stomatal opening.
    (B) Inward K^+ channels are activated after ABA treatment and cytosolic Ca^{2+} elevation
    (C) ABA inhibits plasma membrane anion channels.
    (D) The ABC transporter AtMRP5 is plasma membrane-localized and functions in regulation of S-type anion channels and Ca^{2+} channels in guard cells.

    Which one of the following combination of above statements is true?

    a) A, B and C   b) A, B,C and D
    c) A, B and C   d) A and D

Answer Sheet

Part – B

1.	c	2.	c	3.	b	4.	a	5.	b	6.	b
7.	d	8.	a	9.	b	10.	d	11.	c	12.	c
13.	a	14.	c	15.	a	16.	b	17.	b	18.	d
19.	b	20.	c	21.	b	22.	b	23.	c	24.	b
25.	a	26.	a	27.	d	28.	d	29.	d	30.	c
31.	a	32.	c	33.	c	34.	c	35.	b	36.	b
37.	a	38.	b	39.	c	40.	c	41.	b	42.	c
43.	b	44.	b	45.	b	46.	d	47.	c	48.	d
49.	c	50.	a	51.	a	52.	d	53.	d	54.	c
55.	c	56.	c	57.	d	58.	a	59.	a	60.	b
61.	a	62.	c	63.	d	64.	c	65.	d	66.	b
67.	d	68.	d	69.	b	70.	d	71.	a	72.	c
73.	d	74.	b	75.	c	76.	c	77.	b	78.	c
79.	c	80.	c	81.	c	82.	c	83.	c	84.	c
85.	c	86.	c	87.	c	88.	c	89.	c	90.	d
91.	b	92.	c	93.	b	94.	a	95.	d	96.	b
97.	d	98.	a	99.	b	100.	d	101.	c	102.	b
103.	c	104.	b	105.	d	106.	b	107.	d	108.	a
109.	b	110.	a	111.	d	112.	c	113.	c	114.	b
115.	a	116.	b	117.	d	118.	b	119.	b	120.	a
121.	b	122.	b	123.	c	124.	a	125.	b	126.	b
127.	a	128.	a	129.	a	130.	a	131.	d	132.	c
133.	b	134.	c	135.	d	136.	c	137.	d	138.	b
139.	a	140.	a	141.	d	142.	b	143.	a	144.	d
145.	b	146.	c	147.	a	148.	c	149.	a	150.	b
151.	d	152.	c	153.	c	154.	a	155.	c	156.	c
157.	d	158.	c	159.	d	160.	c	161.	a	162.	c
163.	c	164.	c	165.	d	166.	b	167.	a	168.	b
169.	c	170.	c	171.	a	172.	d	173.	d	174.	d
175.	d	176.	b	177.	d	178.	a	179.	d	180.	d
181.	d	182.	d	183.	d	184.	d	185.	c	186.	b
187.	c	188.	d	189.	c	190.	d	191.	a	192.	b
193.	a	194.	d	195.	a	196.	a	197.	a	198.	c
199.	b	200.	d	201.	b	202.	b	203.	c	204.	c
205.	d	206.	b	207.	a	208.	b	209.	b	210.	b
211.	b	212.	a	213.	a	214.	d	215.	a	216.	a

217.	d	218.	a	219.	b	220.	a	221.	a	222.	d
223.	b	224.	a	225.	d	226.	c	227.	c	228.	c
229.	c	230.	c	231.	a	232.	a	233.	d	234.	a
235.	a	236.	a	237.	a	238.	a	239.	a	240.	d
241.	a	242.	b	243.	c	244.	c	245.	d	246.	c
247.	a	248.	a	249.	a	250.	c	251.	d	252.	c
253.	a	254.	c	255.	d	256.	c	257.	b	258.	d
259.	b										

Part – C

1.	c	2.	d	3.	b	4.	a	5.	b	6.	c
7.	b	8.	d	9.	b	10.	d	11.	d	12.	b
13.	b	14.	c	15.	b	16.	c	17.	d	18.	d
19.	b	20.	d	21.	a	22.	a	23.	b	24.	c
25.	c	26.	c	27.	a	28.	c	29.	d	30.	d
31.	b	32.	d	33.	a	34.	d	35.	a	36.	d
37.	a	38.	c	39.	c	40.	d				

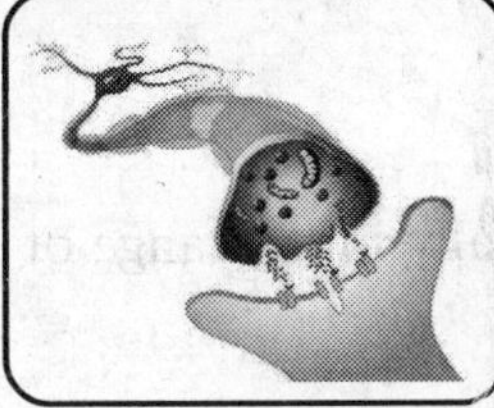

Chapter 7
Animal Physiology

Part B

1. Erythrocytes obtain their energy through
   a) Oxidative phosphorylation
   b) Substrate-level phosphorylation
   c) Fermentation
   d) Pentose phosphate pathway

2. Gluconeogenesis does not occur in muscles and brain because
   a) They have high concentration of glucose
   b) They lack glucose-6-phosphatase
   c) They have substitutes of glucose
   d) They store creatine phosphate

3. Human chronic gonadotropin is produced
   a) Both in males and females
   b) Only in males
   c) Only in females
   d) Only in females during pregnancy

4. In "Rh" factor, Rh name is taken from a monkey found in
   a) India b) Africa
   c) East Asia d) South America
   [CSIR (NET/JRF] Exam. June 2005]

5. RBCs uptake glucose through
   a) Symporter b) Antiporter
   c) Passive Carrier d) ABC transporter

6. Receptors for neurotransmitters are located on the
   a) Cell surface b) Nuclear membrane
   c) Cytosol d) Nucleoplasm

7. Steroid hormones
   a) Bind to receptors in the plasma membrane
   b) Must be actively transported

c) Bind to receptors in the cytosol
d) Change the shape of proteins in the nucleus

8. The concentration of glucose in the blood plasma is usually in the range of
a) 180-200mg/100mL b) 60-70 mg/100mL
c) 65-90 mg/100mL d) 5-50mg/100mL

9. The hormone which is secreted by both hypothalamus and gastrointestine is
a) Gastrin b) Cholecystokinin
c) Somatostatin d) Secretin

[CSIR (NET/JRF) Exam. June 2003]

10. Vertebrates achieved terrestrial habit due to presence of
a) Internal fertilization b) Thermoregulation
c) Amniotic egg d) Vivipary

[CSIR (NET/JRF) Exam. Dec. 2003]

11. Behavioural fever occurs as thermoregulatory control mechanism in
a) Birds and lizards b) Mammals and amphibians
c) Lizards and amphibians d) Fish and humans

12. Chloride cells and pavement cells regulate ion and water balance in
a) Fish b) Reptiles
c) Birds d) Mammals

13. Circulatory system move fluids according to
a) Law of diffusion b) Law of thermodynamics
c) Law of bulk flow d) Henry's law

14. Fish sometimes produce a highly water soluble nitrogen compound which is the characteristic "fish odour". The compound is
a) Ammonia b) Trimethylamine
c) Uric acid d) Derivative of purine

15. For the muscles the major source of energy is
a) ATP b) Phosphocreatine
c) GTP d) Lactic acid

16. Galanin hormone controlling digestion is secreted from
a) Duodenum b) Intestinal nerves
c) Stomach d) Pancreas

17. Green haemoglobin (chlorocruorins) are found in
a) Neurons of vertebrates b) Connective tissues of vertebrates
c) Marine annelids d) Salamander

18. hCG is a hormone which is used in pregnancy test . It is synthesized by
a) Pituitary gland b) Ovary
c) Placenta d) Hypothalamous
[CSIR (NET/JRF) Exam. Dec 2004]

19. Hemerythrins are the respiratory pigments of
a) Arthropods b) Molluscs
c) Brachiopods d) Annelids

20. In a normal kidney, which of the following would cause an increase in GFR?
a) Constriction of the afferent arteriole
b) Decrease in the hydrostatic pressure in the glomerulus
c) Increase in hydrostatic pressure in the Bowman's capsule
d) All of the above.

21. Organisms inhabiting water scarce environment are likely
a) Uricotelic b) Ureotelic
c) Ammonotelic d) to have small kidney size

22. Paneth cells are found in
a) Brain b) Heart
c) Liver d) Small intestine

23. Partially open circulatory system is found in
a) Earthworm b) Lobsters
c) Lamprey d) *Amphioxus*

24. Reptiles are
a) Uricotelic b) Ureotelic
c) Ammonotelic d) None of the above

25. Satellite cells are
a) Absorptive cells of intestine
b) Cells of brain in which ketone bodies are not formed
c) Stem cells of adult muscle
d) Cells having satellite chromosomes

26. Testosterone hormone necessary for spermatogenesis is secreted by
a) Leydig cells b) Sertoli cells
c) Spermatozoa d) Cowpers gland
[CSIR (NET/JRF) Exam. Dec 2004]

27. The effect of which of the following steroid hormone is 'non-genic' while majority of the steroid hormones alter transcription in the target cell?
a) Cortisol b) Testosterone
c) Progesterone d) Aldosterone

28. The excretory waste in birds is uric acid, it suggests that
    a) Birds are more advanced
    b) Birds are omnivores
    c) Birds are adapted for conservation of water
    d) Uric acid is toxic metabolite **[CSIR (NET/JRF) Exam. June 2005]**
29. The hormone containing minimum number of peptides which is secretd by hypothalamus is
    a) TRH b) GnRH
    c) CRH d) ACTH
    [CSIR (NET/JRF) Exam. June 2007]
30. The hormone secreted by developing placenta is
    a) Chorionic gonadotropin b) Estrogen
    c) Relaxin d) ADH
    [CSIR (NET/JRF) Exam. June 2007]
31. The main function of oxytocin is
    a) Relaxation of uterine muscles during pregnancy
    b) Contraction of uterine muscles at birth
    c) Ovulation of egg from ovary
    d) None of the above
32. The maximum amount of air that can be moved into or out of the respiratory system with one breath is called
    a) Tidal volume b) Residual volume
    c) Vital capacity d) Total lung capacity
33. The mechanism of synaptic communication is similar to
    a) Autocrine communication b) Paracrine communication
    c) Endocrine communication d) None of the above
34. Thermogenin is a common integral inner membrane protein in brown fat mitochondria. Its function is to
    a) Increase impermeability of inner membrane
    b) Maintain electron transport chain
    c) Form a channel for the return of pumped protons from the inter membrane space back into the matrix
    d) Enhance ATP synthasis by assisting ATP synthesis
35. Which is a stress hormone?
    a) hCG b) ACTH
    c) Oxytosin d) ADH
    [CSIR (NET/JRF) Exam. Dec 2001]

36. Which of the following can not survive in anaerobic condition?
    a) RBC b) Cornea of eye
    c) Kidney medulla d) Heart muscles

37. Which of the following can not use ketone bodies
    a) Brain b) Heart
    c) Muscle d) Liver

38. Which of the following cannot utilize fatty acids for energy?
    a) Heart b) Skeletal muscle
    c) Liver d) Brain

39. Which of the following component of the vestibular apparatus of the inner ear of mammals is not responsible for the sense of equilibrium?
    a) Utricle b) Saccule
    c) Ampulla d) Cochlea

40. Which of the following enhances the abilities of sperm to swim rapidly and to fuse with the cell membrance of the oocyte?
    a) Acrosomal reaction b) Cortical reaction
    c) Sperm competition d) Capacitation

41. Which of the following hormone is not involved in controlling appetite (the desire to feed)?
    a) Leptin b) Ghrelin
    c) Peptide YY d) Motilin

42. Which of the following hormone is produced during estrous cycle?
    a) Epinephrine b) Vasopressin
    c) Oxytosin d) Progesterone

[CSIR (NET/JRF) Exam. June 2007]

43. Which of the following hormone is used as nutritional supplement to reduce the severity of jet lag?
    a) Corticosteroids b) Melatonin
    c) Inhibin d) Prostaglandins

44. Which of the following hormone regulates the level of Ca^{2+} in the blood.
    a) Aldosterone b) Parathyroid
    c) Epinephrine d) ACTH

45. Which of the following is not related to oxygen transport?
    a) Bohr effect b) Root effect
    c) Haldane effect d) Chloride shift

46. Which one of the following is the only one of all vertebrates that lack blood hemoglobin as adults?
   a) Dolphins b) Icefish
   c) Marine fish d) Sea birds

47. Which of the following macronutrient functions in osmoregulation?
   a) Calcium b) Potassium
   c) Magnesium d) Phosphorus

48. Which of the following part of peripheral nervous system becomes more active during period of stress/physical activity?
   a) Sympathetic b) Parasympathetic
   c) Enteric d) Somatic motor pathway

49. Which of the following part of the brain maintain body posture?
   a) Cerebrum b) Hypothalamus
   c) Medulla oblongata d) Cerebellum

50. Which of the following properties of a neuron does not govern the speed of impulse conduction within an axon?
   a) Membrane resistance b) Length constant
   c) Diameter of axon d) Chemical nature of neurotransmitter

51. Which of the following regulates body temperature?
   a) Hypothalamus b) Supra chiasmatic nuclei
   c) Cerebrum d) Cerebellum

[CSIR (NET/JRF) Exam. June 2008]

52. Which of the following statement is not true for nerve conduction?
   a) The larger the axon's diameter, the faster the conduction.
   b) The larger the axon's diameter, the slower the conduction.
   c) Saltatory conduction can transmit action potential at speeds upto 120m/sec. in myelinated axons.
   d) Myelin sheath increases the axon's diameter and hence effects speed of nerve conduction.

53. Which of the following statements is not correct?
   a) Hippocampus converts short term memories into long term memories.
   b) Amygdala is responsible for sexual urges.
   c) Hypothalamus plays a dominant role in regulating the autonomous nervous system.
   d) Hypothalamus is a component of limbic system.

54. Which of the following statements is not correct?
   a) Synthesis of melatonin increases at night.
   b) In non-mammalian vertebrates pineal complex acts as a 'third eye'.

c) In mammals, the master circadian resides in the paired suprachiasmatic nuclei (SCN)
d) Circadian rhythms appear to occur only in all higher vertebrates and some prokaryotes.

55. During implantation, the blastocyst implants itself in
a) An ovum b) The endometrium
c) The oviduct d) The trophobalst

56. Action potential initiates at
a) Dendrites b) Soma
c) Axon hillock d) Axon

57. Whether a synapse is excitatory or inhibitory depends on
a) Type of neurotransmitter b) Concentration of neurotransmitter
c) Size of the synapse d) Nature of postsynaptic receptors

58. Rhodopsin is integral membrane protein involved in visual transduction. It is active in the form of
a) 11-cis-retinal b) 11-trans-retinal
c) Opsin d) Transducin

59. Which of the following statement is incorrect?
a) All blood cells are formed from a single type of stem cell through a process called hematopoiesis.
b) In adult mammals, blood cells develop from bone marrow only
c) Erythropoietin released from bone marrow is responsible for blood cell differentiation.
d) In reptiles and birds, hematopoiesis can occur in the spleen, liver, kidney and bone marrow.

60. Odorant receptor proteins are
a) G-protein coupled receptor b) Tyrosine kinase coupled receptor
c) Ion-channel linked receptor d) Serine-threonine kinase receptor

61. Pheromones detection in mammal is performed by
a) Olfactory epithelial cells b) Vomeronasal organ
c) Jacobson's organ d) Sensilla cells

62. If we use H^+ lack food, which of the following type of sensation, is not sensitized
a) Salty tastes b) Sour tastes
c) Umami tastes d) Bitter tastes

63. Tactile receptors detect
a) Touch
b) Pressure

c) Vibration on the body surface
d) All of the above

64. Which of the following statement is incorrect ?
a) Outer hair cells of inner ear amplify sounds
b) Inner hair cells of inner ear detect sounds
c) Vestibular apparatus of the inner ear detects movements in body position and responsible for the sense of equilibrium
d) The outer ear is the organ of equilibrium in vertebrates

65. Blood pressure is maintained by
a) Heart b) Kidney
c) Liver d) Hypothalamus

66. It you destroy the neurons in the suprachiasmatic nuclei
a) Circadian rhythms disappear
b) Melatonin secretion disappear
c) Individual not suffered with jet lag
d) All of the above

67. In a typical mammalian kidney, the net glomerular filteration rate is about
a) 60 mm Hg b) 45 mm Hg
c) 30 mm Hg d) 15 mm Hg

68. Seminal fluid is mainly composed of
a) Glucose b) Fructose
c) Maltose d) Galactose

69. Inhibin hormone is released by
a) Hypothalamus b) Anterior pituitary
c) Corpus luteum d) Placenta

70. Which of the following is correct for thyroid hormone?
a) It is a derivative of thyroglobulin protein.
b) Collectively, T3 and T4 are called the thyroid hormones.
c) It plays an important role in setting metabolic rate and body temperature
d) All of the above

71. Which of the following channel is responsible for the hyper polarization of the neuron
a) Voltage gated Ca^{++} channel
b) Voltage gated Na^{+} channel
c) Voltage gated K^{+} channel
d) Ligand gated Ca^{++} channel

72. The ability of an axon to generate new action potential during the phases of action potential is
   a) Absolute refractory period by normal stimulus
   b) Relative refractory period by normal stimulus
   c) Absolute refractory period by strong stimulus
   d) Relative refractory period by strong stimulus

73. Action potential generally occurs in
   a) Dendrite b) Cell body
   c) Axon d) All of the above

74. The pumping of the ventricle pushes blood into the pulmonary artery is due to
   a) Ventricular diastole b) Ventricular systole
   c) Atrial diastole d) Atrial systole

75. Which of the following part of brain regulates breathing, heart rate and blood pressure of mammal
   a) Hypothalamus b) Medulla oblongata
   c) Pons d) Cerebellum

76. HCO_3^- is moved out of the red blood cells by
   a) Chloride shift b) H^+/HCO_3^- antiporter
   c) Na^+-HCO_3^- symporter d) H^+/HCO_3^- symporter

77. If we increase the P_{50} then
   a) Oxygen affinity decreases with hemoglobin
   b) Oxygen affinity increases with hemoglobin
   c) Oxygen not available for tissues
   d) Oxygen transport is not affected

78. Animals have thermoreceptors that monitor internal and environmental temperature, they are located in
   a) Hypothalamus b) Cerebrum
   c) Cerebellum d) Medulla oblongata

79. Salt glands are present in
   a) Uricoteles b) Ammonioteles
   c) Ureoteles d) Both (a) and (b)

80. In the urea cycle, urea is formed from
   a) Glutamine b) Citrulline
   c) Ornithine d) Arginine

81. Ventral nerve cord and tubular heart is present in
   a) Annelida and arthropoda b) Annelida and mollusca
   c) Arthropoda and mollusca d) Coelentreta and mollusca

82. Which statement about angiotensin is true?
   a) It is released by the posterior pituitory when blood pressure falls
   b) It stimulates thirst
   c) It increases the permeability of the collecting ducts to water
   d) It decreases glomerular filteration rate when blood pressure rises

83. Which of the following neurotransmitter act as a major inhibitory neurotransmitter
   a) Acetylcholine b) Glutamate
   c) Glycine d) All of the above

84. Epinephrine is secreted by
   a) anterior pituitory b) posterior pituitory
   c) Adrenal medulla d) Adrenal cortex

85. Which organ convert glucose into the polysaccharide glycogen
   a) Liver b) Muscle
   c) Adipose tissue d) Both (a) and (b)

86. Excretory organ in insects is
   a) Antennal organ b) Flame cells
   c) Protonephridia d) Malpighian tubule

87. The mechano-gated channels are found in
   a) membranes of retina
   b) stereocilia on the hair cells of the inner ear
   c) kidney
   d) muscle cells

88. Sperm motility develops within
   a) Vas deferens b) Seminal vesicles
   c) Epididymis d) Seminiferous tubules

89. The ion-channel responsible for the mechano-receptor response was identified by screenings for mutations in Drosophila. It is a member of transient receptor potential (TRP) channel family. Most stretch-activated channels are permeable to
   a) Na^+ b) Ca^{++}
   c) Cl^- d) Na^+ and K^+

90. The vertebrate eye focuses light into retinal rods and cones, and light entry is governed by
   iris b) pupil
   c) cornea d) Aqueous humor

91. Which of the following statement is incorrect for photoreceptor response to turn off?
   a) Phosphorylation of rhodopsin by rhodopsin kinase.

b) Release of arrestin protein from phosphorylated rhodopsin.
c) The phosphodiesterase (PDE) activity must be reinhibited to prevent further hydrolysis of cGMP.
d) The decreased Ca^{++} levels lead to disinhibition of guanylyl cyclase, allowing more rapid cGMP synthesis.

92. A shark's blood is isotonic to the surrounding sea water because of the reabsorption of
a) Ammonia b) Urea
c) Uric acid d) NaCl

93. Diureties are drugs that can be used to treat high blood pressure by increasing urinary output. Possible mechanisms of action in the kidney include
a) increasing ADH secretion.
b) inhibition of NaCl reabsorption from the loop of Henle or the proximal tubule.
c) increasing permeability of the collecting duct.
d) increasing NaCl reabsorption in the proximal tubule.

94. Caffine inhibits the secretion of ADH. What would happen if you take large coffee?
a) greater water reabsorption from the collecting duct.
b) less water reabsorption from the collecting duct.
c) an increase in reabsorption of glucose from the proximal convoluted tubule.
d) a decrease in reabsorption of glucose from the proximal convoluted tubule.

95. Which of the following is the correct sequence of events that controls the reabsorption of sodium ion when blood pressures falls?
1. Aldosterone is released.
2. Kidney tubules reabsorb Na^+
3. Renin is released
4. Juxtaglomerular apparatus recognizes a drop in blood pressure.
5. Angiotensin II is produced.
a) 1, 3, 5, 2, 4 b) 4, 2, 3, 1, 5
c) 4, 3, 5, 1, 2 d) 2, 4, 3, 1, 5

96. You are studying renal function in different species of mammals that are found in very different environments. You look at species from a desert environment and compare them with ones from a tropical environment. The desert species would be expected to have
a) shorter loops of henle that the tropical species
b) larger loops of henle than the tropical species.

c) shorter proximal convoluted tubule than the tropical species.
d) longer distal convoluted tubules than the tropical species.

97. Which of the following organ regulate the blood volume of the animal's body?
a) Heart
b) Kidney
c) Medula oblongata
d) Hypothalamus

98. Which of the following force determine net glomerular filtration pressure
a) Glomerular capillary hydrostatic pressure
b) Bowman's capsule hydrostatic pressure
c) Net oncotic pressure
d) All of the above

99. Excretory cells of Annelids are
a) Flame cells
b) Protonephridia
c) Metanephridia
d) Malpighian tubules

100. Which of the following enzyme is not used in ornithine-urea cycle?
a) Carbamoyl phosphate synthase-I (CPS-I)
b) CPS-II
c) CPS-III
d) Arginase

101. A person eat protein-rich diets, what would happen?
a) urea production rate increases
b) urea production rate decreases
c) no effect as urea production
d) person faces metabolic problem.

102. A capillary network that surrounds the loop of Henle, called
a) peritubular capillary
b) vasa recta
c) efferent arteriole
d) afferent arteriole

103. Which of the following restricts blood flow to specific vessels with in the capillary network, regulating blood pressure with in the glomerulus to control filteration?
a) podocyte
b) mesangial cells
c) foot processes
d) efferent arteriole

104. NH_4^+ secretion occurs at
a) proximal tubule
b) distal tubule
c) Loop of Henle
d) Collecting duct

105. Ectotherms
a) Cannot regulate their body temperatures.
b) Regulate their internal temperature using metabolic energy

c) Can regulate temperature using behavior.
d) Regulate temperature by dissipating but not generating heat.

106. Mammalian thermoregulation is controlled by
a) Medulla oblongata b) Cerebrum
c) Cerebellum d) Hypothalmus

107. Insulation is modulated by adjustments of the hair or feathers, under control of the sympathetic nervous system. In mammals, this response is termed
a) Pilomotor responses b) Ptilomotor responses
c) Vasomotor responses d) Postural responses

108. Cellulose is an an important nutrient for many animals, although most species require the help of symbiotic organisms which provides cellulase enzyme that is capable of breaking the cellulose by breaking
a) α-1, 4-glycosidic bond
b) α-1,6-glycosidic bond
c) β-1, 4 - glycosidic bond
d) α-,1,4 and β-1,4-glycosidic bond

109. During periods of high glucose concentrations in the lumen, glucose transport by facilitated diffusion is mediated by
a) SGLT - 1 b) GLUT - 5
c) GLUT - 2 d) GLUT - 1

110. Chylomicron is large lipoprotein complex that carries lipid from the digestive tract through the circulation to processing and target tissues. Lipids are absorbed in the
a) Stomach b) Small intestine
c) Cecum d) Large intestine

111. Antimicrobial molecules into the lumen is secreted by
a) Enterocytes b) Paneth cells
c) Goblet cells d) Interepithelial lymphocytes

112. Peristalsis is controlled by the intrinsic myogenic activity of the smooth muscle cells, but also influenced by pacemaker cells that is
a) Myenteric plexus b) Interstitial cell of Cajal
c) Meissner's plexus d) All of the above

113. How is the digestion of fats different from that of proteins and carbohydrates?
a) Fat digestion occurs in the small intestine, and the digestion of proteins and carbohydrates occurs in the stomach.
b) Fats are absorbed into cells as fatty acids and monoglycerides but are then modified for absorption; amino acids and glucose are not modified further.

c) Fats enter the hepatic portal circulation, but digested proteins and carbohydrates enter the lymphatic system.
b) Digested fats are absorbed in the large intestine, and digested proteins and carbohydrates are absorbed in the small intestine.

114. After being absorbed through the intestinal mucosa, glucose and amino acids are
a) Absorbed directly into the systemic circulation.
b) Used to build glycogen and peptides before being released to the body cells.
c) Transported directly to the liver by the hepatic portal vein.
d) Further digested by bile before release into the circulation.

115. Insulin
a) Increases blood glucose level by the hydrolysis of glycogen.
b) Increases blood glucose level by stimulating glucagon production.
c) Decreases blood glucose level by forming glucagon.
d) Increase blood glucose level by promoting cellular uptake of glucose.

116. Which of the following is related with the extreme obesity in human?
a) Insulin b) Ghrelin
c) Neuropeptide Y d) Leptin

117. Orexins hormone is produced by
a) Liver b) Kidney
c) Hypothalamus d) Placenta of pregnant female mammal

118. Leptin is released by
a) Hypothalamus b) Base osteoblasts
c) White adipose tissue d) Brown adipose tissue

119. Which of the following is not correct for the stress response in mammals?
a) Mobilizing stored energy
b) Enhancing cardiovascular and respiratory functions.
c) Increasing alertness and cognition.
d) Increasing energy storage.

120. Which of the following is incorrect?
a) Antidiuretic hormone conserve water.
b) The rennin-angiotensin-aldosterone system conserve sodium.
c) Atrial natriuretic peptide promotes excretion of sodium and water.
d) Cl^- typically follows Na^+ actively.

121. Acromegaly is caused by
a) Excessive secretion of TSH

b) Excessive secretion of GH
c) Deficiency of GH
d) Deficiency of TSH

122. In humans fetal blood-hemoglobin molecule consists of
a) One α-globin and one β-globin
b) Two α-globin and two β-globin
c) One α-globin and are γ-globin
d) Two α-globin and two γ-globin

123. Which of the following is incorrect for hemerythrins?
a) Hemerythins do not contain heme.
b) They do contain iron and each O_2 binding site contain one iron atom.
c) Hemerythrins are colorless when deoxygenated but turn reddish-violet when oxygenated.
d) Hemerythrins occur in many brachiopods.

124. The respiratory pigment of Arthropods is
a) Chlorocruorins
b) Hemocyanins
c) Hemerythrins
d) Hemoglobin

125. Which of the following is incorrect for hemocyanin?
a) Hemocyanins are found in just two phyla-the arthropods and the molluscs.
b) Hemocyanins do not contain heme, iron, or porphyrin structures
c) Hemocyanins contain copper which bound directly to the protein
d) Each O_2-binding site of a hemocyanin contains four copper atoms.

126. Erythropoietin is a glycoprotein hormone, which accelerates erythropoiesis and it is released by
a) Posterior pituitary gland
b) Anterior pituitary gland
c) Kidney
d) Liver

127. Which of the following is correct for RBCs?
a) The RBCs of mammals are essentially devoid of cell organelles.
b) The RBCs of all other vertebrates and all the respiratory pigment containing blood cells of invertebrates are nucleated.
c) Erythropoietin is synthesized by secretory cells in the interstitial tissue located between nephron tubules in kidney.
d) All of the above.

128. Which of the following is correct for Bohr effect?
a) Oxygen affinity depends on the partial pressure of CO_2 and pH.
b) Affinity for O_2 decreases as blood pH decreases, the oxygen-equilibrium curve shifts to the right.

c) Affinity for O_2 decreases as the CO_2 partial pressure of the blood increases.
d) All of the above

129. Which of the following inorganic ions modulate the O_2 affinity to respiratory pigments in ruminant mammals?
a) Ca^{++} b) Mg^{++}
c) Cl^- d) HCO_3^-

130. The carbon dioxide equilibrium curve of an animal's blood commonly changes with the state of oxygenation of the respiratory pigment in the blood; this phenomenon is named as
a) The root effect b) The Bohr effect
c) The Haldane effect d) The thermal effect

131. The liver produces most of the plasma proteins. Which of the following protein serve as carriers of lipid and steroid hormones?
a) Globulins b) Albumin
c) Fibrinogen d) All of the above

132. Platelets are cell fragments that are pinched off from larger cells in the bone marrow. The cells which form platelets are
a) Promyelyocytes b) Megakaryocyte
c) Proerythroblast d) Monoblast

133. Which of the following hormone play important role in the negative regulation of blood volume?
a) Anti diuretic hormone b) Aldosterone
c) Atrial natriuretic hormone d) Nitric oxide

134. Electrocardiograms (ECG) are measurements over time of voltage difference of the cardiac muscle cell of atrium and ventricle. The repolarization of ventricles generates
a) P-wave b) Q-wave
c) R- wave d) T- wave

135. The highest pressure attained at the time of cardiac contraction is termed
a) The systolic pressure b) The diastolic pressure
c) The mean pressure d) Arterial pressure

136. Contraction of the smooth muscle layers of the arterioles
a) increases the frictional resistance to blood flow.
b) May be a way of increasing heat exchange through the skin.
c) Can increase blood flow to an organ
d) All of the above

137. In vertebrate hearts, atria contracts from the top, and ventricles contract from the bottom. How is this accomplished?
   a) Depolarization from the SA node proceeds across the atria from the top; depolarization from the AV node is carried to the bottom of the ventricles before it emanates over ventricular tissue.
   b) The depolarization from the SA node is initiated from motor neurons coming down from our brain; depolarization from the AV node is initiated from motor meurons coming up from our spinal cord.
   c) Gravity carries the depolarization from the SA node down from the top of the heart; contraction of the diaphragm forces depolarication from the AV node from the bottom up.
   d) This statement is false; both contract from the bottom.

138. The difference between the amphibian and mammal hearts is that
   a) In the amphibian heart, oxygenated and deoxygenated blood mix compeletely in the single ventricle.
   b) In the amphibian heart, there are two SA nodes so that contractions occurs simultaneously throughout the heart.
   c) In the ventricle in the amphibian heart, internal channels reduce mixing of blood.
   d) In the amphibian heart, only the left aorta pumps oxygen obtained by diffusion through the skin.

139. An ECG measures
   a) Changes in electrical potential during the cardiac cycle.
   b) Ca++ concentration of the ventricles in diastole.
   c) The force of contraction of the atria during systole.
   d) The volume of blood being pumped during the contraction cycle.

140. Systole is vitally important to heart function and begins in the heart with the
   a) Activation of the AV node.
   b) Activation of the SA node.
   c) Opening of the voltage gated potassium channel
   d) Opening of the semilunar valves.

141. The lymphatic system is like the circulatory system in that they both
   a) Have nodes that fitter out pathogens.
   b) Have a network of arteries.
   c) Have capillaries.
   d) Are closed systems.

142. The fish heart consists of four chambers arranged in series. The main propulsive force is developed by
   a) Sinus venosus
   b) Atrium

c) Ventricle
d) Conus/Bulbus arteriosus.

143. The heart of *Protopterus* (lung fish) is very different from that of most fish in
   a) The atrium and ventricle are partly divided into right and left halves by septa.
   b) The conus arteriosus possesses two longitudinal ridges that project toward each other from opposite sites of its lumen, partially dividing the lumen into two channels.
   c) The four pairs of afferent branchial arteries arise immediately from the anterior end of the conus arteriosus
   d) All of the above

144. Which of the following animal have closed circulatory system?
   a) Octopus
   b) Crayfish
   c) Lobsters
   d) Crabs

145. In adult decapod crustaceans blood enters the heart not through vessels, but through slits in the heart wall, called
   a) Lacunae
   b) Sinuses
   c) Pericardial sinus
   d) Ostia

146. Fick's law of diffusion states the rate of diffusion is directly proportional to
   a) The area differences between the cross section of the blood vessel and the tissue.
   b) The pressure differences between the two sides of the membrane and area over which the diffusion occurs.
   c) The pressure differences between the inside of the organism and the outside.
   d) The temperature of the gas molecule.

147. Cutaneous respiration requires
   a) Moist and highly vascularized skin
   b) The absence of gills and lungs
   c) An environment rich in oxygen.
   d) Low temperatures

148. In Arthropods, respiratory organ is
   a) Spiracles
   b) Tracheae
   c) Operculum
   d) Branchial chambers

149. In mammal, during inhalation, the thoracic volume is increased through
   a) Contraction of the external intercostal muscles.
   b) Relaxation of diaphragm.
   c) Relaxation of the external intercostal muscle.
   d) Both b and c.

150. Respiration is controlled by the respiratory control center present in
   a) Cerebellum
   b) Medulla oblongata
   c) Pons
   d) Cerebrum

151. A rise in Pco2 causes
   a) An increased production of carbonic acid.
   b) Lowers the blood pH
   c) The stimulation of increased breathing
   d) All of the above

152. Hyperventilation occurs
   a) As a result of breathing rapidly.
   b) When oxygen levels become low.
   c) When tidal volume are unusually low.
   d) When the partial pressure of carbon dioxide is low.

153. In mammalian ear, the sounds are detected by
   a) Cochlea
   b) Organ of carti
   c) Hair cells
   d) Basilar membrane

154. Podocyte is a specialized epithelial cell present in the
   a) Liver
   b) Kidney
   c) Intestinal inner wall
   d) Pancreas

155. Nephron is a functional unit of kidney. Which of the following have mammalian-type nephorns?
   a) Amphibia
   b) Reptiles
   c) Birds
   d) All of the above

156. Green glands are present in
   a) Decapod crustaceans
   b) Pisces
   c) Amphibia
   d) Reptiles

157. A complex multi-ionic equilibrium state that tends to be reached by the interacting diffusion of multiple permeating ions and water across a cell membrane when there is a set of nonpermeating ions that are more abundant an one side than on the other, is called.
   a) Electrochemical equilibrium
   b) Electrical gradient
   c) Donnan equilibrium
   d) Concentration gradient

158. Which of the following transporter mediates the secondary active transport of glucose across the apical membrane?
   a) GLUT-2
   b) GLUT-5
   c) SGLT-1
   d) GLUT-7

159. Which of the following is correct for the peak of an action potential?
   a) Na^+ channels open and K^+ channels close
   b) Na^+ channels close and K^+ channels close
   c) Na^+ channels close and K^+ channels open
   d) Na^+ channels open and K^+ channels open

160. Electrical synapses send signals
   a) through synaptic clefts
   b) through gap junctions
   c) using neurotransmitters
   d) All of the above

161. The "all or none" law in regard to action potentials means
   a) all refractory periods are absolute
   b) refractory periods determine the direction of the propagation of an action potential
   c) a stronger triggering event results in a larger action potential
   d) once triggered, an action potential always goes to a maximal height

162. In the peripheral nervous system (PNS) of vertebrates
   a) the afferent division carries information from the CNS
   b) the afferent division carries information to the CNS
   c) the afferent division carries information to effector organs
   d) the afferent division carries information to sensory organs

163. The widely prescribed drug Prozac acts as an antidepressant, because it
   a) blocks the reuptake of transporters for released dopamine
   b) supplements low levels of norepinephrine
   c) prolongs the activity of serotonin
   d) binds dopamine

164. Long-term memory storage involves
   a) CREB and CREB2
   b) activation of specific genes
   c) formation of new synaptic connections
   d) All of the above

165. Which of the following vertebrate brain structures has changed least over evolutionary time?
   a) cerebrum
   b) cerebral cortex
   c) brain stem
   d) fore brain and diencephalon

166. The ability to adjust strength of the lens so that both near and far light sources can be focused on the retina is known as
   a) refraction
   b) photo transduction
   c) light adaptation
   d) accommodation

167. In our ear, which structure encounters sound waves first?
   a) the organ of corti   b) the incus
   c) the oval window   d) the tympanum

168. Which of the following would lead to the perception of a salty taste?
   a) Citric acid   b) Na^+
   c) K^+ d) Glutamate

169. Which of the following is a part of the vertebrate brain that is important in establishing biological rhythms?
   a) Pineal gland   b) Sinus glands
   c) Pituitary gland   d) Hypothalamus

170. The dominant hormones responsible for glucose homeostasis are
   a) Cortisol and corticosterone
   b) Insulin and glucagon
   c) Epinephrine and thyroid hormone
   d) None of the above

171. Which of the following methods of initiating action potentials is used by cardiac muscle?
   a) Receptor potential   b) Slow-wave potential
   c) Summation of EPSPs   d) Pacemaker potential

172. Which of the following ions play a major role in cardiac muscle physiology?
   a) Ca^{++}, Cl^- and K^+ b) Ca^{++}, Na^+ and Mg^{++}
   c) Ca^{++}, Na^+ and K^+ d) Na^+, Ca^{++} and I^+

173. Blood clots are slowly dissolved by
   a) Plasminogen   b) PDGF
   c) Hageman factor   d) Plasmin

174. In the mammalian cardiac cycle, stroke volume
   a) is also known as end-systolic volume
   b) is also known as end-diastolic volume
   c) causes rupturing of vessels
   d) is equal to end-diastolic volume minus end-systolic volume

175. The Frank-starling law of the heart states that
   a) increased venous return results in decreased stroke volume
   b) increased venous return results in increased stroke volume
   c) stroke volume is determined by sympathetic activity
   d) stroke volume always exceeds venous retum volume

176. Antimicrobial peptides are
   a) found only in vertebrates b) found only in plants
   c) found only in insects d) found in plants and animals

177. For hemoglobin (Hb) a high P50 value
   a) means that the Hb has a high affinity for O2
   b) makes it more difficult to unload O2 at tissues
   c) means that the Hb has a reduced affinity for O2
   d) would likely be found in species adapted to living at high altitudes

178. Which of the following hormone is secreted by epithelial cells in the stomach when it is empty?
   a) Cholecystokinin b) Ghrelin
   c) Gastric inhibitory peptide d) PYY3-36

179. In mammals interleukin -1 (IL-1)
   a) acts on the thermoregulatory center to lower the setting of the thermostat
   b) helps the body maintain normal temperature
   c) raises the lower critical temperature
   d) acts on the thermoregulatory center to raise the setting of the thermostat

180. A range of environmental temperatures in which the animal does not need to expend significant energy for thermoregulation is called
   a) critical temperature zone b) lower critical temperature
   c) thermoneutral zone d) upper critical temperature

181. In a normal human eye, for sharp image formation on the retina, maximum dioptric power is provided by the
   a) retina
   b) cornea
   c) anterior surface of the lens
   d) posterior surface of the lens

[CSIR (NET/JRF) Exam. Dec. 2011]

182. Which of the following waves is likely to be absent in a normal frog ECG?
   a) P b) Q
   c) T d) R

[CSIR (NET/JRF) Exam. Dec. 2011]

183. In this flow diagram name the chemicals A, B, C and D in proper sequence.
   a) Renin, Angiotensin II, Angiotensin I, Angiotensinogen
   b) Angiotensin I, Angiotensinogen, Angiotensin II, Renin
   c) Renin, Angiotensin I, Angiotensin II, Angiotensinogen
   d) Renin, Angiotensinogen, Angiotensin I, Angiotensin II

[CSIR (NET/JRF) Exam. Dec. 2011]

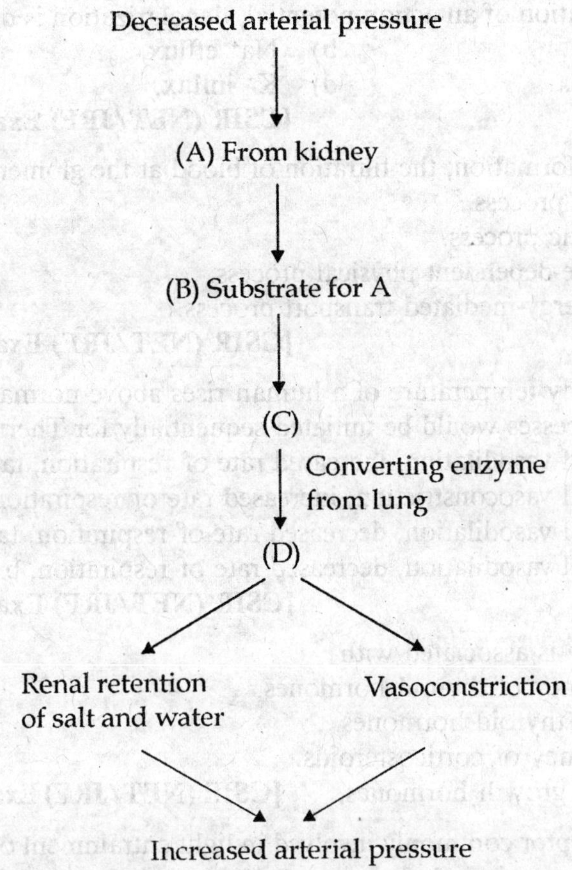

184. Stercobilin is the major pigment of
   a) Urine b) Blood
   c) Faeces d) Lymph

185. Hemoglobin is a better long-distance oxygen transporter than myoglobin because
   a) It has quaternary structure.
   b) It can bind four oxygen molecule.
   c) It has the ability to change its affinity for oxygen under different conditions.
   d) It can circulate very easily in blood vessels.

186. Polar bears maintain their body temperature because they have more of
   a) transducin protein. b) uncoupling protein.
   c) myoglobin protein. d) F_0F_1 ATPase.

[CSIR (NET/JRF) Exam. June 2011]

187. During generation of an action potential, depolarization is due to
   a) K^+ efflux. b) Na^+ efflux.
   c) Na^+ influx. d) K^+ influx.

[CSIR (NET/JRF) Exam. June 2011]

188. During urine formation, the filtration of blood at the glomerulus is
   a) an active process.
   b) an osmotic process.
   c) a pressure-dependent physical process.
   d) a non energy-mediated transport process.

[CSIR (NET/JRF) Exam. June 2011]

189. If the core body temperature of a human rises above normal, which of the following processes would be initiated sequentially for Thermo-regulation?
   a) Peripheral vasodilation, increased rate of respiration, tachycardia.
   b) Peripheral vasoconstriction, increased rate of respiration, bradycardia.
   c) Peripheral vasodilation, decreased rate of respiration, tachycardia.
   d) Peripheral vasodilation, decreased rate of respiration, bradycardia.

[CSIR (NET/JRF) Exam. June 2011]

190. Graves disease is associated with
   a) insufficiency of thyroid hormones.
   b) excess of thyroid hormones.
   c) insufficiency of corticosteroids.
   d) excess of growth hormones. **[CSIR (NET/JRF) Exam. June 2011]**

191. The photoreceptor commonly involved in light entrainment of the biological clock in flies, moulds and plants is
   a) phytochome. b) rhodopsin
   c) carotenoid. d) cryptochrome

[CSIR (NET/JRF) Exam. June 2011]

192. Name the ectothermic animal that can thermoregulate by behavioral means rather than by physiological means.
   a) Bumble bee in an orchard. b) Tuna fish in the Ocean.
   c) Lizard in a desert. d) Flatworm in a pond.

[CSIR (NET/JRF) Exam. June 2011]

193. Animal that generate much heat internally and have good thermal insulation are called
   a) Endotherms b) Ectotherms
   c) Ect-endotherms d) Isotherms

194. Which of the following groups of poikilothermic animals have members showing endothermy?

a) Mammals
b) Aves
c) Reptiles
d) Amphibia

195. Which pump is responsible for initiating muscle contraction through depolarization of muscle cell membrane?

a) Na^+ pump.
b) K^+ pump.
c) Ca^{2+} pump.
d) Mg^{2+} pump.

[CSIR Model Paper 2011]

196. Unidirectional propagation of electrical signal in nervous system is

a) proportional to the length of axon.
b) due to chemical synapse.
c) due to electrical synapse.
d) proportional to myelination.

[CSIR Model Paper 2011]

197. A myasthenia gravis patient develops muscle paralysis because

a) the nerve terminal at the neuromuscular junction fails to release acetylcholine.
b) although enough acetylcholine is released at the neuromuscular junction, it is destroyed by acetylcholinesterase.
c) the patient develops immunity against his own acetylcholine receptor.
d) the patient develops antibody against his own acetylcholine.

[CSIR Model Paper 2011]

198. Inhibin from sertoli cells of testes selectively inhibits

a) luteinizing hormone.
b) follicle stimulating hormone.
c) thyroid stimulating hormone.
d) growth hormone.

[CSIR Model Paper 2011]

199. Hawk's retina possesses a large number of

a) rods.
b) melanocytes.
c) cones.
d) kuffer cells.

[CSIR Model Paper 2011]

200. If a man is lacking hearing capacity. Which part of the brain is probably affected?

a) Cerebrum
b) Cerebellum
c) Hypothalamus
d) Spinal cord

201. If a person is unablc to write properly which part of the brain is most probably abnormal?
a) Cerebellum
b) Cerebrum
c) Medula oblongata
d) Frontal lobe

202. Ganglionic nervous system is found in
a) Cockroach
b) Reptiles
c) Birds
d) Monkey

203. Which of the following is the result of damage of myelin sheath?
a) Brain tumor
b) Meningitis
c) Tay sach's disease
d) Multiple sclèrosis

204. Outer most covering of human brain is
a) Arachnoid
b) Piamater
c) Duramater
d) Choroid

205. Which of the following is the centre of reflex action?
a) Peripheral nervous system
b) Medula
c) Spinal cord
d) None of the above

206. The hormone erythropoietin which is involved in erythrocyte formation is produced by
a) Liver
b) Poserior pituitary gland
c) Kidney
d) Pancreas

207. In ECG depolarization of ventricles is represented by
a) P wave
b) T wave
c) S wave
d) Q R S complex

208. Which of the following is **NOT** a true fish?
a) Cat fish
b) Rat fish
d) Saw fish
d) Cuttle fish

209. Peacock worm belongs to the class
a) Arachnida
b) Insecta
c) Polycheta
d) Nematoda

Part C

1. Which of the following is incorrect for conduction speed of action potential
   a) Myelination and increasing the diameter of axon increases the speed of action potential.
   b) High membrane resistance resulting in greater dissipation of the axonal current with distance.
   c) When the length constant is large, the change in membrane potential degrades less with distance.
   d) A neuron that uses only electronic current flow would transmit signals very rapidly.

2. ADH is believed to control the permeability of the amphibian distal convoluted tubule to water by controlling the insertion and retrieval of aquaporin proteins in cell membranes in parts of the tubular epithelium.
   When the level of ADH is high:
   A) Aquaparins are retrieved from the cell membranes, and osmosis through the epithelium is impeded.
   B) Permeability of the wall of the distal convoluted to water is low.
   C) The wall of the late distal convoluted tubule to become relatively permeable to water.
   D) Aquaporins are inserted into the cell membranes, and water can pass through the epithelium relatively readily by osmosis.

   Which of the following combination is true?

   a) A and B b) A and C
   c) B and D d) C and D

3. If an amphibian experiences excess water influx as can occur during immersion in fresh water:
   A) Secretion of ADH is reduced and the glomerulus filteration rate is relatively high.
   B) Secretion of ADH is increased and the GFR is relatively decreases.
   C) Distal tubule reabsorption of water is relatively low, and a voluminous, dilute urine results.
   D) An increase in NaCl reabsorption.

   Which of the following combination is correct?

   a) A, C and D b) Only A
   c) Only B d) A and C

4. Fish eating cone snails incapicitate their prey in part using toxins that block the channels. One of the most potent of a cone snail's conotoxins is α-conotoxins, which specifically binds to the receptor sites on muscle cell.

A) α-conotoxin blocks ligand-gated Na^+/K^+ channel.
B) α-conotoxin preventing the receptors from binding with or responding to acetylcholine.
C) α-conotoxin blocks the voltage-gated Na^+ ion channel.
D) α-conotoxin binds to the swimming muscle cells receptor and promptly blocked from responding to nervous stimulation and the fish becomes paralyzed.

Which of the following combination is correct?

a) A and B b) B and C
c) B, C and D d) A, B and D

5. An isolated carotid sinus was prepared so that the pressure may be regulated by a pump and the resulting discharge in single carotid sinus nerve fibre could be recorded. The following are the possible observations.
   A. No discharge when carotid sinus perfusion pressure was below 30mm Hg.
   B. Linear increase in discharge frequency when carotid sinus perfusion pressure was gradually increased from 70 to 110 mm Hg.
   C. Increase in discharge frequency was more prominent in greater pulsatile changes of carotid sinus pressure keeping the mean pressure identical in all cases.
   D. Increase in discharge was more prominent in the falling phase of pulsatile change of carotid sinus pressure than in the rising phase.

   Which one of the following is correct?

   a) A, B and C b) A and C
   c) B and D d) D only

   [CSIR (NET/JRF) Exam. Dec. 2011]

6. For a normal heart, the time taken for atrial systole and diastole are As and Ad seconds, respectively, while the same for ventricular systole and diastole are Vs and Vd. Which one of the following equations is correct?

   a) $As + Ad = Vs + Vd$ b) $As + Ad < Vs + Vd$
   c) $As + Ad - Vs + Vd = 0$ d) $As + Ad > Vs + Vd$

   [CSIR (NET-JRF) Exam. Dec. 2011]

7. A nerve impulse or action potential is generated from transient changes in the permeability of the axon membrane to Na^+ and K^+ ions. The depolarization of the membrane beyond the threshold level leads to Na^+ flowing into the cell and a change in membrane potential to a positive value. The K^+ channel then opens allowing K^+ to flow outwards ultimately restoring membrane potential to the resting value. The Na^+ and K^+ channels operate in opposite directions because

a) there is an electrochemical gradient growth generated by proton transport
b) there is a difference in Na^+ and K^+ concentrations on either side of the membrane
c) Na^+ is a voltage-gated channel, whereas K^+ is ligand-gated
d) Na^+ is dependent on ATP whereas K^+ is not

[CSIR (NET/JRF) Exam. Dec. 2011]

8. A monkey undergoes cerebellectomy. After the post-operative recovery, the monkey was given a task to press a bar. The possible observations are:
   A. Its hand would overshoot the target while reaching the bar.
   B. It would be unable to move forelimbs.
   C. It would show intention tremor while trying to press the bar.
   D. It would press the bar with mouth instead of hand.

   Which one of the following is correct?

   a) A and C b) B only
   c) D only d) B and D

[CSIR (NET/JRF) Exam. Dec. 2011]

9. During the spanish conquest of the Inca Empire at the high altitude in Peru, many soldiers fell sick. It was found that the sickness was due to low partial pressure of O_2 in the atmosphere at that altitude. To determine the reason, blood was collected from those patients. The circulating erythropoietin (EPO) level were estimated and the O_2-dissociation curve of haemoglobin were drawn and compared with the same in native people as depicted below.

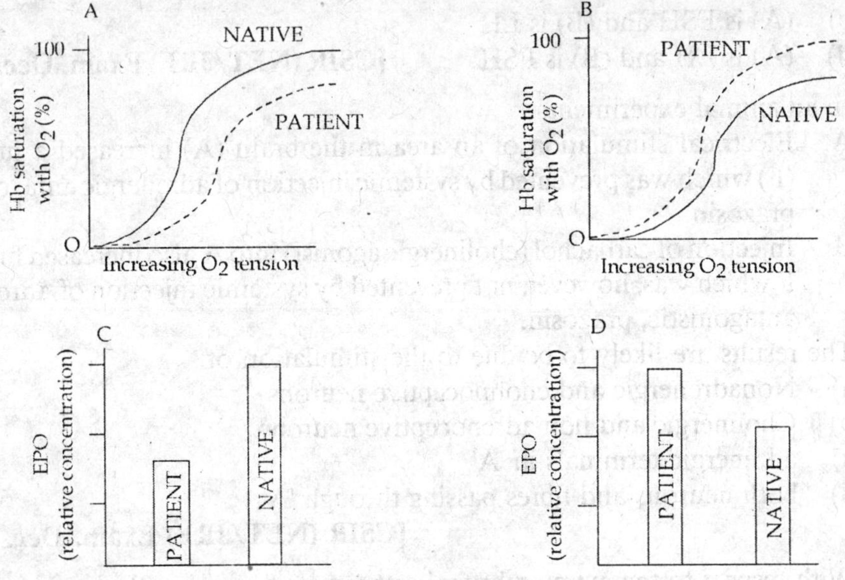

Which one of the following combinations is logically correct?

a) A and C
b) A and D
c) B and C
d) B and D

[CSIR (NET/JRF) Exam. Dec. 2011]

10. The graph represents relative plasma concentration of hormones (A and B) during reproductive cycle in a normal female. Which one of the following

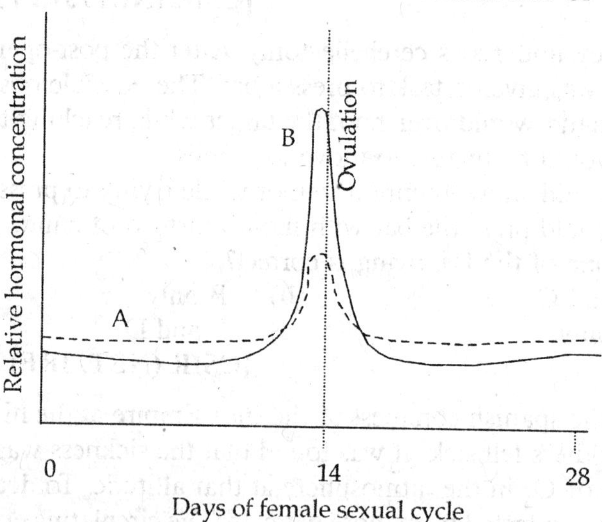

combinations is correct?

a) (A) is FSH and (B) is estrogen
b) (A) is estrogen and (B) is LH
c) (A) is FSH and (B) is LH
d) (A) is LH and (B) is FSH

[CSIR (NET/JRF) Exam. Dec. 2011]

11. In an animal experiment;

A. Electrical stimulation of an area in the brain (A) increased a function (F) which was prevented by systemic injection of adrenergic antagonistic, prazosin.

B. Injection of carbachol (cholinergic agonist) into A also increased function F which was, however, not prevented by systemic injection of adrenergic antagonistic, prazosin.

The results are likely to be due to the stimulation of

a) Nonadrenergic and cholinoceptive neurons.
b) Cholinergic and non-adrenoceptive neurons.
c) adrenergic terminals in 'A'.
d) both neurons and fibres passing through 'A'.

[CSIR (NET/JRF) Exam. Dec. 2011]

12. With respect to the extra embryonic structures formed in the mammals, the

possible functional attributes have been designated:

A. Allantoin stores urinary waste and helps mediate gas exchange. It is derived from splanchnopleure at caudal end of the primitive streak.

B. Amnion is a water sac and protects the embryo and its surrounding amniotic fluid. This epithelium is derived from somatopleure.

C. Chorion is essential for gas exchange in amniote embryos. It is generated from the splanchnopleure.

D. Yolk sac is the last embryonic membrane to form and is derived from somatopleure.

Which of the above statements are correct?

a) A and B b) A and C
c) B and C d) A and D

[CSIR (NET/JRF) Exam. Dec. 2011]

13. From among the five animals listed below, match the two attributes-amniotic egg and endothermy, with the correct animal(s):

A. Fish B. Frog
C. Crocodile D. Pigeon
E. Zebra

a) Amniotic egg : B, C, D; Endothermy : D, E
b) Amniotic egg : C, D, E; Endothermy : D, E
c) Amniotic egg : A,B, C, D; Endothermy : C, D, E
d) Amniotic egg : B, C, D; Endothermy : C, D, E

[CSIR (NET/JRF) Exam. Dec. 2011]

14. An organism having heart for circulation, excretes through green glands. It has several ganglia and tactile organs on its body and its larval form is very different that its adult form. This organism is most likely to respire by:

A. exchanging oxygen and carbon dioxide through an extensive tracheal system.

B. gaseous exchange over thinner areas of cuticle or by gills.

C. an efficient tracheal system that delivers oxygen directly to the tissues.

D. a double transport system, where the circulating fluid contains a dissolved respiratory pigment.

Choose the correct option.

a) A and C b) Only D
c) Only B d) B and D

[CSIR (NET/JRF) Exam. June 2011]

15. Spinal cord of an animal was transected at C1/C2 level. The respiration of the animal stopped and it needed artificial respiration. However, the heart continued to beat although at a slower rate. Some of the explanations given

were:

A. respiration regulatory centre is located in the medulla.
B. respiration regulatory centre is located above the C1/C2 cut.
C. heart regulatory centre is above the C1/C2 cut.
D. heart has autoregulation.

Which one of the following is most appropriate?

a) A only b) B and C only
c) A, B and D only d) B, C and D only.

[CSIR (NET/JRF) Exam. June 2011]

16. In a stressful condition, ACTH secretion was increased and as a result glucocorticoid concentration was elevated in blood. One or a combination of the following changes most likely taking place in this condition:

A. Decreased circulating eosinophils and basophils.
B. Reduced IL2 release.
C. Potentiated inflammatory response to tissue injury.
D. Increased mitotic activity of lymphocytes in lymph nodes.

The correct answer is

a) B and C. b) A and B
c) B and D d) C and D

[CSIR (NET/JRF) Exam. June 2011]

17. Which one of the following graphs represents a normal sexual cycle in a normal human female?

— estrogen
-- progestrone

a)

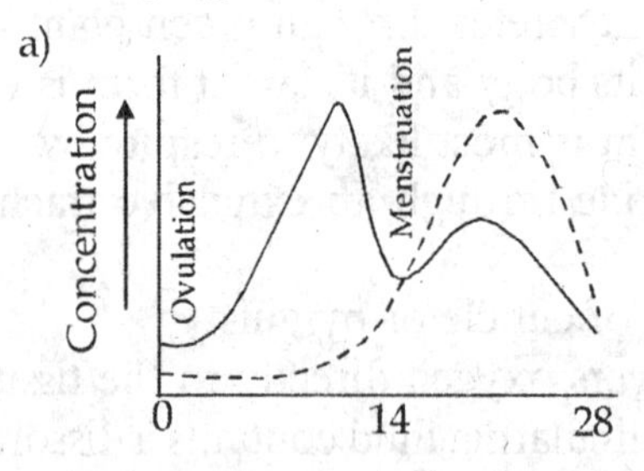

b)

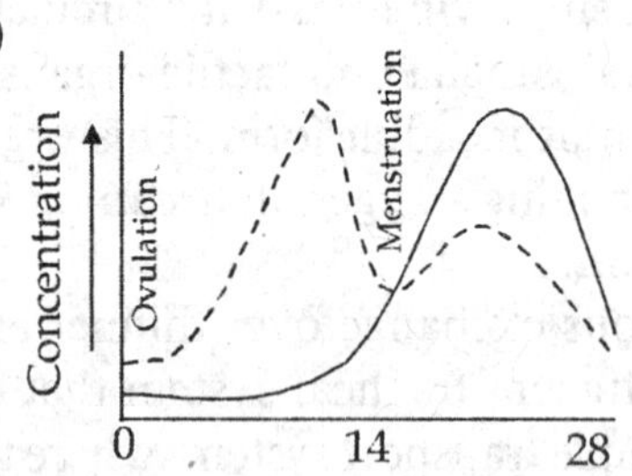

c)

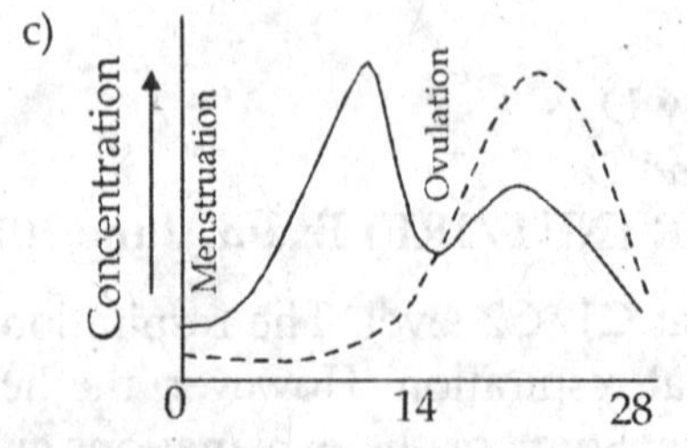

d)

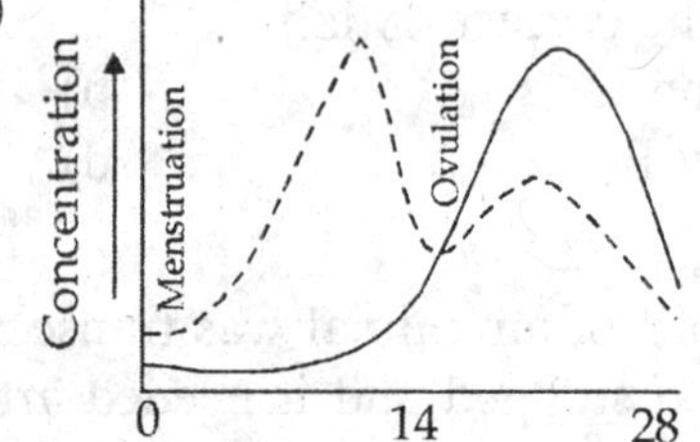

[CSIR (NET/JRF) Exam. June 2011]

18. The time taken for atrial systole and diastole in a normal heart are tas and tad seconds, respectively. If ventricular systole takes tvs seconds, calculate the ventricular diastolic time (seconds).
    a) (tas + tad) - tvs b) (tas - tad) + tvs
    c) (tad - tas) - tvs d) (tas + tad) × tvs

[CSIR (NET/JRF) Exam. June 2011]

19. Carbon dioxide can be carried in the blood as dissolved CO2 as HCO3-, or bound to proteins such as hemoglobin. Following statements are related with CO_2 transportation.
    A. Blood CO_2, HCO_3^-, and pH are interrelated via the carbonic anhydrase equilibrium reaction.
    B. Blood oxygenation affects CO_2 transport by altering hemoglobin CO_2 binding.
    C. Blood oxygenation does not affects the blood pH.
    D. The majority of the CO_2 is transported via the hemoglobin protein.
    Which of the following statement is not correct?
    a) A and C b) D only
    c) C and D d) B and C

20. Kidney function is regulated at multiple levels. The following statements explain mechanism of kidney function.
    A. Glomerular filteration pressure is affected by the hydrostatic pressure and oncotic pressure gradients between the glomerulus and Bowman's capsule
    B. Vasopressin alters the permeability of the loop of Henle.
    C. Aldosterone regulates sodium and potassium balance.
    D. Atrial natriuretic peptide also plays a role in potassium balance.
    Which of the following combination is correct?
    a) A and B b) A and C
    c) A, C and D d) A, B and C

21. In most vertebrates, the nervous and endocrine systems can control heart rate by altering the rate of pacemaker potentials in the cells of the sinoatrial node or sinus venosus. The following statements are related to heart beat regulation
    A. Norepinephrine binds with b1 adrenergic receptors and activate cAMP mediated pathway that opens the Na^+ and Ca^{+2} channels and increasing the rate of depolarization of cell which ultimately increses heart rate.
    B. Epinephrine binds with b1 adrenergic receptors and activate cAMP mediated pathway which ultimately decreses heart rate.

C. Acetylcholine binds to muscarinic receptors (G-protein coupled receptors) on the pacemaker cells of the heart, and increases the K^+ permeability causing hyperpolarization of the cells which ultimately decreases heart rate.
D. The herbal supplement ephedra can bind to adrenergic receptors and cause a rapid heart rate.

Which of the following combination is correct?

a) A, B and C b) A, C and D
c) A, B and D d) B, C and D

22. The depolarization of cardiac muscles produce a strong electrical signal that travels through the body can be detected by electrocardiograph. This instrument is used electrodes applied to various areas on the surface of the body to generate an electrocardiogram. The following statements explain about electrocardiograph.

A. The small P wave is the result of the spread of depolarization through the atria.
B. The large QRS complex is the result of atrial repolarization.
C. The T wave is caused by ventricular repolrization.
D. The deflections on the chart are markers of the electrial activity of the heart as a whole.

Which of the following combination is correct?

a) A, B and C b) A, C and D
c) B, C and D d) A and C

23. Many animals can control the blood flow through their organs by changing the radius of the blood vessesl leading to those organs. During vasoconstriction

A. The radius of the blood vessel decreases
B. Resistance of the blood vessel increases
C. Reducing the flow through the blood vessel
D. Blood pressure of the vessel decreases

Which of the following combination is true

a) A and B b) A, B and C
c) B, C and D d) A, C and D

24. What would happen if the connection between the AV node and the bundle of His were blocked?

A. The depolarization spreads more slowly through the contractile cells of the atrium via gap junctions, causing the atrium contraction.
B. Contraction of ventricle is not possible
C. Purkinje fibres spreads the coming signal from AV node to the ventricular myocardium

D. The contraction of the ventricle begins at the bottom.

Which of the following combinations is correct?

a) A only b) B only
c) A, C and D d) C and D

25. During digestion, a large amout of H+ is secreted into the stomach, which results in the so called alkaline tide, a large metabolic alkalosis in which blood pH increse. What is the likely response of the respiratory system to this increased oxygen demand and pH disturbance?

A. Carbonic anhydrase reaction shifts to the right increasing [H+] and decreasing pH.
B. The carbonic anhydrase reaction shifts to the left and increase the pH.
C. Inducing the respiratory acidosis
D. Increased ventilation

Which of the following statement is correct?

a) A only b) B only
c) A, C and D d) B, C and D

26. A number of mammalian species, including human have colonized high altitude habitats. These poulation uses a different strategy for coping with high altitude. They have.

A. Barrel chested
B. Higher lung capacity
C. High hemoglobin levels
D. Reduced levels of 2, 3-DPG in their red blood cells

Which of the following combination is correct?

a) A and D b) C and D
c) Only D d) A, B, C and D

27. Polar bear lives in extremely cold condition and reduced the deleterious effects of temperature by changing the composition of their membranes. They possess:

A. Phospholipid with short chain fatty acids
B. High amout of unsaturate fatty acid in their plasma membrane
C. Phosphatidylcholine is more common in membranes of cold-acclimated animals.
D. Cholesterol tend to preven phospholipids from solidifying

Which of the following combination is correct?

a) A, B, C and D b) A, B and C
c) A, B and D d) B, C and D

28. Control of body temperature in endothermic animals requires coordination of multiple physiological systems. Animals must be able to monitor body temperature in critical anatomical neurons is received and interpreted by a

thermostat within central nervous system. The central thermostat triggers the appropriate behavioral and physiological response

A bird lives in a tundra region which of the following physiological or behaviour response they follow-

A. Regulate heat loss by changing the orientation of the hair or feathers.
B. Regulation of the amount of blood following into the vasculature.
C. Counter current exchangers in the vasculature
D. Increase ventilation frequency
E. Gular flattering behaviour

Which of the following combination is correct?

a) A, B and C
b) A, B, C and D
c) A, B and E
d) A, B, C and E

29. The glomerular membrane is more than 100 times more permeable than capillaries present elsewhere in the body. The basement membrane of glomerulus is composed of collagen and glycoproteins. The collagen provides structural strength and the glycoprotein discourage the filteration of small plasma protein. The glycoproteins are strongly negatively charged and it repels albumin and other plasma proteins, and are almost completely excluded from the filtrate.

If we disrupt the negative charges with in the glomerular membrane, then what would be the effect on protein filteration?

a) No effect on the protein filteration because plasma proteins consist of both positively and negatively charged proteins.
b) Highly permeable due to pore size increasement.
c) Membrane more permeable to albumin even though the size of the pores remains constant.
d) Membrane permeability does not depend on the protein charges.

30. The hormones that regulate molting have been intensively studied in the insects, and one of the most important is a steroid hormone called ecdysone. Ecdysone can stimulate an insect larvae to form a larger larva, a pupa, or an adult. Depending on the level of an additional hormone. Some statements are given below related to the ecdysone.

(A) Ecdysone is regulated by a neurohormone called prothoracicotropichormone (PTTH) produced by the insect brain.
(B) When juvenile hormone levels are high, ecdysone stimulates molting from one larval stage to another.
(C) When juvenile hormone levels are low, ecdysone triggers the formation of pupa.
(D) When juvenile hormone is absent, ecdysone triggers the emergence of the adult insect.

Which of the following combination is correct?

a) Aand B b) Aand C
c) A and D d) A, B, C and D

31. Most neurons have a resting membrane potential of approximately-70 mV, and it is maintained by the movement of the charged ions across the membrane. Some statements are given below about the membrane potential of nerve cell.
(A) Either positively charged ions entering the cell or negatively charged ions moving out of the cell, causing depolarization.
(B) Either negatively charged ions entering the cell or positively charged ions moving out of the cell, causing hyperpolarization.
(C) Stimulating Na^+, Ca^{+2} and Cl^- channels typically depolarizes the neuron cell.
(D) Stimulating K^+ channel typically hyperpolarizes the neuron cell.

Which of the following combination is correct?
a) Only A b) A and D
c) B, C and D d) A, B, C and D

32. Signaling in a vertebrate motor neuron depends on the charge of membrane potential of the cell. The following statements correlate nerve conduction via neurons.
(A) The neuron will fire an action potential in the axon only if the combination of all the graded potentials in the dendrites and cell body causes the axon hillock to depolarize beyond threshold.
(B) During the absolute refractory period, the axon is capable of generating a new action potential by very large stimulus.
(C) During the relative-refractory period, the axon is capable of generating a new action potential by normal stimulus.
(D) Voltage gated Na^+ channels prevent backward transmission of action potentials.

Which of the following combination is correct?
a) A and B b) A, B and D
c) A and D d) A, B and C

33. The current flow in the nerve cell is similar the current flow in capacitors? In the case of the cell membrane intracellular fluid and extracellular fluid are the conducting layers of the capacitor, while the phospholipids of the cell membrane are the insulating layers. Some statements are given below related to the current flow in a cell.
(A) When membrane resistance is high, current flow across the membrane will be low, and less charge will be lost.

(B) When membrane resistance is low, current flow across the membrane will be large, and more charge will be lost.
(C) When the length constant is large, the change in membrane potential degrades more with distance.
(D) When the length constant is small change in membrane potential degrades less with distance.
Which of the following combination is true?
a) A, B, C and D
b) A, B, and C
c) A, B and D
d) A and B

34. Signal conduction in nerve cells depends on the nature of the neurotransmitter. The following statements explain the mode of action of neurotransmitters
(A) Inhibitory neurotransmitter generally causes repolarization, making the post synaptic cell less likely to generate an action potential.
(B) Excitatory neurotransmitter generally causes depolarization making the post synaptic cell more likely to generate an action potential.
(C) Metabotropic receptors tend to cause slower-acting changes in the postsynaptic cell than ionotropic receptors.
(D) Acetylcholine receptors can be nicotinic receptor or muscarinic receptors.
Which of the following combination is correct?
a) A, B and C
b) B and C
c) B, C and D
d) A, B, C and D

35. Cardiac muscles use a process called Ca^{+2}-induced Ca^{+2} release to link dihydropyridine receptor (DHPR) and ryanodine receptor (RyR) activation. Once DHPR open, extracellular Ca^{+2} enters the cell, it triggers the opening of cardiac muscle RyR, and the sarcoplasmic reticulum Ca^{+2} stores are released into the muscle cytoplasm that induce contraction.
If cardiac muscle is bathed in Ca^{+2} free media, then what would happen?
a) Depolarization and activation of the DHPR induces a muscle contraction.
b) Depolarization and activation of the DHPR does not induce a muscle contraction.
c) Depolarization of DHPR is not possible.
d) Affects the storation of Ca^{+2} in sacrcoplasmic reticulum of cardiac muscle cell.

36. Mechanoreception is important for cell volume control, and the senses of touch, hearing and balance, and it plays a critical role in regulating blood pressure in the vertebrates. Mechanoreceptors are specialized cells or organs that can transform mechanical stimuli into electrical signals. The following statements are related to mechanoreceptors.
(A) Baroreceptors are interoceptors that detect pressure changes in the walls

of blood vessels.

(B) Tactile receptors are interoceptors that detect touch, pressure and vibration on the body surface.

(C) Proprioceptors monitor the position of the body and are found only in vertebrates.

Which of the following combination is true?

a) Only A b) A and B
c) A and C d) A, B and C

37. The G cells secrete the hormone gastrin into the blood in response to protein products in the stomach lumen. Gastrin stimulates the parietal cells and promoting secretion of HCl. Some explanation are given below related to the HCl secretion.

(A) The H^+ is secreted into the stomach lumen by H^+-K^+ ATPase.

(B) Cl^- is secreted passively to maintaining the concentration gradient of the parietal cells.

(C) Carbonic anhydrase activity is high in the parietal cells.

(D) Chloride shift is necessary process for the secretion of HCl by parietal cells.

Which of the following combination is correct?

a) A and B b) A, B and D
c) A, C and D d) A, B and C

38. Absorption is most important process for the survival of organism after digestion. Following statements related to the absorption of biomolecules are given below.

(A) Glucose and galactose are both absorbed by secondary active transport with Na^+ from the lumen.

(B) Amino acids are absorbed across the intestinal cells by secondary active transport.

(C) Monoglycerides and free fatty acids actively transfers from the micelle into the epithelial cells.

(D) Water soluble vitamin absorbed passively while the fat soluble vitamins absorbed actively in the epithelial cells of intestine.

Which of the following combination is correct?

a) A and B b) A, B and C
c) A, B and D d) A, B, C and D

39. The glial cells are not nerve cells, which serve as the connective tissue of the CNS and support physically and metabolically. Glial cells are four major types present in the CNS as astrocytes, oligodendrocytes, epenedymal cells and microglia. Some characteristic features of glial cells are given below.

(A) Astrocytes serve as a scaffold to guide neurons to their proper final destination during fetal brain development.

(B) Astrocytes induce the small blood vessels of the brain to establishment of blood-brain barrier.

(C) Microglia is the immune defense cells of the CNS, and it is maturated in bone marrow of the organism.

(D) Ependymal cells serve as neural stem cells with the potential of forming all glial cells and nerve cell also.

(E) Oligodendrocytes form the insulating myelin sheaths around axons in the axon, and abundant in white matter.

Which of the following combination is correct?

a) A, B and C b) B, D and E
c) A, B, C and D d) A, B, D and E

40. Which of the following is correct sequence of blood circulation?

a) Left auricle → Left ventricle → Pulmonary artery
b) Right auricle → Right ventricle → Carotic systemic aorta
c) Left auricle → Left ventricle → Pulmonary vein
d) Left auricle → Left ventricle → Carotic systemic aorta

Answer Sheet

Part – B

1.	b	2.	b	3.	d	4.	b	5.	c	6.	a
7.	c	8.	b	9.	c	10.	c	11.	c	12.	a
13.	c	14.	b	15.	b	16.	b	17.	c	18.	c
19.	c	20.	d	21.	a	22.	d	23.	c	24.	a
25.	c	26.	a	27.	a	28.	c	29.	b	30.	a
31.	b	32.	c	33.	b	34.	c	35.	b	36.	d
37.	d	38.	d	39.	d	40.	d	41.	d	42.	d
43.	b	44.	b	45.	c	46.	b	47.	b	48.	a
49.	d	50.	d	51.	a	52.	b	53.	b	54.	d
55.	b	56.	c	57.	d	58.	b	59.	c	60.	a
61.	b	62.	b	63.	d	64.	d	65.	b	66.	d
67.	d	68.	b	69.	c	70.	d	71.	c	72.	d
73.	c	74.	b	75.	b	76.	a	77.	a	78.	a
79.	a	80.	d	81.	a	82.	b	83.	c	84.	c
85.	d	86.	d	87.	b	88.	c	89.	d	90.	a
91.	b	92.	b	93.	b	94.	b	95.	c	96.	b
97.	b	98.	d	99.	c	100.	b	101.	a	102.	b
103.	b	104.	d	105.	c	106.	d	107.	a	108.	c
109.	c	110.	b	111.	b	112.	b	113.	b	114.	c
115.	c	116.	d	117.	c	118.	c	119.	d	120.	d
121.	b	122.	d	123.	b	124.	b	125.	d	126.	c
127.	d	128.	d	129.	c	130.	c	131.	a	132.	b
133.	c	134.	d	135.	a	136.	a	137.	a	138.	c
139.	a	140.	b	141.	c	142.	c	143.	d	144.	a
145.	d	146.	b	147.	a	148.	b	149.	a	150.	b
151.	d	152.	d	153.	c	154.	b	155.	c	156.	a
157.	c	158.	c	159.	c	160.	b	161.	d	162.	a
163.	c	164.	d	165.	c	166.	d	167.	d	168.	b
169.	d	170.	b	171.	d	172.	c	173.	d	174.	d
175.	b	176.	d	177.	c	178.	b	179.	d	180.	c
181.	d	182.	c	183.	d	184.	c	185.	c	186.	b
187.	c	188.	c	189.	d	190.	b	191.	d	192.	c
193.	a	194.	c	195.	c	196.	b	197.	c	198.	b
199.	c	200.	a	201.	a	202.	a	203.	d	204.	c
205.	c	206.	c	207.	d	208.	d	209.	c		

Part - C

1.	b	2.	d	3.	d	4.	d	5.	a	6.	a
7.	b	8.	b	9.	a	10.	c	11.	b	12.	a
13.	b	14.	c	15.	a	16.	b	17.	c	18.	a
19.	c	20.	b	21.	b	22.	b	23.	b	24.	b
25.	c	26.	d	27.	c	28.	a	29.	c	30.	d
31.	b	32.	c	33.	d	34.	c	35.	b	36.	a
37.	c	38.	a	39.	d	40.	d				

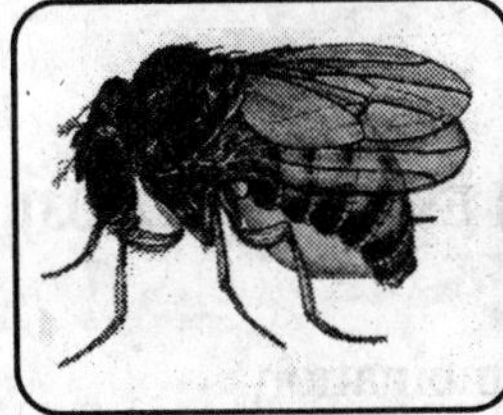

Chapter 8 Genetics

Part B

1. "Chromosome diminution" in somatic cells can be displayed by
   a) *Drosophila*
   b) Yeast
   c) *Ascaris*
   d) *Caenorhabditis elegans*

2. Balance of two X linked genes in Drosophila is achieved by
   a) Hyperactivation of paternal X chromosome
   b) Hypoactivation of paternal X chromosome
   c) Hyperactivation of maternal X chromosome
   d) Hypoactivation of maternal X chromosome

   [CSIR (NET/JRF) Exam. June 2005]

3. Crossing over is not found in
   a) Female *Drosophila*
   b) Male *Drosophila*
   c) Maize
   d) Evening primrose

4. Dicentric bridges are formed in
   a) Paracentric inversion
   b) Pericentric inversion
   c) Reciprocal translocation
   d) Terminal deletion

5. DNA fossils are
   a) Inactive transposons in human genome
   b) DNA extracted from fossils
   c) Very primitive sequences of DNA
   d) None of the above

6. Down's syndrome result in mental retardation in humans. This condition is characterized by having
   a) Trisomy for chromosome 21
   b) Monosomy for 21
   c) Trisomy for chromosome X
   d) Trisomy for chromosome 18

7. Holiday junctions are formed during
   a) Chromosomal aberration b) DNA replication
   c) Recombination d) DNA repair

[CSIR (NET/JRF) Exam. Dec. 2003]

8. Holiday structure is used to explain
   a) Gene transfer b) Homologous recombination
   c) Site specific recombination d) Nonhomologous recombination

9. How many linkage groups are found in human male
   a) 23 b) 22
   c) 24 d) 25

[CSIR (NET/JRF) Exam. Dec 2005]

10. Hybrid dysgenesis in Drosophila is caused by
    a) Copia element b) Gypsy element
    c) P-element d) None of the above

11. In Drosophila, sex is determined by the dosages of autosomes and sex-chromosomes. This means that sex determination in Drosophila males carrying only one X chromosome is based on
    a) Presence of Y-chromosome
    b) Hyper activation of the male X chromosome
    c) Balance of two sets of autosomes with a single X chromosome
    d) Balance of one set of autosomes with a single X chromosome

12. Individuals having Down's syndrome at older age show symptoms of
    a) Kuru disease b) Chronic schizophrenia
    c) Alzheimer's disease d) Adison's disease

13. Karyotype shows 45 chromosome appear normal male, due to
    a) Deletion b) Inversion
    c) Translocation d) Non disjunction

[CSIR (NET/JRF) Exam. June 2005]

14. Pattern of shell coiling in freshwater snails is an example of
    a) Mendelian inheritance b) Cytoplasmic inheritance
    c) Maternal effect d) Infectious inheritance

15. Pseudodominance is caused by
    a) Deletion b) Inversion
    c) Translocation d) Duplication

16. Pseudolinkage is caused by
    a) Translocation b) Deletion
    c) Inversion d) Duplication

17. The genetic event that results in Down's syndrome can be described as
    a) Non-reciprocal crossing over
    b) Non-disjunction
    c) Chromosomal duplication
    d) Uniparental disomy

18. The maximum frequency of recombination of genes at two loci is
    a) 25% b) 75%
    c) 50% d) 100%

19. The primary cause of aneuploidy in an organism is
    a) Pericentric inversion b) Translocation
    c) Non-disjunction d) Double fertilization

20. Transposons cause mutations in plants, animal and bacteria. These are
    a) Infective protein molecules b) Mutagenic viruses
    c) Retroviruses d) Mobile genetic elements

21. Which is crossing over suppressor?
    a) Deletion b) Translocation
    c) Inversion d) Duplication

22. Which of the following kind of chromosomal aberration may lead to independent assortment of linked genes?
    a) Duplication b) Deletion
    c) Inversion d) Translocation

23. Which of the following plays a vital role in determination of sex in Drosophila ?
    a) Trans splicing b) RNA editing
    c) Polyadenylation d) Alternative splicing

24. Which of the following statement is not correct for transposable elements?
    a) They were discovered in maize
    b) They create flanking repeats at their insertion site
    c) Sometimes they have terminal inverted repeats at both ends
    d) They are selfish DNA and have freezed the host genome evolutionarily

25. Which of the following statement is not true?
    a) Barr bodies are always found in somatic cells
    b) Dosage compensation in Drosophila is achieved by hyperproduction
    c) Dosage compensation in Drosophila is achieved by hypoproduction
    d) Male Drosophila has five linkage groups

26. Which of the following types of chromosomal aberration can change linkage pattern of genes?
    a) Inversion b) Translocation
    c) Duplication d) Deletion

27. Haploinsufficient gene may be resulted due to
    a) Deletions b) Inversion
    c) Translocation d) Duplication

28. Loss of both members of a homologous pair of chromosomes causes
    a) Monosomy b) Trisomy
    c) Tetrasomy d) Nullisomy

29. The pattern of genomic imprinting is maintained from one generation to another by
    a) Phosphorylation of DNA b) Methylation
    c) Acetylation d) Glycosylation

[CSIR (NET/JRF) Exam. June 2007]

30. When a genotype has the capacity to produce different phenotypes, suitable for different environmental conditions, the phenomen is called
    a) Phenocopy effect b) Genetic erosion
    c) Genotypic plasticity d) Phenotypic plasticity

31. Which of the following type of chromosomal aberrations can affect the independent assortment of alleles?
    a) Pericentric inversion b) Duplication
    c) Deletion d) Translocation

32. Tsix gene plays a vital role in
    a) Sex determination b) Genetic imprinting
    c) Dosage compensation d) Self-incompatibility

33. Barr bodies in somatic cells of mammalian females indicate that
    a) Mammalian females are XO
    b) One of their two X-chromosomes is genetically inactive
    c) They have an extra X chromosome
    d) Mammalian females are XX

34. Which of the following statement is not correct?
    a) *Sxl* gene is the master regulator of the sex determination pathway in *Drosophila*.
    b) In addition to regulating the sex determination pathway *Sxl* also regulates dosage compensation
    c) X/A ratio controls the expression of the Sxl gene
    d) *Sxl* is Y linked gene

35. Complementation test predicts
    a) Allelism b) Allelic exclusion
    c) Gene interaction d) Gene conversion

36. Crossing over is not found in
    a) Zebra fish b) *C. elegans*
    c) *Spirulina* d) Maize

37. During transposition transposons are excised by
    a) Nuclease b) Transposase
    c) Topoisomerase d) Exonuclease

38. For dosage compensation hypoactivation of X-linked genes occur in
    a) *Drosophila* b) Mammals
    c) *C. elegans* d) Zebra fish

39. If a genetic disorder occurs in males more often than females, it would be suspected to be
    a) Autosomal recessive b) Autosomal dominant
    c) Sex-linked recessive d) Y-linked

40. In *Drosophila* XO are male and XXY are female while in humans XX are female and XY are male. On the basis of given information which statement is not true?
    a) In *Drosophila* sex determination is based on number of X chromosome to sets of auto somes
    b) Y chromosome is Sex determinant in humans
    c) In humans sex determination is based on number of X chromosome to sets of autosomes
    d) Y chromosome do not play any role in sex determination of *Drosophila*

41. In mammals effective dosage of genes of two sexes is made equal by
    a) Elimination of X chromosome in females
    b) Hypoactivation of X chromosome in males
    c) Inactivation of X chromosome in females
    d) Hypoactivation of X chromosome in females

42. Linkage map is based on
    a) Segregation of alleles b) Interaction of alleles
    c) Recombination of alleles d) Interaction of genes

43. Lod score is used in
    a) Gene mapping b) Gene sequencing
    c) Gene manipulation d) Tetrad analysis

44. Major cause of evolution of genes and protein is
    a) Point mutation b) Chromosomal aberrations
    c) Sexual reproduction d) Gene duplication and divergence

45. Merozygotes are formed in
   a) Drosophila b) *Neurospora*
   c) Yeast d) Bacteria

46. Pseudoautosomal genes are those that are -
   a) Duplicated copies of autosomal genes
   b) Sex-linked
   c) Involved in sex determination
   d) Found on both X and Y chromosomes.

47. Sex chromosome-based dosage compensation in humans is brought about by
   a) Inactivation of one X-chromosome in females
   b) Hyperactivity of single X-chromosome in males
   c) Hyperactivation of both X-chromosomes in females
   d) Hyperactivation of autosomes in females

48. Sex determination in Drosophila is based on ratio of number of X chromosome to
   a) Number of autosomes b) Sets of total chromosomes
   c) Set of autosomes d) Sets of autosomes

49. SRY gene plays a vital role in sex determination in humans because
   a) It produces testosterone
   b) It forms receptor for TDF
   c) It produces mullerian inhibitory substance
   d) It produces TDF

50. The degree to which one cross over interferes with additional crossovers in the some region is termed
   a) Recombination frequency b) Interference
   c) Coefficient of coincidence d) None of the above

51. A plant of the genotype AaBb is selfed. The two genes are linked and are 50 map units apart. What proportion of the progeny will have the genotype aabb?
   a) ½ b) ¼
   c) 1/8 d) 1/16

[CSIR (NET/JRF) Exam. Dec. 2011]

52. The probability of a son to be colour blind for parent with colour blind father and normal homozygous mother would be
   a) 25% b) 75%
   c) 50% d) 0%

53. The somatic cell hybridization of human and mouse cell can effectively carried out by using
a) Dextron b) PEG
c) Enzymatic treatment d) Inactivated sendai virus

54. Two point test cross ratio is
a) 9:3:3:1 b) 1:1
c) 9:3:4 d) 1:1:1:1

55. Which of the following is not correctly matched?
a) Phenotypic and genotypic ratio equal : codominance
b) Genomic imprinting : monoallelic expression
c) Sequential hermaphrodism : honey bees
d) Operon : *C. elegans*

56. Which of the following statement is not correct?
a) Sex influenced traits are found on autosomes
b) Maternal effect genes are found in nucleus
c) Female *Drosophila* has five linkage groups
d) Any diploid individual can have only two alleles for a particular locus

57. Yeast with petite colony when crossed with wild type generates no petite colony. The most probable mode of inheritance is
a) Chloroplast b) Mitochondria
c) Episomal d) Nuclear

58. What kind of aneuploid gametes will be generated if meiotic non-disjunction occurs at first division? (n' represents the haploid number of chromosomes)
a) only n+1 and n b) only n-1 and n
c) both n+1 and n-1 d) either n+1 or n-1

[CSIR (NET/JRF) Exam. Dec. 2011]

59. Androgen receptor is located on
a) small arm of Y chromosome
b) large arm of Y chromosome
c) p arm of X chromosome
d) q arm of X chromosome

60. Diploid housefly has eight chromosomes. Which one of the following terms should NOT be used to describe housefly with sixteen number of chromosome?
a) Polyploid b) Aneuploid
c) Euploid d) Tetraploid

61. Corn growing in a field had a lysine content of 2.0%, with a variance of 0.16. When grown in the greenhouse under controlled and uniform conditions, the mean lysine content was again 2.0%, but the variance was 0.09. What measure of heritability can you calculate?
    a) 0.16
    b) 0.7
    c) 0.56
    d) 0.25

62. Criss-cross inheritance is shown by
    a) Sex linked traits
    b) Sex influenced traits
    c) Sex limited traits
    d) Autosomal traits

63. *Drosophila* with chromosome complements XXXY/AA would be
    a) Meta male
    b) Meta female
    c) Normal male
    d) Inter sex

64. When two mutants having the same phenotype were crossed, the progeny obtained showed a mutant-type phenotype. Thus the mutations are
    a) Non-allelic
    b) Allelic
    c) Segregating from each other
    d) Independently assorting

65. An animal has diploid chromosome number of 12. An egg cell of that animal has 5 chromosomes. The most probable explanation is
    a) Deletion of chromosomes.
    b) Non-disjunction of mitosis.
    c) Non-disjunction of meiosis I.
    d) Non-disjunction of meiosis I and II.

66. Any type of inheritable state or change that is not encoded in the DNA base sequence, but which affects the expression state of the DNA is called
    a) Somaclonal variation
    b) Somatic mutagenesis
    c) Epigenetic
    d) Phenotypic plasticity

67. Which of the following histone proteins is involved in dosage compensation in humans?
    a) H2AX
    b) H2A2
    c) H2ABbd
    d) All of the above

68. Sometimes XX humans develop as males even though they have no SRY gene because
    a) In humans sex is primarily determined by hormones.
    b) SRY can be replaced by another gene Sox 9 in testis formation.
    c) 2A+XX embryos may develop into male by chance due to abnormal splicing of some genes during early development.
    d) Concentration of aromatase is high in 2A+XX embryos that can result in development of male in some circumstances.

69. Repair of double strand breaks made during meiosis in the yeast Saccharo-*myces cerevisiae*
    a) occurs mostly by non-homologous end joining.
    b) occurs mostly using the sister chromatid as a template.
    c) occurs mostly using the homologous chromosome as a template.
    d) is associated with a high frequency of mutations.

70. Plasmids differ from transposons because plasmids
    a) Become inserted into chromosome
    b) Can self-replicate outside the cell
    c) Move from chromosome to chromosome
    d) Carry genes for antibiotic resistance

71. Recombination is thought to be the primary source of variations which are "spice" of evolution because
    a) It creats new alleles
    b) It creats new genes
    c) It creats new combination of genes
    d) It creats new combination of alleles

72. Sexual reproduction is called as "master piece of nature" because it involves gamete formation through meiosis. What property of the meiosis justifies the above saying?
    a) Pairing of homologous chromosomes
    b) Independent assortment of alleles during Anaphase I
    c) Recombination of alleles during meiosis
    d) Separation of homologous chromosomes during gamete formation

73. What is the fate of most duplicated genes?
    a) Gene activation
    b) Gain of a novel function through subsequent mutation
    c) They are transferred to a new organism using lateral gene transfer
    d) They become orthologous

74. A mother of blood group O has a group O child. The father could be of blood type
    a) A or B or O. b) O only.
    c) A or B. d) AB only

[CSIR (NET/JRF) Exam. June 2011]

75. The following is the biochemical pathway for purple pigment production in flowers of sweet pea:

$$\text{Colourless Precursor 1} \xrightarrow{\text{Allele A}}$$
$$\text{Colourless Precursor 2} \xrightarrow{\text{Allele B}} \text{Purple pigment}$$

Recessive mutation of either gene A or B leads to the formation of white flowers. A cross is made between. two parents with the genotype : AaBb x aabb. Considering that the two genes are not linked, the phenotypes of the expected progenies are

a) 9 purple : 7 white.
b) 3 white : 1 purple.
c) 1 purple : 1 white.
d) 9 purple : 6 light purple : 1 white.

[CSIR (NET/JRF) Exam. June 2011]

76. Aneuploid females with only one X chromosome is a characteristic of individuals with
   a) Cri du chat syndrome.
   b) Klinefelter syndrome.
   c) Down syndrome.
   d) Turner syndrome

   [CSIR (NET/JRF) Exam. June 2011]

77. A mechanism that can cause a gene to move from one linkage group to another is
   a) crossing over
   b) inversion
   c) translocation
   d) duplication

   [CSIR (NET/JRF) Exam. June 2011]

78. Inversion may lead to crossing over suppression because
   a) It inhibits formation of Holiday junction
   b) Inversion genes are completely linked
   c) Recombinant gametes are inviable
   d) Disjunction of sister chromatids is prevented

79. Which of the following statements is not true for transposable element system?
   a) It consists of both autonomous and non-autonomous elements.
   b) Dissociation elements are autonomous in nature.
   c) Transposase is transcribed by the central region of autonomous elements.
   d Certain repeats in the genome remain fixed even after the element transposes out.

   [CSIR Model Paper 2011]

80. When two mutants having the same phenotype were crossed, the progeny obtained showed a wild-type phenotype. Thus the mutations are
   a) non-allelic.
   b) allelic.
   c) segregating from each other.
   d) independently assorting.

   [CSIR Model Paper 2011]

81. Two varieties of maize averaging 48 and 72 inches in height, respectively, are crossed. The F1 progeny is quite uniform averaging 60 inches in height. Of the 500 F2 plants, the shortest 2 are 48 inches and the tallest 2 are 72 inches. What is the probable number of polygenes involved in this trait?
a) Four.
b) Eight.
c) Sixteen.
d) Thirty two **[CSIR Model Paper 2011]**

82. If an F1 plant having genotype (Rr) round seed is back crossed to the parent with round seeds, what proportion of the progeny will have wrinkled seeds?
a) 1/2
b) 1/4
c) 3/4
d) 0

83. A useful tool for analyzing genetic crosses is the testcross in which
a) One individual of unknown genotype is crossed with another individual with a homozygous recessive genotype
b) One individual of unknown genotype is crossed with another individual with either homozygous recessive or homogygous dominant genotype.
c) An individual with an unknown genotype is crossed with another individual which have same morphological characters.
d) Individual of F1 generation is crossed with either of the parental genotypes

84. In humans, what would be the phenotype of a person with XXXY sex chromosome?
a) Down syndrome
b) Klinefelter syndrome
c) Turner syndrome
d) Poly-X female

85. How many Barr bodies can be seen in a human male having XXXYY genotype?
a) 1
b) 2
c) 3
d) No Barr bodies present in male cells

86. Which of the following is not correct for X-linked recessive trait?
a) Males show the phenotypes of all X-linked traits
b) It shows cris-cross inheritance
c) Exceptionally some females also suffer from X-linked recessive traits
d) Males inherit X-linked traits from their mother pass X-linked traits to all of their descendents.

87. Which of the following statement is incorrect for sex-influenced characters?
a) These characters are determined by autosomal genes, whose expression is limited to one sex.
b) Inherited according to Mendel's principles.
c) The trait has higher penetrance in one of the sexes.
d) Expression of genes depends on the sexes of organisms.

88. When the offspring's phenotype is determined not by its own genotype but by the genotype of its mother it is called
   a) Cytoplasmic inheritance b) Genetic maternal effect
   c) Mitochondrial effect d) Genomic imprinting

89. The influence of multiple genes on the expression of a single characteristic is called
   a) Phenocopy effect b) Synteny
   c) Polygeny d) Pleiotropy

90. Autosomal recessive traits often appear in pedigrees in which there have been consanguine matings, because these traits
   a) Tend to skip generations.
   b) Appear only when both parents carry a copy of the gene for the trait, which is more likely when the parents are related.
   c) Usually arise in children born to parents who are unaffected.
   d) Appear equally in males and females.

91. A male is affected with an X-linked dominant trait. What proportion of offspring would be affected with the trait?
   a) 1/2 sons and 1/2 daughters
   b) 3/4 daughters and 1/4 sons
   c) All daughters and no sons
   d) All sons and no daughters

92. A trait which passed from father to all sons is
   a) X-linked dominant b) Autosomal dominant
   c) X-linked recessive d) Y-linked

93. Human male has Klinefelter syndrome, having XXY genotype. How many linkage groups are present in this male?
   a) 24 b) 25
   c) 46 d) 47

94. For single crossover, the frequency of recombinant gametes is half the frequency of crossing over because
   a) A test cross between a homozygote and heterozygote produces 1/2 heterozygous and 1/2 homozygous progeny.
   b) The frequency of recombination is always 50%.
   c) Each crossover takes place between only two of the four chromatics of a homologous pair.
   d) Crossovers occur in about 50% of meioses.

95. Conjugation between an F^+ and an F^- cell usually results in
   a) Two F^+ cells b) Two F^- cells
   c) An F^+ and an F^- cell d) An Hfr cell and an F^+ cell

96. In gene mapping experiments using generalized transduction, bacterial genes that are cotransduced are
    a) For apart on the bacterial chromosome
    b) On different bacterial chromosome
    c) Close together on the bacterial chromosome
    d) On a plasmid

97. The transfer of bacterial genes located near the site of prophase insertion is called
    a) Generalized transduction b) Specialized transduction
    c) Conjugation d) Transformation

98. How does maternal inheritance of mitochondrial genes differ from sex linkage?
    a) Mitochondrial genes do not contribute to the phenotype of an individual.
    b) Because mitochondria are inherited from the mother, only females are affected,
    c) Since mitochondria are inherited from the mother, females and males are equally affected.
    d) Mitochondrial genes must be dominant while sex-linked traits are typically recessive.

99. Principle of independent assortment states that
    a) Alleles at same loci separate independently of one another.
    b) Alleles at different loci separate independently of one another.
    c) Genes at same loci separate independently of one another.
    d) Genes at different loci separate independently of one another.

100. If we were to isolate four sperm cells from the testes of a mouse. How could we identify the sperms are the resultant of single or more meiotic division
    a) Minute map b) Tetrad analysis
    c) QTL mapping d) Lod score

101. Which of the following method is not used to determine the physical location of genes on a chromosome?
    a) Deletion mapping b) Somatic cell hybridization
    c) QTL mapping d) Direct DNA sequencing

Part C

1. An F^+, marked at 10 loci, gives spontaneously to HFr progeny wherever the F factor becomes incorporated into the chromosome of the F+ strain. The F factor can integrate into the circular chromosome at many points, so that the resulting HFr strains transfer the genetic markers in different orders. For any HFr strain, the order of markers entering a recipient cell can be determined by interrupted mating experiments. From the following data for several HFr strains derived from the same F^+, determine the order of markers in the F^+ strain

HFr Strain	Markers donated in orders
1	-Z-H-E-R →
2	-O-K-S-R →
3	-K-O-W-I →
4	-Z-T-I-W →
5	-H-Z-T-I →

a) Z H E R S K O W I T   b) O W K S R R E I T Z H
c) K O W S R E H Z T I   d) H Z T I E R S K O W

2. Groups of alleles associated with the lactose operon are as follows (in order of dominance for each allelic series) : repressor, I^s (superrepressor), I^+ (Inducible), and I^- (constitutive), operator, O^c (constitutive cis-dominant) and O^+ (inducible, cis-dominant); structural Z^+, Y^+ which of the following genotypes will produce β-galactosidase and β-galactoside permease if lactose is absent?

$I^+ O^+ Z^+ Y^+$ $I^- O^c Z^+ Y^+$ $I^S O^C Z^+ Y^+$ $I^S O^+ Z^+ Y^+$ $I^- O^+ Z^+ Y^+$

a) 2,3,4   b) 1,2,3
c) 1,4,5   d) 3,4,5

3. The lac operon consists of three structural genes, *lac* Z, *lac* Y and *lac* A. These genes encode three enzymes that are involved in lactose metabolism. If strains of E. coli having only anyone mutated copy of the genes are cultured, colony of which of the following strains would you find to grow?
a) Strain 1: lac Z^+, lac Y and lac A
b) Strain 2: lac Z, lac Y^+ and lac A
c) Strain 3: lac Z, lac Y and lac A^+
d) None of the above

4. Assuming a 1:1 sex ratio, what is the probability that three children from the same parents will consist of two daughters and one son?
a) 0.375 b) 0.125
c) 0.675 d) 0.75
[CSIR (NET/JRF) Exam. Dec. 2011]

5. Consider the following crosses involving grey (wild-type) and yellow body colour true-breeding Drosophila:

	Cross	F_1 progeny	F_2 progeny
Cross 1	Grey female X yellow male	All males : grey All females : grey	Grey females : 98 Yellow males : 45 Grey males : 49
Cross 2	Yellow females X grey males	All males : Yellow All females : grey	?

Assuming 200 F2 offsprings are produced in cross 2, which one of the following outcome is expected?
a) 97 grey males, 54 yellow females, 49 grey males
b) 102 yellow males, 46 yellow females, 52 grey females
c) 52 grey males, 49 yellow males, 48 yellow females, 51 grey females
d) 98 grey males, 94 yellow females, 2 yellow males, 6 grey females
[CSIR (NET/JRF) Exam. Dec. 2011]

6. The ABO blood type in human is under the control of autosomal multiple alleles. Colour blindness is recessive X-linked trait. A male with a blood type A and normal vision marries a female who also has blood type A and normal vision. The couple's first child is a male who is colour blind and has O blood group. What is the probability that their next female child has normal vision and O blood group?
a) 1/4 b) 3/4
c) 1/8 d) 1
[CSIR (NET/JRF) Exam. Dec. 2011]

7. In E.coli four Hfr strains donate the following genetic markers in the order shown below:
Strain 1 : L Q W X Y
Strain 2 : M T A D Y
Strain 3 : E C M T A
Strain 4 : W Q L E C
Which of the following depicts the correct order of the markers and the site of integration (▸) of the F-factor in the four Hfr strains?

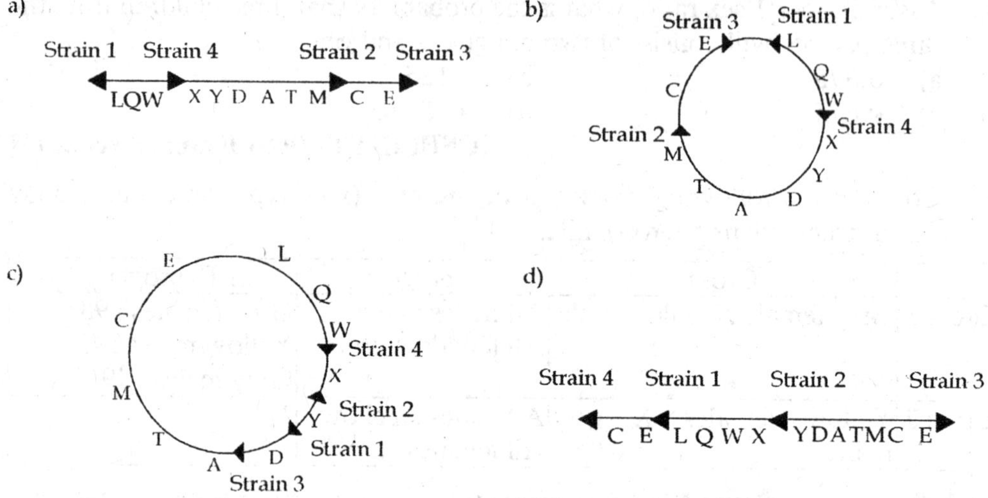

[CSIR (NET-JRF) Exam. Dec. 2011]

8. The following figure depicts the relationship between a genetic map for four genes (A, B, C and D) and their corresponding physical map:

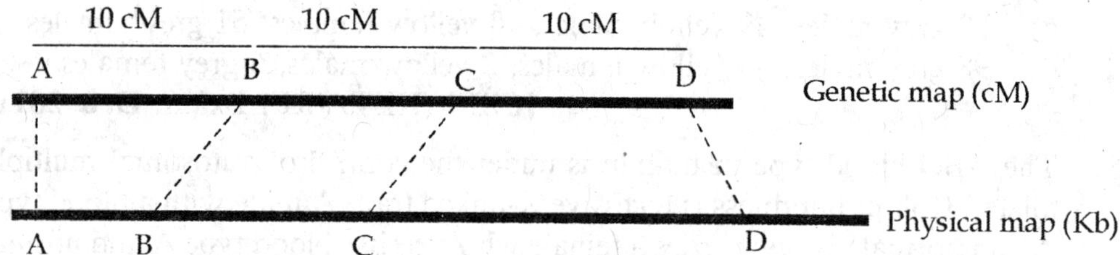

The following statements are made to explain this relationship.

A. More number of recombination events occur between A and B as compared to B and C.
B. Lesser number of recombination events occur between C and D as compared to B and C.
C. Although the physical distance between A and B is less than that between C and D, the region between A and B is more recombinogenic.
D. The physical distance between A and B is less than that between C and D, and thus the region between A and B is less recombinogenic.
E. Although the physical distance between C and D is more than that between B and C. the region between C and D is less recombinogenic.
F. Although the physical distance between C and D is more than B and C, the region between C and D is more recombinogenic.

Which statements are correct?

a) A and B
b) C and E
c) D and F
d) A, C and E

[CSIR (NET/JRF) Exam. Dec. 2011]

9. The frequencies of two alleles p and q for a gene locus in a population at Hardy-Weinberg equilibrium are 0.3 and 0.7, respectively. After a few generations of inbreeding, the heterozygote frequency was found to be 0.28. The inbreeding coefficient in this case is

a) 0.42 b) 0.28
c) 0.33 d) 0.67

[CSIR (NET/JRF) Exam. Dec. 2011]

10. A conjugation experiment is carried out between F+ his+ leu+ thr+ pro+ bacteria and F- his- leu- thr- pro- bacteria for a period of 25 minutes. At this time the mating is stopped, and the genotypes of the recipient F- bacteria are determined. The results are shown below:

Genotype	Number of colonies
his$^+$	0
leu$^+$	15
thr$^+$	28
pro$^+$	8

What is the probable order of these genes on the bacterial chromosome?

a) thr, leu, pro, his
b) pro, leu, thr and the position of his cannot be determined.
c) thr, leu, pro, and the position of his cannot be determined.
d) his, pro, leu, thr

11. In E. coli, four Hfr strains donate the following genetic markers, shown in the order donated:

Strain 1: Q W D M T
Strain 2: A X P T M
Strain 3: B N C A X
Strain 4: B Q W D M

All these Hfr strains are derived from the same F$^+$ strain. What is the order of these markers on the circular chromosome of the original F$^+$?

a) Q W D M T P X A C N B
b) A X P T M Q W D M T
c) B N C A P X Q W D M T
d) M D W Q B A X P T C N

12. In Neurospora a cross between the genotypes 'A' and 'a' results in an ascus with ascospores of genotypes as shown below:

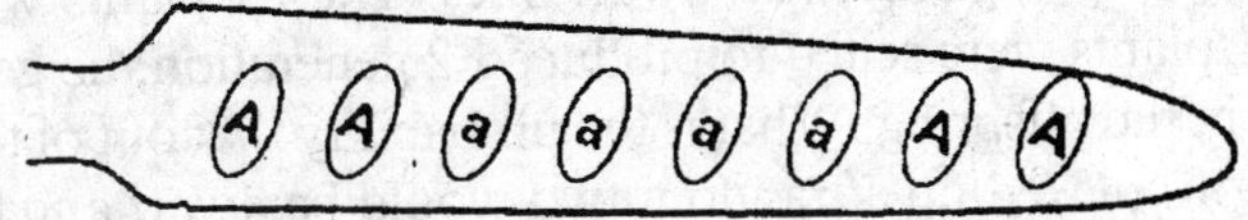

Statements A to D are events that could have occurred during meiosis.
A. Crossing over between the centromere and the gene.
B. Segregation of alleles 'A' and 'a' in meiosis I.
C. Segregation of alleles 'A' and 'a' in meiosis II.
D. Assortment of alleles 'A' and 'a'.
Which of the above events could correctly explain the observation shown in the figure?
a) A followed by C
b) A followed by B
c) C alone
d) D alone

[CSIR (NET/JRF) Exam. June 2011]

13. When F_1 female *Drosophila* of the genotype $a^+ab^+bc^+c$ is test crossed, the following progenies were obtained :

Progeny classes*	No. of progenies
$a^+ b^+ c^+$	22
$a^+ b^+ c$	28
$a\ b\ c^+$	26
$a\ b\ c$	24
$a^+ b^+ c^+$	230
$a^+ b\ c$	220
$a\ b^+ c^+$	225
$a\ b^+ c$	225
Total	1000

*The progeny has been shown as classes derived from the female gamete.
Statement A to F as given below are conclusions derived from the above result.
A. Genes *a* and *b* are linked in *cis*.
B. Genes *a* and *b* are linked in *trans*.
C. Genes *a* and *b* are linked in cis while *b* and *c* are linked in *trans*.
D. The genotype of the parents are $a^+a^+b^+b^+$ and *aabb*
E. The genotype of the parents are a^+a^+bb and aab^+b^+.
F. Genes *a* and *b* are 10cM apart.
Which of the above statements are correct?
a) C alone
b) A, E and F.
c) B, E and F
d) A, D and F.

[CSIR (NET/JRF) Exam. June 2011]

14. Mendel crossed tall pea plants with dwarf ones. The F1 plants were all tall. When these F1 plants were selfed to produce F2 generation, he got a 3:1 tall to dwarf ratio in the offspring. What is the probability that out of three plants (of F2 generation) picked up at random two would be dwarf and one would

be tall?

a) 3/4 b) 3/8

c) 9/64 d) 9/32

[CSIR (NET/JRF) Exam. June 2011]

15. The following is a hypothetical pathway for the development of wild type (red)eye colour in an insect:

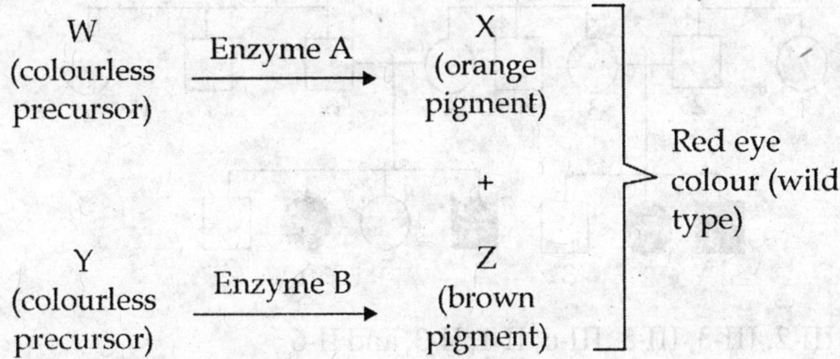

Enzymes A and B are encoded by the genes a+ and b+, respectively. The following statements are made regarding inheritance of the genes in volved in the development of eye colour:

A. When two heterozygous individuals of the genotype a+ ab+ b are mated, progenies with red, orange, brown and white eye colour will be observed irrespective of whether the genes are independently assorting or showing incomplete linkage.

B. When two heterozygous individuals of the genotype a+ ab+ b are mated, progenies with red, orange, brown and white eye colour will be observed in a ratio of 9:3:3:1, when the genes are independently assorting.

C. When an heterozygous individual of the genotype is test crossed, progenies with red and white eye colour will be more in number.

D. When an heterozygous individual of the genotype is test crossed, progenies with orange and brown eye colour will be more in number.

Which of the above statements is TRUE?

a) A and C b) B and C

c) A, B and C d) A, B and D

[CSIR (NET/JRF) Exam. June 2011]

16. Affected individuals from the pedigree given below are suffering from albinism, an autosomal recessive disease. Identify the confirmed carrier individuals in this pedigree assuming that the members coming from outside the family are homozygous for the dominant allele.

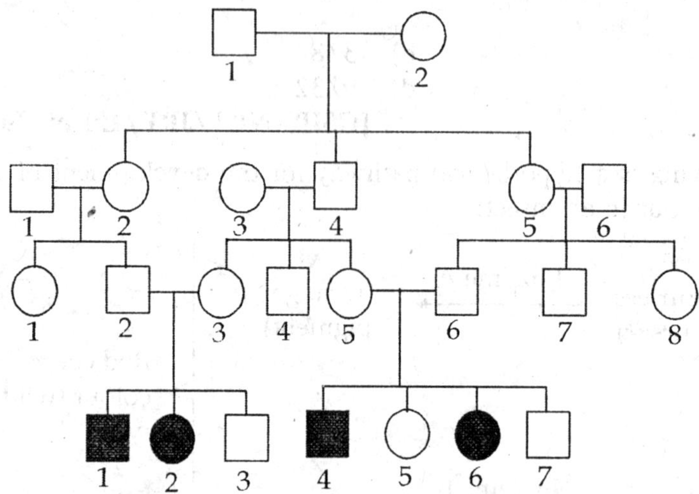

a) III-2, III-3, III-5, III-6, II-1, II-3, and II-6
b) III-2, III-3, III-5, III-6, II-2, II-4, II-5 and I-2
c) III-2, III-3, III-5, III-6, II-2, II-4 and II-5
d) III-1, III-4, III-7, II-2, II-4 and II-5

[CSIR (NET/JRF) Exam. June 2011]

17. The total variance in a phenotypic character can be split into two components-genetic (VG) and environmental (VE). The heritability of a phenotypic trait can be expressed quantitatively as heritability coefficient (h2) which is calculated as h2 =

a) VG - VE
b) VE/VG
c) $\frac{V_G}{(V_G + V_E)}$
d) $\frac{V_G}{(V_G - V_E)}$

[CSIR (NET/JRF) Exam. June 2011]

18. Upon studying a considerable number of different crosses in *Drosophila*, Morgan reached the conclusion that all genes of this fly were clustered into four linked groups corresponding to the four pairs of chromosomes. Further studies revealed that linkage is not absolute and it is broken frequently. It is broken in prophase by a process called

a) Recombination.
b) Jumping of genes.
c) Integration.
d) Mutation. **[CSIR Model Paper 2011]**

19. Mismatch of blood in parents many result in erythroblastosis fetalis in a new born. Match the correct cause (left column) and usual treatment (right column). Commonest cause

A. Mother Rh(+) and father Rh(-)
B. Mother Rh (-) and father Rh (+)
Used treatment
C. replacement of neonate's blood with Rh(-) blood.
D. replacement of neonate's blood with Rh(+) blood.

a) A and C b) A and D
c) B and C d) B and D **[CSIR Model Paper 2011]**

20.

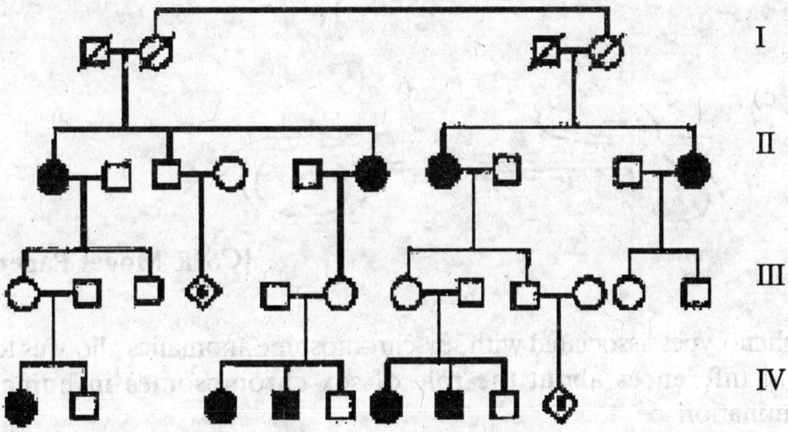

I
II
III
IV

Find the pattern of inheritance of the trait showing incomplete penetrance from the figure shown above.

a) Autosomal dominant. b) Autosomal recessive.
c) Mitochondrial inheritance. d) X-linked recessive.

[CSIR Model Paper 2011]

21. Which of the following assumption support the Hardy-Weinberg Equilibrium?
a) Presence of Natural Selection.
b) Random mating.
c) Genetic Drift.
d) Assortative mating. **[CSIR Model Paper 2011]**

22. If the probability of being blood type A is 1/8 and the probability of blood type O is 1/2, what is the probability of being either blood type A or blood type O?
a) 1/2 b) 1/8
c) 1/16 d) 5/8

23. Which of the following illustrations explain the correct pairing preceeding recombination between a chromosome (ABC•DEFG/ABC•DEFG) and its inverted homologue (ABC•DGFE/ABC•DGFE). The dot in genotype represent the centromere.

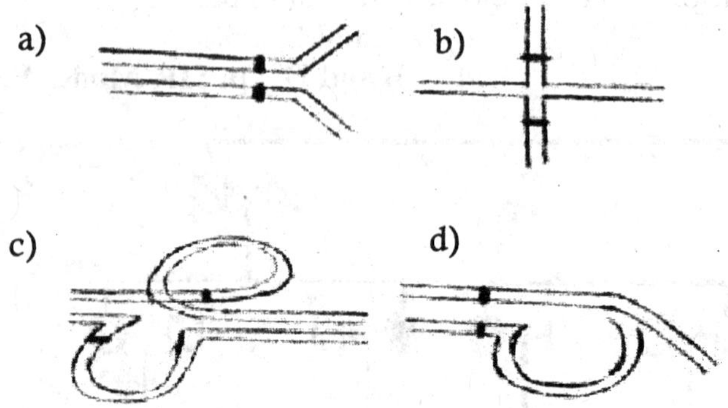

[CSIR Model Paper 2011]

24. The phenotypes associated with sex-chromosome anomalies allow us to make several inferences about the role of sex chromosomes in human sex-determination

Following statements relate to some characteristic features of sex chromosomes

a) The X-chromosome contains genetic information essential for both sexes.
b) The male-determining gene SRY and their receptor is located on the Y chromosome
c) Additional copies of the X-chromosome cannot upset normal development in both males and females.
d) A female usually needs at least two copies of the X-chromosome to be fertile

Which of the following combination is **NOT** correct?

a) A and B
b) B and C
c) A, B and C
d) A and D

25. A chromosomally normal woman and a chromosomally normal man have a son whose sex-chromosome constitution is XYY. Which of the following explanation of this observation is correct?

a) Non-disjunction took place in father during the first meiotic division
b) Non-disjunction took place in mother during first meiotic division
c) Non-disjunction took place in father during second meiotic division
d) Non-disjunction took place in mother during second meiotic division

26. Among sibships consisting of size children, and assuming a sex ratio of 1:1, what is the proportion with no girls and exactly two girls, respectively?
    a) 1/64 and 15/64 b) 42/64 and 20/64
    c) 6/64 and 1/64 d) 15/64 and 42/64

27. A cross in corn is carried out with three linked genes in triply heterozygous genotype for the allele pairs (A, a), (D, d), and (R, r). The dominant A allele results in red leaves; aa plants have green leaves. The dominant D allele results in tall plants; dd plants are dwarfed. The dominant R allele results in ragged leaf margin; rr plants have smooth leaf margins. The triply heterozygote is crossed with homozygous recessives for all three alleles, and the following phenotypes of progeny are observed. Assume that interference in each interval is complete, so that the map distance in centiMorgans (cM) corresponds to the percent recombination,

red, tall, ragged	265
red, tall, smooth	24
red, dwarf, ragged	120
red, dwarf, smooth	90
green, tall, ragged	70
green, tall, smooth	140
green, dwarf, ragged	16
green, dwarf, smooth	275
Total	1000

    What is the order of genes and the shortest map distance between adjacent genes?
    a) A D R and 20 cM b) D A R and 30 cM
    c) A R D and 40 cM d) A R D and 20 cM

28. The data in the accompanying table show 1000 gametes observed from a triply heterozygous parent in a three-point test cross to determine the genetic map of three linked genes. Neither the parental genotype of the heterozygous parent nor the order of the genes is known.

M	N	R	14
M	N	r	41
M	n	R	393
M	n	r	50
m	N	R	64
m	N	r	413
m	n	R	33
m	n	r	2

What is the correct linear order of the genes and the expected number of double crossovers?

a) M N R and 6.9 b) M R N and 9.6
c) R M N and 0.08 d) M N R and 9.6

29. A trait have following characteristics:
 (A) Only males show the trait
 (B) Affected male do not pass the trait to their sons
 (C) Unaffected females producing both affected and unaffected sons
 (D) Affected male producing unaffected female

 The trait is

a) X-linked dominant b) X- linked recessive
c) Autosomal dominant d) Autosomal recessive

Answer Sheet

Part B

1.	c	2.	a	3.	b	4.	a	5.	a	6.	a
7.	c	8.	b	9.	c	10.	c	11.	c	12.	c
13.	c	14.	c	15.	a	16.	a	17.	b	18.	c
19.	c	20.	d	21.	c	22.	d	23.	d	24.	d
25.	c	26.	b	27.	a	28.	d	29.	b	30.	d
31.	d	32.	c	33.	b	34.	d	35.	a	36.	c
37.	b	38.	c	39.	c	40.	c	41.	c	42.	c
43.	a	44.	d	45.	d	46.	d	47.	a	48.	d
49.	d	50.	b	51.	d	52.	d	53.	d	54.	d
55.	c	56.	c	57.	b	58.	c	59.	c	60.	b
61.	c	62.	a	63.	b	64.	b	65.	d	66.	c
67.	b	68.	b	69.	c	70.	c	71.	d	72.	c
73.	b	74.	a	75.	b	76.	d	77.	c	78.	c
79.	a	80.	a	81.	a	82.	d	83.	a	84.	b
85.	b	86.	d	87.	a	88.	b	89.	c	90.	b
91.	c	92.	d	93.	a	94.	c	95.	a	96.	c
97.	b	98.	c	99.	b	100.	b	101.	c		

Part – C

1.	a	2.	a	3.	c	4.	a	5.	c	6.	c
7.	b	8.	c	9.	c	10.	a	11.	a	12.	a
13.	a	14.	c	15.	a	16.	b	17.	c	18.	a
19.	c	20.	b	21.	b	22.	d	23.	c	24.	b
25.	c	26.	a	27.	d	28.	d	29.	b		

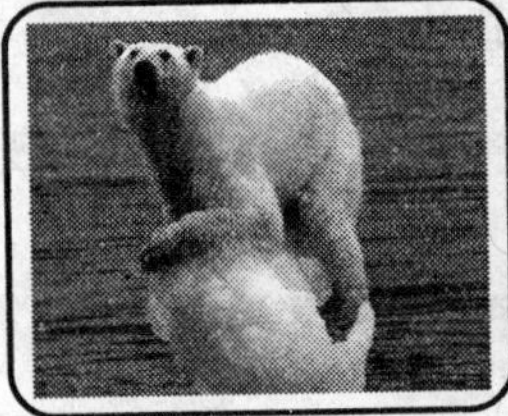

Chapter 9
Ecological Principles

Part B

1. "Dancing deer" is the main species of
   a) Kaziranga National Park b) Keibul Lamjao National Park
   c) Bannerghatta National Park d) Dachigam National Park

2. "Lee Boot Effect" is seen in
   a) Honey Bees b) Birds
   c) Lion d) Drosophila

3. In which of the following habitats would you expect a high incidence of wingless insect species?
   a) Deserts b) Savanna
   c) Tropical alpine habitats d) Temperate rain forests

4. A group of interconnected food chains is called
   a) Pyramid of energy b) Complex food chain
   c) Food web d) Food cycle

5. A J-shaped growth curve should be associated with
   a) exponential growth
   b) biotic potential
   c) no environmental resistance and rapid population growth
   d) All of these

6. A keystone species is one that
   a) has a higher likelihood of extinction than a non-keystone species
   b) exerts a strong influence on an ecosystem
   c) causes other species to become extinct
   d) has a weak influence on an ecosystem

7. A population inhabiting in a highly dynamic environment will have the following except
   a) Low reproductive potential b) High juvenile death.
   c) Low competitor. d) J-shaped growth curve.

8. A population with a larger proportion of older individuals than younger individuals will likely
   a) Grow larger then decline rapidly
   b) Continue to grow larger indefinitely
   c) Grow smaller and may stabilize at a smaller population size
   d) Not experience a change in population size.

9. A population with lower survivourship at old ages will follow survivourship
   a) Pattern I b) Pattern II
   c) Pattern III d) None of the above

10. A predation series linking animals to ultimate plant food is called
    a) Food web b) Trophic level
    c) Food cycle d) Food chain

11. A researcher has found a biome having characters like presence of evergreen trees, low biodiversity, with only a two-layered forest community, very slow turn over rate of nutrients and trees are heavily dependent upon mycorrhizal association.
    a) Tropical rain forest b) Taiga
    c) Temperate forest d) Tundra

12. A species is susceptible to extinction having all of the following characteristics except
    a) Endemic b) Specialized habitat requirement
    c) Geographically widespread d) K-strategist

13. A species that has repeated reproductive events, but suffers a crash due to the weather is exemplifying
    a) r-selection
    b) K-selection
    c) a mixture of both r-selection and K-selection
    d) density dependent and density independent regulation

14. Acid rain is chiefly due to atmospheric pollution by
    a) NO_2 b) SO_2
    c) H_2S d) HCl

15. All of the following imparts diversity except
    a) Stable ecosystem
    b) Controlled climatic conditions
    c) Stable forest and ocean ecosystem
    d) Decreasing population growth rate and trophic specialization

16. All the living organisms of the Earth constitute
    a) Biosphere b) Community
    c) Biome d) Ecosystem

17. Allochthonus input is common in
    a) Lotic ecosystem b) Lentic ecosystem
    c) Tundra d) Estuaries

18. Altruism is common where
    a) $r b > c$ b) $r b < c$
    d) $r b = c$ c) $r b = 0$

19. Amensalism can be represented as
    a) + - b) 0 -
    c) 0 0 d) - -

20. Among the following which equation denotes the population growth where resources are not limiting?
    a) Nt = N0e-rt b) Nt/Nt = Nt - N0
    c) dN/dt = Krt d) dN/dt = rN

21. Among the following which has highest productivity/biomass ratio?
    a) Grassland b) Large lakes
    c) Open ocean d) Rain forest

22. Among the following which is global cycle ?
    a) Phosphorus b) Nitrogen
    c) Carbon d) Sulphur

23. Among the following which is not a characteristic feature of r-selected species
    a) Maturity at later stage b) Large clutch size
    c) Small size of offspring d) Maturity at early stage life

24. Among the following which trend shows the decreasing population?
    a) Less individual in pre-reproductive stage and more in reproductive stage
    b) Less individual in reproductive stage and more in pre-reproductive stage
    c) More individual in reproductive stage
    d) More individual in post-reproductive stage

25. Among the vertebrates the maximum biodiversity occurs in
    a) Pisces b) Mammals
    c) Aves d) Reptiles

[CSIR (NET/JRF) Exam. June 2001]

26. An endemic species is
    a) One found naturally in just one geographic area
    b) One found naturally in many different geographic area

c) One found only on Islands
d) One that has been introduced to a new geographic area

27. Areas rich in plant or animal species are considered as hot spots of biodiversity if they
   a) Support 1500 endemic plant species and the region have lost 65% of its original habitat
   b) Support 2100 endemic plant species and the region have lost 70% of its original habitat
   c) Support 3300 endemic plant species and the region have lost 70% of its original habitat
   d) Support 1500 or more endemic plant species and the region have lost 70% of its original habitat

28. Areas with annual cool temperature and almost constant rate of precipitation throughout year is
   a) Poles
   b) Temperate deciduous
   c) Tundra
   d) Tropics

29. As one goes from the tropics to the temperate regions of the earth biological diversity
   a) Increases
   b) Decreases
   c) Stays constant
   d) Fluctuate in an unpredictable manner

30. Asiatic elephant can be differentiated with African elephant by having
   a) Much larger ears than African elephant
   b) Trunk ending with only one lip
   c) Larger tusks and seldom found in male
   d) Trunk ending with two lips of equal length

31. Benthic organisms of lakes/sea are usually
   a) Detritivores
   b) Herbivores
   c) Carnivores
   d) Producers

32. Biological magnification is maximum in human. It proves that human is
   a) More susceptible
   b) Top consumer in food chain
   c) Most efficient in storage of reserve food
   d) None of the above

33. Biotic potential of a species is
   a) Intrinsic rate of natural increase
   b) Theoretical maximum production of new individuals
   c) Difference between the intrinsic rate and the rate that occurs in a actual field condition
   d) Instaneous coefficient of population growth

34. Chain extinction indicates that
    a) Ecosystems are self regulating systems.
    b) Extinction of a species promotes the extinction of another species.
    c) No one species is exclusively independent in an ecosystem.
    d) Extinction is a natural process.

35. Chain extinction occurs
    a) Due to catastrophic events.
    b) When habitat is modified due to "ecosystem engineers".
    c) Due to loss of keystone species which may favour survival of many other species.
    d) When many species are lost in a series due to environmental stochasticity.

36. Character displacement spells out all of the following except
    a) Niche diversification.
    b) Low competition among individuals.
    c) Resource partitioning.
    d) Migration.

37. Coevolution is not seen in
    a) Mutualism b) Parasitism
    c) Commensalism d) Antibiosis

[CSIR (NET/JRF) Exam. June 2007]

38. Commensalism is represented by
    a) + + b) + 0
    c) - - d) + -

39. Communal suckling is common in some groups of animals. It can be explained with the help of
    a) Kin selection b) Reciprocal altruism
    c) Group selection d) Individual selection

40. Communal suckling of young ones is found in
    a) Cats b) Dogs
    c) Lions d) Humans

41. Competing species can coexist when
    a) Both are provided with a realized niche by their habitat
    b) Both are provided with a fundamental niche by their habitat
    c) One is provided with a realized niche and other with fundamental niche
    d) Their habitats are different

42. Competitive exclusion principle which states that 'complete competitors cannot coexist' is related to:
    a) Intra specific competition b) Inter specific competition
    c) Scramble competition d) Contest competition

43. Conservation hotspots are best described as
    a) Areas with large number of endemic species that are disappearing rapidly
    b) Areas where people are particularly active supporters of biological diversity
    c) Islands that are experiencing high rates of extinction.
    d) Areas where native species are being replaced with introduced species

44. Coral reefs are most abundant in
    a) Colder fresh water b) Warmer fresh water
    c) Colder marine water d) Warmer marine water

45. Critically endangered animal is
    a) Asiatic wild ass b) Lion-tailed macaque
    c) Spotted civet d) Asiatic Elephant

[CSIR (NET/JRF) Exam. June. 2008]

46. Cryopreservation is not possible for
    a) Fast dividing cells b) Mature cells
    c) Frost sensitive cells d) Stem cells

47. Cryopreservation may employ
    a) Over solid carbon dioxide (At -79°C)
    b) Low temperature deep freezers (At -80°C)
    c) In vapour phase nitrogen (at-150°c) and in liquid nitrogen (at -196°C)
    d) All of the above

48. Cryopreservaton is the preservation of plant material at
    a) Mild temperature b) Very high temperature
    c) Very low temperature d) Between 45oC-65oC

49. Dachigam National Park is famous for conservation of
    a) Cheetal b) Hangul
    c) Musk deer d) Barasingha

50. Decomposition rate is high in
    a) Warm temperature and dry conditions
    b) Low temperature and moisture conditions
    c) Low temperature and dry conditions
    d) Warm temperature and moisture conditions

51. Diversity in range of communities due to replacement of species with the change in community habitat is
    a) α diversity b) β diversity
    c) γ diversity d) None of these

52. During succession the bare rock is first colonized by
    a) Fungi   b) Algae
    c) Lichens   d) Bacteria

53. Each Biosphere reserve has the following zones except
    a) Core zone   b) Transvertion zone
    c) Buffer zone   d) Transition zone

54. Early successional species are characterized by all of the following except
    a) High degree of dispersal
    b) Smaller size.
    c) High rates of population growth.
    d) Slower growth rates.

55. Ecological efficiency of energy as it passes from one trophic level to another is about
    a) 50%   b) 1%
    c) 10%   d) 0.1%

56. Ecological isolation among species is the result of
    a) Rich resources   b) Coexistence
    c) Low biotic potential   d) Niche overlap

57. Ecosystem may be defined as
    a) Group of plants which act as the energy suppliers
    b) Group of organisms which form population
    c) Functional unit for ecological studies
    d) None of the above

58. Edge species are those which are
    a) found on islands   b) found at ecotone
    c) more prone to extinction   d) found at the edge of a community

59. Endemic flowering plants recorded in India includes
    a) 33%   b) 55%
    c) 18%   d) 28%

60. Endemic species
    a) Grow in a large geographical area
    b) Can grow in a particular soil type
    c) Grow in a small geographical area
    d) Are able to survive in different environmental conditions

61. Endemism is shown by
    a) Mountain ranges   b) Plateaus
    c) Grassland   d) Island

[CSIR (NET/JRF) Exam. Dec. 2004]

62. Energy flow in an ecosystem follows
    a) First law of thermodynamics
    b) Second law of thermodynamics
    c) Third law of thermodynamics
    d) None of the above

63. Energy flow in the ecosystem is a unidirectional process because
    a) Autotrophic production is more
    b) Heterotrophic production is more
    c) Autotrophic respiration is more
    d) Heterotrophic respiration is more

64. Exotic weed which has proved very harmful for wetlands is
    a) Eichhornia b) Salvia
    c) Verbenia d) Eupatromia

[CSIR (NET/JRF) Exam. June 2003]

65. Exponential growth is characteristic of populations
    a) Inhabiting resources rich environment at low population densities
    b) Having low ecological densities
    c) Growing in the habitat where environmental stochasticity is common
    d) None of the above

66. For climax community which statement is incorrect?
    a) Species diversity decreases
    b) Dependency on detritus food chain increases
    c) Vertical stratification of community increases
    d) Exploitation competition is more than normal competition

67. Frequent use of nitrogenous fertilizers has adversely affected the soil by
    a) Making them alkaline
    b) Leaching many essential elements
    c) Enhancing dentrification
    d) Desertification

68. Gause's Competitive Exclusion Principle states that
    a) If any two competitors are grown together, one will always exclude the other
    b) If two species consume each other's limiting resources, one will always competitively exclude the other
    c) If two species consume same resources that is essential for the survival of both, one will eventually exclude the other
    d) If two competitors permanently coexist, they must have different limiting resources

69. Gause's exclusion principle can not explain
    a) Speciation
    b) Extinction
    c) Succession
    d) Character displacement

70. Generally the largest animals are found in aquatic habitat because
    a) There is more food available
    b) Gravity effects are minimized by buoyancy
    c) Temperature fluctuations are less drastic
    d) It is easier to maintain homeostasis

71. Generally, when populations approach their carrying capacity, negative feed-back occurs. But sometimes, growth rates increase with population size. This phenomenon is referred to as the
    a) Edge effect
    b) Sues effect
    c) Allee effect
    d) Kreb's effect

72. Genetic diversity can not be determined by
    a) RFLP
    b) RAPD
    c) Allozymes
    d) Molecular probes

73. Gir National Park is related to
    a) Lion
    b) Elephant
    c) Deer
    d) Rhinoceros

74. Global climate change is the result of the imbalanced
    a) Carbon cycle
    b) Phosphorus cycle
    c) Nitrogen cycle
    d) Sulphur cycle

75. Global warming is due to which of the following?
    a) Green house gases absorb to both visible and infrared radiation
    b) Infrared radiation is absorbed by green house gases where as visible radiation is not
    c) Infrared radiation is not absorbed by green house gases whereas visible radiation is
    d) Earth is slowly coming closer to the sun

76. Golden langurs are found in
    a) Corbett National Park
    b) Manas National Park
    c) Ranthambaur National Park
    d) Kaziranga National Park

77. Grasslands where trees are also present along with grasses are called
    a) Pampas
    b) Steppe
    c) Prairie
    d) Savanna

[CSIR (NET/JRF) Exam. Dec. 2006]

78. Groups of species that exploit a common resource in a similar fashion are termed
    a) Demes
    b) Guilds
    c) Subspecies
    d) Edge species
79. Hemipteran queens show 75%, similarity to sisters but 50% to daughter. It can be explained in the light of
    a) Eusocialism
    b) Genic balance theory
    c) Kin selection
    d) Absence of crossing over in male
80. High level of nitrate in drinking water may cause human health problem because it
    a) Causes haemolysis
    b) Promotes thrombosis in arteries and veins
    c) Causes decrease in intestinal microbial flora which synthesize many essential vitamins.
    d) Causes formation of methaemoglobin.
81. Highest species diversity is of
    a) Amphibians
    b) Pisces
    c) Mammals
    d) Birds
82. Historically, Island species have tended to become extinct faster than species living on a mainland, which of the following reasons cannot be used to explain this phenomenon ?
    a) Island species have often evolved in the absence of predators and have no natural avoidance strategies
    b) Humans have introduced diseases and competitors to Islands, which negatively impacts Island populations
    c) Island's populations are usually smaller than mainland populations
    d) Island populations are usually less fit than mainland populations
83. Honey bee shares more its genes with sister (75%) as compare to its daughter (50%). It can be explained with the help of
    a) Coefficient of coincidence
    b) Coefficient of relatedness
    c) Inclusive fitness
    d) Social behaviour
84. Hoolock gibbon, the only ape found in India, can easily be seen in
    a) Manas National Park
    b) Sanjay Gandhi National Park
    c) Kaziranga National Park
    d) Belta National Park · **[CSIR (NET/JRF) Exam. Dec. 2001]**

85. How many species of birds are found in India-
   a) 1200 b) 3200
   c) 500 d) 5700

[CSIR (NET/JRF) Exam. Dec. 2005]

86. Humans are an example of an organism with a type-I survivorship curve. This means
   a) Mortality rates are highest for younger individuals
   b) Mortality rates are highest for older individuals
   c) Mortality rates are constant over the life span of individuals
   d) The population growth rate is high

87. Hydrography plays a significant role in the production of
   a) Tropical rain forest b) Open ocean
   c) Grass land d) Tundra

88. If a species has been eliminated, the species is
   a) Exotic b) Endemic
   c) Extinct d) Threatened

89. If the organism carrying the gene survives to reproduce and also helps the borne who carry many of the same genes survive to reproduce, the phenomenon is termed as
   a) Reproductive fitness b) Survival fitness
   c) Darwinian fitness d) Inclusive fitness

90. In a stable ecosystem the food chain mostly contains
   a) 3-5 links b) 2 links
   c) 6 links d) 7 links

91. In an ecosystem phytoplanktons follow
   a) Type I survivourship curve
   b) Type II survivourship curve
   c) Type III survivourship curve
   d) None of the above

92. In an ecosystem, fixed carbon has accumulated in the form of organic matter derived from dead plants and animals. Which one of the following is the best explanation for the observation?
   a) Secondary consumers are absent from the ecosystem
   b) Primary consumers are absent from the ecosystem
   c) Producers have been utilizing sunlight inadequately
   d) Decomposers activity is low

93. In Birds waste material is solid due to
    a) Less water storage
    b) High metabolic rate
    c) Low metabolic rate
    d) Due to formation of electrolytes

CSIR (NET/JRF] Exam. June 2005]

94. In describing biological diversity the Shanon-Wiener index takes into consideration:
    a) Species richness alone
    b) Equitability alone
    c) Both species richness and quitability
    d) Simpson's index

95. In ecology, the second law of thermodynamics explains the
    a) Adaptation of animals to cold climates
    b) Progressive loss of energy at each trophic level
    c) High species diversity of the tropics
    d) Increase in average body size of related species

96. In global warming the dangerous gas next to CO_2 is
    a) CH_4 b) SO_2
    c) NO_2 d) water vapour

[CSIR (NET/JRF) Exam. Dec. 2006]

97. In India maximum biodiversity is seen at
    a) Eastern Himalayas and Andaman and Nicobar Islands
    b) Eastern and Western Ghats
    c) Eastern and Western Himalayas
    d) Eastern Himalayas & Western Ghats

[CSIR (NET/JRF) Exam. June 2003]

98. In many species mating occurs with no strong pair-bonds or pair-lasting relationships. This type of mating relationship is called
    a) Monogamous b) Polygamous
    c) Promiscuous d) None of the above

99. In Ranunkiaer's life forms trees come under
    a) Cryptophytes b) Therophytes
    c) Chamaeophytes d) Phanerophytes

100. In the evolution of life histories of populaitons living in uncertain and catastrophic environments,
    a) Earlier age at maturity and high fecundity
    b) Earlier age at maturity and low fecundity

c) Later age at maturity and high fecundity
d) Late age at maturity and low fecundity

101. In the nutrient recycling of which ecosystem is the role of detritivores maximum
a) Grassland b) Open sea
c) Temperate lake d) Tropical rain forest

102. In which interaction is the realized niche of one partner greater than its fundamental niche ?
a) Amensalism b) Competition
c) Commensalism d) Mutualism

[CSIR (NET/JRF) Exam. June. 2008]

103. In which of the following terrestrial biomes does the variety of life reach its culmination?
a) Tropical rain forests
b) Tropical grasslands
c) Temperate deciduous forests
d) Northern coniferous forests

104. Indian fauna has maximum endemic vertebrate species of
a) Mammalia b) Pisces
c) Aves d) Reptiles

105. Indian fauna has maximum vertebrates species of
a) Amphibia b) Reptiles
c) Aves d) Pisces

106. Indian flora has maximum species of
a) Algae b) Fungi
c) Bryophyta d) Angiosperm

107. Individuals of the same species in a particular locality constitute
a) Population b) Community
c) Flora d) Fauna

108. Inverted pyramid of biomass is often seen in
a) Parasitic food chain b) Ecosystem by a single tree
c) Open-water sea d) Forest ecosystems

109. Island populations show maximum extinction rate because
a) They are fast evolving populations.
b) Nutrient availability is very poor on islands.
c) These populations can easily be affected by demographic & environmental stochasticity.
d) Inbreeding depression is absent.

110. J-shaped growth curve is obtained when density of organism
   a) Increases rapidly and stops abruptly
   b) Increases rapidly and decreases slowly
   c) Decreases rapidly and suddenly increases
   d) None of these

111. Kin selection is
   a) The mating between relatives
   b) The recognition of relatives in societal groups
   c) The adoption of young by generally unrelated adults
   d) A behaviour that increases the survivorship of an individual's relatives

112. K-selected species would be common in
   a) Developing community b) Mature community
   c) Pioneer community d) All of these

113. Langur monkey when occupy harem starts infanticide because
   a) To remove alleles of dominant gene
   b) To maintain the constant population
   c) For reproductive advantage
   d) They does not want child of earlier dominant male to survive

[CSIR (NET/JRF) Exam. June 2004]

114. Lantana camara, an exotic species, was introduced in India from
   a) China b) Sri Lanka
   c) West Bengal d) Bhutan

115. Law of tolerance is proposed by
   a) Leibig b) Shanon
   c) Shelford d) Lindman

116. Lichen growing on the surface of rocks provides an example of
   a) Tolerance b) Facilitation
   c) Inhibition d) Secondary succession

117. Logistic growth is common in
   a) Limited environment b) Unlimited environment
   c) Catastrophic conditions d) Pioneer communities

118. Lotka -voltera model explains
   a) Competition b) Herbivory
   c) Predation d) Mutualism

119. Mammals from colder climates tend to have shorter ears and limbs, it supports
   a) Bergmann's rule b) Gloger's rule
   c) Allen's rule d) Rensche's rule

120. Manas National Park is situated in
   a) Gujarat
   b) Uttar Pradesh
   c) Assam
   d) Uttaranchal

121. Mangroves are highly productive ecosystems but they are rich only in bird diversity because
   a) More number of predators that feed on birds are found here
   b) Rich in food diversity
   c) Lack of structural diversity
   d) Lack of breeding place

122. Many areas of ocean that receive the greatest intensity of solar radiation have the lowest biological activity because
   a) oxygen is in limiting amount.
   b) salt content is very high.
   c) they are limited by shortage of mineral nutrients.
   d) none of the above.

123. Many short-lived and rapidly reproducing species show boom-and-bust cycles. Which of the following is not characteristic of these species?
   a) Their growth is exponential
   b) Their survivourship curve is concave
   c) They are found in unlimited environment
   d) They are better competitior

124. Maximum biodiversity occurs at
   a) Equator
   b) Tropics
   c) Temperate
   d) Poles

125. Maximum number of hotspots of biodiversity have been reported from
   a) Africa
   b) North America
   c) South America
   d) Asia Pacific

126. Maximum number of species extinction has occurred on Island because
   a) Island populations have high rate of mortality
   b) Island populations are poor in genetic diversity
   c) Island populations experience high rate of predation
   d) Island populations are fast evolving

127. Maximum species of insects are found in
   a) Diptera
   b) Hymenoptera
   c) Coleoptera
   d) Hemiptera

[CSIR (NET/JRF) Exam. Dec. 2006]

128. Metapopulations have all of the following characters except
   a) Synchronized dynamics.   b) Interdemic extinction.
   c) Recolonization.   d) Rescue effect.

129. Mimicry in which both mimic and model are distasteful is
   a) Batesian mimicry   b) Mullerian mimicry
   c) Counter shading   d) Aposematic colouration

130. Mimicry in which model has benefit is called
   a) Aggressive mimicry   b) Batesian mimicry
   c) Mullerian mimicry   d) Both (b) and (c)

131. Monal pheasant is found in
   a) Western Ghat   b) Eastern Ghat
   c) Himalayas   d) Gir Forests

132. Most frequently used cryoprotectant is
   a) Glycerol   b) praline
   c) Ethylene   d) DMSO

133. Most suitable material for cryopreservation is
   a) embryo   b) Endosperm
   c) Ovules & seeds   d) Meristematic cells

134. Mullerian mimicry can be represented by
   a) + -   b) + +
   c) + 0   d) - -

135. Musk deer is found in
   a) Garhwal Himalaya   b) Kumaun Himalaya
   c) North-East Himalaya   d) Western Himalaya

[CSIR (NET/JRF) Exam. Dec. 2006]

136. Mutualism may be best defined as
   a) A relationship between two species
   b) A relationship between two symbionts
   c) A relationship which is favourable to both and obligatory
   d) A relationship which is favourable to both but not obligatory

137. Mycorrhizal association helps trees in obtaining
   a) Nitrate from soil   b) Phosphorus from soil
   c) Sulphate from soil   d) Zinc from soil

138. Mycorrhizal association is an example of
   a) Amensalism   b) Cannabalism
   c) Mutualism   d) Protocooperation

139. Number of individuals surviving to reproductive stage is termed as
a) Fecundity b) Reproductive mortality
c) Net reproductive rate d) Survivourship

140. Nutrient cycling occurs slowly in
a) Corals b) Tropical rain forest
c) Grasslands d) Temperate rain forests

141. On islands the large numbers of endemic species are mainly evolved due to
a) Niche diversification to overcome competition.
b) Generalists species are more common on islands.
c) They are rich in resources.
d) Usually island formation is a time taking process and this provides species more time to evolve.

142. One of the major pollutants implicated in the process of eutrophication of fresh water bodies is
a) Lead b) Mercury
c) Iron d) Phosphorus

143. One of the most important functions of botanical gardens is that
a) They allow ex-situ conservation of germplasm
b) One can observe tropical plants there
c) They provide the natural habitat for wild life
d) They provide a beautiful area for recreation

144. Organisms that produce fewer young at one time and repeat reproduction throughout their life time are
a) Iteroparous and r-selected b) Iteroparous and K-selected
c) Semelparous and r-selected d) Semelparous and k-selected

145. Ozone depletion is frequent on
a) Equators b) Antarctica
c) Himalayas d) Tundra

146. Ozone hole means
a) holes in ozone layer
b) thining of ozone layer
c) damaging effects of ozone in troposphere
d) absence of ozone layer in some parts of stratosphere

147. Ozone protects from
a) Infra-red b) UV rays
c) Heat d) Far red

CSIR (NET/JRF] Exam. June 2005]

148. Periyar National Park is famous for
a) Tiger b) Rhinoceros
c) Elephant d) Chinkara

149. Pest resurgense is
a) Increase in pest population after application of narrow-range pesticides
b) Increase in pest population after application of broad-range pesticides
c) Evolution of pest resistance species after application of pesticides
d) Control of pests by means of IPM

150. Pilots of jets aircraft prefer to fly in the stratosphere because
a) Ozone layer is present in the stratosphere.
b) It is relatively stable and free from weather fluctuations.
c) Temperature is very cold.
d) None of the above.

151. Polar bears have recently been considered as threatened species because of
a) Habitat destruction caused by deforestation
b) Habitat destruction caused of melting of glaciers
c) Increased coldness
d) Lack of food

152. Population growth is the function of
a) Natality, mortality, emigration b) Natality, mortality, immigration
c) Natality, mortality, dispersion d) Natality, mortality

153. Population of plants within a species adapted genetically to a particular habitat but able to cross freely with other plants of the same species is called
a) Ecophene b) Ecad
c) Ecotype d) Ecotone

154. Production of nitrate ions by microorganism is called
a) Biological nitrogen fixation b) Ammonification
c) Denitrification d) Nitrification

155. Which one of the following would be positioned at the top of a typical ecological pyramid?
a) Producers
b) Trophic level with the least numbers
c) Trophic level with the greatest biomass
d) Trophic level with the most energy

156. Pygmy hog, the smallest wild boar in the world is found in
a) Kaziranga National Park b) Kanha National Park
c) Manas National Park d) Corbet National Park

157. Pyramid of energy can never be inverted. It can be explained with the help of
a) Farlow's assumptions on dinosaur physiology.
b) Energy flow in tundra biome.
c) Second law of thermodynamics.
d) All of the above.

158. Pyramid of energy is often seen to be inverted in
a) Tundra b) Tropics
c) Deserts d) Grasslands
[CSIR (NET/JRF) Exam. June 2004]

159. Rainbow is formed in
a) Stratosphere b) Mesosphere
c) Ionosphere d) Troposphere

160. Rajaji National Park is famous for
a) Tiger b) Rhinoceros
c) Elephant d) Musk deer
[CSIR (NET/JRF) Exam. Dec. 2002]

161. Rapid nutrient cycling occurs in
a) Ocean b) Grassland
c) Coral reefs d) Desert

162. Rescue effect is the
a) Increase in diversity in ecotone
b) Prevention of extinction of a species in metapopulation
c) Protective mechanism of a prey
d) Result of character displacement.

163. Resource partitioning does not result in
a) Coexistence b) Speciation
c) Coevolution d) Extinction

164. Resource partitioning pertains to
a) niche specialization b) character displacement
c) increased species diversity d) All of these

165. r-selected species is represented by the equation
a) $\frac{dN}{dt} = rN\left(1 - \frac{N}{K}\right)$ b) $\frac{dN}{dt} = \frac{N}{r}\left(1 - \frac{N}{K}\right)$
c) $\frac{dN}{dt} = rN$ d) $\frac{dN}{dt} = \frac{rN}{(1-K)}$

166. Sariska National Park is situated in
a) Tamil Nadu b) Maharashtra
c) Rajasthan d) Orissa

167. Shanon and Simpson's indexes are related to
a) Numerical taxonomy
b) Biodiversity
c) Environment Impact Assessment
d) Water pollution

168. Some organisms may alter the environment through their behaviour or by virtue of their large collective biomass; ecological view point, these are called
a) Dominant species b) Keystone species
c) Invasive stone species d) Ecosystem engineers

169. Some plants and animals devote energy and resources only to growth and development for and extended period, and then expend huge amounts in a single reproductive effort. Which statement is not correct for them?
a) They are better competitor b) They follow semelparity
c) They are r-strategist d) They follow J-shaped growth curve
[CSIR (NET/JRF) Exam. Dec. 2006]

170. Sometimes a group of sympatric species, often from different taxa, share a common warning pattern, this phenomenon is known as
a) Adaptive radiation b) Coevolution
c) Competitive exclusion d) None of the above

171. Species diversity between two communities is called as
a) Alfa diversity b) Beta diversity
c) Gamma diversity d) Pattern diversity
[CSIR (NET/JRF) Exam. Dec. 2005]

172. Species diversity cannot be measured by
a) Brillion index b) Simpson's index
c) Shanon's index d) Sex index

173. Species extinction is more frequent on islands because
a) Small population size. b) Less variation in habitat.
c) Inbreeding depression d) All of the above.

174. Species richness can be measured by
a) Shanon index b) Grieger Mullar Counter
c) Survivourship curves d) None of the above

175. Spring over turn and fall over turn are common phenomenon in some larger lakes. It is essential
   a) for nutrient cycling
   b) to eliminate polluted water from the system.
   c) to maintain temperature constant.
   d) for mixing of nutrients and oxygen to reach them at deep water.

176. Stem nodules in Sesbania rostrata are formed due to the presence of
   a) Sinorhizobium b) Bradyrhizobium
   c) Azorhizobium d) Mesorhizobium

177. Supersonic aircraft may contribute massively to reduce the level of atmospheric ozone because it produces
   a) Methane b) CFCs
   c) Ozone d) Nitric oxide

178. Taxidermy (skin trade) is one of reasons of
   a) Loss of biodiversity b) Origin/generation of diversity
   c) Mass extinction d) Natural extinction

179. Taxonomy, in which every character is of equal weight in creating natural taxa is
   a) Chemotaxonomy b) Morphotaxonomy
   c) Numerical taxonomy d) Molecular taxonomy

[CSIR (NET/JRF) Exam. Dec. 2006]

180. The 'J' shaped population growth curve is related to
   a) Unstable environment b) Stable environment
   c) High species composition d) Low species composition

181. The "spring bloom" of the phytoplankton in temperate freshwater lakes is caused by
   a) Eutrophication b) Salinization
   c) Turbulence d) Thermal stratification

182. The amount of energy reaching a higher trophic level is determined by
   a) Net primary production
   b) Net primary production and the efficiencies with which food energy is converted to biomass
   c) gross primary production
   d) gross primary production and the efficiencies with which food energy is converted to biomass

183. The best definition of biodiversity is variability
   a) Within species only
   b) Between species only

c) Both within and between species
d) Within species, between species and of ecosystem

184. The biokinetic zone generally lies between
a) 0-45°C b) 20-45°C
c) 0-35°C d) 10-45°C

185. The burning of fossil fuels have severely affected
a) Sulphur cycle b) Phosphorus cycle
c) Carbon cycle d) Nitrogen cycle

186. The concept of r or K selection was given by
a) Dobzansky b) Gause
c) Arthur and Wilson d) Odum

187. The correlation between species richness and productivity is
a) Species richness directly increases as increase in productivity
b) Species richness has inverse relation to productivity
c) Species richness and productivity are independent
d) Species richness is maximum at intermediate levels of productivity

188. The entire range of factors an organism is able to exploit in its environment is its
a) Community b) Realized niche
c) Fundamental niche d) Ecological release

189. The first National Park established in India was
a) Rajaji National Park b) Jim Corbett National Park
c) Gir National Park d) Kaziranga National Park

190. The genetic relatedness between an uncle and his nephew in an outbreed human population is expected to be
a) 1.0 b) 0.75
c) 0.50 d) 0.25

191. The growth of population in the logistic growth model is maximum, when
a) It is less than carrying capacity
b) It is equal to the carrying capacity
c) It is greater than carrying capacity
d) It is exactly half the carrying capacity

[CSIR (NET/JRF) Exam. June. 2005]

192. The headquarters of IUCN is located in
a) England b) Belgium
c) Switzerland d) New York

193. The highest percentage of endemics in the world is found at
a) Hawaian Islands b) New Caledonia

c) New Zealand d) Galapagos Islands

194. -diversity is defined as diversity
   a) Between two different ecosystem
   b) Overall large area
   c) Within a sampling area
   d) Total species richness

195. The inherent capacity of an organism to increase in numbers under ideal condition is known as
   a) Growth rate b) Biotic potential
   c) Reproductive potential d) Population explosion

196. The intrinsic rate of population increase is high
   a) For a population consisting of more juveniles
   b) For a population consisting of more reproductive females
   c) For a population consisting of more reproductive males
   d) For a population consisting of more senescent individuals

197. The largest and most continuous region of rain forest in the world is in the
   a) Amazon basin of South America
   b) Southeast Asia
   c) West Africa
   d) Northeastern coast of Australia

198. The largest biogeographical region of India is
   a) Western Ghats b) Gangetic Plain
   c) Deccan Peninsula d) Eastern Himalayas

199. The largest extinction event in the history of life occurred during which geological period?
   a) Jurassic b) Cretaceous
   c) Permian d) Precambrian

200. The largest food chain can be recognized in which of the following ecosystems?
   a) Deserts b) Lakes
   c) Open ocean d) Savanna

201. The largest number of species are to be found amongst
   a) Beetles b) Flowering plants
   c) Fungi d) Birds

202. The logistic population growth model, describes a population's growth when

an upper limit to growth is assumed. This upper limit to growth is known as the populations' ________, and as N gets larger, dN/dt________.

a) Biotic potential/increases
b) Biotic potential/decreases
c) Carrying capacity/increases
d) Carrying capacity/decreases

203. The major pollution in lake by effluents coming from cloth industry containing high detergents is

a) Phosphates
b) Nitrates
c) Silicate
d) Sulphates

[CSIR (NET/JRF) Exam. Dec. 2004]

204. The maximum number of individuals of a species that can be accommodated in a particular patch of habitat is known as the

a) Ecological amplitude
b) Carrying capacity
c) Niche saturation
d) Fecundity

205. The most drastic extinction event occurred during

a) Ordovician
b) Cretaceous
c) Permian
d) Devonian

[CSIR (NET/JRF) Exam. June. 2008]

206. The most productive ecosystem in the biosphere is

a) Estuary
b) Open ocean
c) Coral reef
d) Tundra

207. The net primary productivity is highest in

a) Tropical forests
b) Temperate forests
c) Open oceans
d) Marshes

208. The number of "hottest spots" of diversity around the globe are

a) 10
b) 25
c) 33
d) 8

209. The number of links in a food chain depends upon the

a) number of organism in an ecosystem
b) number of producers in an ecosystem
c) length of food chain in an ecosystem
d) length of day

210. The only animal in the world that has four horns is a/an

a) Deer
b) Antelope
c) Wild buffalo
d) Wild sheep

211. The only Floating National Park is situated in
a) West Bengal b) Manipur
c) Kerala d) Nagaland

212. The only non leguminous plant in which Rhizobia is found as symbiont is
a) Casuarina b) Rice
c) Sugarcane d) *Parasponia*

213. The organism that produce very large numbers of offspring but provide little or no care have
a) Type I survivourship curve
b) Type II survivourship curve
c) Type III survivourship curve
d) Both (a) and (c) **[CSIR (NET/JRF) Exam. Dec. 2007]**

214. The organism with high parental care will also show
a) Semelparity b) Iteroparity
c) Maturation at early stage d) Small sized offsprings
[CSIR (NET/JRF) Exam. Dec. 2006]

215. The phenomenon known as character displacement is associated with
a) Allopatric speciation b) Sympatric speciation
c) Competitive exclusion d) Succession

216. The principal source of water is
a) rainfall b) ground water
c) ocean d) rivers and streams

217. The rich diversity of large, grazing animals and their predators is found in
a) Tropical rain forest. b) Savanna
c) Temperate forests d) Cold & hot deserts.

218. The second most severe mass extinction next to the Permian occurred at the end of
a) Devonian b) Triassic
c) Ordovician d) Cretaceous/Tertiary

219. The species replacement that occurs over very large geographic region is described as
a) Alpha diversity b) Beta diversity
c) Gamma diversity d) Point diversity

220. The survivorship curve for Hydra is
a) Convex b) Concave
c) Diagonal d) Horizontal

221. The symbiotic relationship in which one partner receives benefit while the other is unaffected is called
   a) Mutualism b) Commensalism
   c) Parasitism d) None of the above

222. The tallest trees in the world are found in
   a) Tropical rain forest. b) Temperate rain forest.
   c) Tropical seasonal forest. d) Temperate evergreen forest.

223. The taxa in danger of extinction is termed as
   a) Extinct b) Rare
   c) Vulnerable d) Endangered

224. There are three groups of species which show J-shaped growth curve, S-shaped growth curve and diagonal growth curve respectively. Which of these groups of species will have the highest fitness?
   a) group of species showing S-shaped growth curve
   b) group of species showing J-shaped growth curve
   c) group of species showing diagonal growth curve
   d) All groups of species will have equal fitness

225. Thermal stratification is characteristic of
   a) Larger temperate lakes. b) Larger tropical lakes.
   c) Rivers and streams. d) Algal beds and reefs.

226. Tiger project is a holistic approach for the conservation of
   a) Ecosystem b) Tiger
   c) Deer d) Plant communities

227. To conserve whole "ecological region" which of the following is more efficient?
   a) Project Lion b) Project Elephant
   c) Ramsar sites d) Biosphere reserve

[CSIR (NET/JRF) Exam. June. 2008]

228. Transducers of ecosystem are
   a) Fungi b) Plants and Microbes
   c) Animals d) All of the above

229. Tropical rain forests are richest in diversity among all the terrestrial biomes because
   a) Location on the globe is favoured by solar radiation and they receive very little light throughout the year.
   b) Their soil is leached due to high rainfall.
   c) High productivity, spatial heterogeneity and stable environment is favourable for speciation

d) These forests face climatic variations and very harsh changes in climates with Increasing rate of speciation.

230. Tropical rainforest cover only 7% of land area but are the richest in biodiversity because
a) They are stable ecosystem
b) They experience intermediate disturbances
c) They experience climatic variations
d) All of the above

231. Twelve mega diversity countries together hold upto
a) 80% of the diversity b) 70% of the diversity
c) 60% of the diversity d) 50% of the diversity

232. Two important hot spots of India are
a) Eastern Himalayas and Western Ghats
b) North Himalayas and Western Ghats
c) Eastern Himalayas and Shivalik
d) Upper Gangetic Plain **[CSIR (NET/JRF) Exam. Dec. 2005]**

233. Type III survivourship curve is applicable to
a) Fruit flies
b) Birds
c) Lizards
d) Pelagic marine fishes **[CSIR (NET/JRF) Exam. Dec. 2007]**

234. What is not true about coral reefs?
a) They resemble rain forests in their high species diversity
b) They generally inhabit nutrient rich waters
c) Loss of their symbiotic algae cause coral bleaching
d) Geologically, they are associated with oil repositories

235. What would happen if there were no green house gases in the atmosphere?
a) The Earth's temperature would become zero
b) The Earth's temperature would become very less than zero
c) There would be no global warming
d) The Earth's temperature would remain constant

236. What would happen if we release the high BOD water into fresh lake?
a) Number of organisms will decrease
b) Number of organisms will increase
c) Amount of dissolved oxygen will decrease
d) No effects

237. When a large population suddenly experiences a severe, temporary reduction in size for whatever reasons, the phenomenon may results

a) Genetic drift b) Founder effect
c) Inbreeding depression d) Bottleneck effect

[CSIR (NET/JRF) Exam. Dec. 2006]

238. When a population is allowed to grow in a limited environment it shows

a) Exponential growth b) Logistic growth
c) Geometric growth d) None of these

239. When a species expands its niche in response to the removal of a competitor, the phenomenon is called

a) Antibiosis b) Mutual inhibition
c) Competitive release d) Resource partitioning

240. When amount of resources available to a trophic level controls the productivity of that trophic level, the phenomenon is called

a) top-down control b) bottom-up control
c) Antagonism d) Allelopathy

241. When evolution of an organism is coordinated with the evolution of another organism the phenomenon is called

a) Mimicry b) Coevolution
c) Adaptive radiation d) Mutualism

242. When individuals in a population experience very high juvenile mortality their survivourship curve appears as:

a) Convex b) Concave
c) Diagonal d) Zig-zag

243. When new male lions take over a pride, they often engage in infanticide. The reason attributed for the same is

a) The females of the pride are brought to estrous by killing of suckling infants
b) The infants interfere with hunting
c) They hate the former males of the pride and therefore kill their infants
d) To prove their dominance in the pride

244. When organisms are restricted to certain area and they are found nowhere else they are called

a) Cosmopolitan b) Sibling species
c) Ecotypes d) Endemic

245. When predatory populations control the diversity of prey species the ecological term used is
a) bottom up control b) top down control
c) escalation d) coevolution

246. When two or more organisms use a portion of the same resource simultaneously, it may result in all of the following except
a) Niche overlap b) Competition
c) Migration d) Coexistence

247. When two similar species co-exist in a dynamic equilibrium, it is usually through the
a) Competitive exclusion b) Character displacement
c) Resource partitioning d) Intraspecific competition

248. When two species live in the same niche, it is called
a) Hyper volume niche b) Niche width
c) Niche overlap d) Population outbreak

249. Where would you expect to find the highest biomass of mammals?
a) Tropical savannas b) Tropical rainforests
c) Tropical deserts d) Tropical mountains

250. Which group of organisms are generally used to name a community
a) Plant b) Animals
c) Fungi d) None of the above

251. Which of the following animals may face extinction due to inability to switch over to alternative food
a) Red panda b) Cheetah
c) Asiatic Lion d) Elephant

252. Which of the following biomes is an example of aqua-terrestrial ecotonal biome?
a) Wetland b) Grassland
c) Estuaries d) Lakes

253. Which of the following can be considered as a "keystone" species in ecological terms?
a) Sandalwood tree b) Teak tree
c) Fig tree d) Pine tree

254. Which of the following can be regarded as a major "greenhouse gas"?
a) Ozone b) Carbon monoxide
c) Methane d) Water vapor

255. Which of the following can not be resultant of competitive exclusion?

a) Migration
b) Character displacement
c) Speciation
d) Formation of metapopulation

256. Which of the following can not favour coexistence?
a) Niche differentiation
b) Character displacement
c) Ecological release
d) Unlimited resource

257. Which of the following can not result in co-evolution?
a) +/-
b) +/+
c) -/-
d) + / 0

258. Which of the following characterises climax stage of succession ?
a) Linear food chain
b) High rate of community production
c) High resilience
d) Narrow niche and speciation

[CSIR (NET/JRF) Exam. June. 2008]

259. Which of the following does not eat dead matter?
a) Detritivore
b) Saprophytes
c) Sarcophagous
d) Coprophagous

260. Which of the following does not govern distribution of biodiversity?
a) Spatial heterogeneity
b) Competition
c) Productivity
d) High disturbances

261. Which of the following ecosystem is characteristic of the alpine Himalayas?
a) Coniferous forests
b) Meadows
c) Evergreen forests
d) Deciduous forests

262. Which of the following ecosystems has the nutrient rich soil
a) Tropical rain forest
b) Temperate forest soil
c) Desert soil
d) Tundra soil

263. Which of the following ecosystems have the highest productivity?
a) Temperate deciduous forest
b) Tropical rain forest
c) Estuary
d) Open ocean

264. Which of the following factors does not determine the growth rate of a population?
a) The population's sex ratio
b) The species generation time
c) The age structure of the population
d) The optimal temperature at which an organism can reproduce.

265. Which of the following factors is not involved in increasing biodiversity?
a) Spatial heterogeneity
b) Intermediate disturbance
c) High productivity
d) Global warming

266. Which of the following habitats despite of perpetual cold and continual darkness exhibits great diversity.
a) Lake bottom b) River bottom
c) Ocean floor d) Dense forests

267. Which of the following has been listed as one of the global biodiversity hot spot?
a) Chilka lake b) Silent valley
c) Western ghats d) Eastern ghats

268. Which of the following has richest soil?
a) Prairie grassland. b) Coniferous forest.
c) Savanna grassland. d) Temperate forests.

269. Which of the following holds a place between the deer and the antelopes?
a) Sambhar b) Barasingha
c) Black buck d) Musk Deer

270. Which of the following is a character of mature community?
a) P/R> 1
b) Broad niche, high entropy and high species diversity
c) P/R< 1
d) Predominantly detritus food chain

271. Which of the following is a permafrost biome?
a) Temperate grassland b) Taiga
c) Tundra d) All of the above

272. Which of the following is called as "Bird Continent"?
a) North America b) South America
c) Australia d) Africa

273. Which of the following is correct ?
a) High disturbance high diversity
b) Mild disturbance high diversity
c) No disturbance high diversity
d) Low disturbance high diversity

[CSIR (NET/JRF) Exam. June 2005]

274. Which of the following is currently considered as the leading cause of extinction?
a) Overexploitation of species
b) Habitat loss
c) Competition from introduced species
d) Pollution

275. Which of the following is not a characteristic feature of K-selected species?
    a) High biotic potential b) Logistic growth
    c) More prone to extinction d) Large body size

276. Which of the following is NOT a factor which increases biodiversity?
    a) High productivity
    b) More heterogeneity
    c) High disturbance
    d) Stable environment and climatic variations.

277. Which of the following is not a monogamous bird?
    a) Swans b) Eagles
    c) Geese d) Praire chickens

278. Which of the following is not a secondary pollutant?
    a) Ozone b) PAN
    c) Smog d) SO_2

279. Which of the following is not an attribute of hotspots of biodiversity?
    a) Areas extremely rich in species
    b) Have high endemism
    c) Species are under constant threat
    d) High extinction rate

280. Which of the following is not an endangered?
    a) Indian Python b) Indian wild as
    c) Indian Pangolin d) Indian Cheetah

281. Which of the following is not an example of a density dependent effect on population growth?
    a) An extremely cold winter
    b) Competition for food resources
    c) Stress-related illness associated with overcrowding
    d) Competition for nesting sites.

282. Which of the following is not an example of ex situ conservation?
    a) Seed banks b) Cryopreservation
    c) Botanical gardens d) National parks

283. Which of the following is not an example of palaeoendemic?
    a) Ginkgo biloba b) Piper nigrum
    c) Sequoiadendron giganteum d) Degeneria vitiensis

284. Which of the following is not an exotic weed?

a) Eichhornia b) Lantana
c) Xanthium d) Chenopodium

285. Which of the following is not characteristic of r-strategists?
a) High fecundity b) Short life span
c) Small body size d) Specialist niche

286. Which of the following is not cryoprotectant?
a) Dimethyl Sulphoxide b) Proline
c) Sucrose d) Alanine

287. Which of the following is not responsible for decrease in biodiversity?
a) Habitat loss and fragmentation.
b) Invasive species.
c) Global climate change.
d) Adaptive radiation.

288. Which of the following is not the characteristic feature of K-strategist species?
a) Large body size. b) Low birth rate.
c) Logistic growth. d) High juvenile death rate.

289. Which of the following is not threatened species
a) Critically endangered b) Endangered
c) Vulnerable d) Extinct

290. Which of the following is not true for smaller animals but true for larger animals?
a) Short generation time b) Large clutch
c) Later stage matureness d) Exponential growth

291. Which of the following is the most fragile ecosystem?
a) Open ocean b) Desert
c) Rain forest d) Tundra

292. Which of the following is the most stable ecosystem?
a) Forest b) Grassland
c) Ocean d) Desert

293. Which of the following is the second most important factor next to the habitat destruction, which is responsible for species extinction?
a) Over consumption b) Introduction of invasive species
c) Pollution d) Climate change

294. Which of the following marine ecosystem is highest in biodiversity?
a) Coastal areas b) Mangrooves
c) Coral reefs d) Estuary

[CSIR (NET/JRF) Exam. Dec. 2005]

295. Which of the following not severely affected species extinction?
a) Habitat destruction b) Invasive species
c) Over exploitation d) Environmental pollution
[CSIR (NET/JRF) Exam. Dec. 2007]

296. Which of the following oxide of nitrogen catalyzes the formation of photochemical smog?
a) Nitrogen dioxide b) Nitrous oxide
c) Nitric oxide d) Nitrite and Nitrate

297. Which of the following pairs is not correct
a) Rhinoceros - Kaziranga b) Ranthambore - Bengal Tiger
c) Bandipur - Elephant d) Rajaji - Hoolock Gibbon
[CSIR (NET/JRF) Exam. June. 2007]

298. Which of the following plant community is commonly referred to as "kidney" of the ecosystem?
a) Coral reefs b) Mangroves
c) Estuaries d) Amazon valley forests

299. Which of the following provides an example of an inverted pyramid of numbers?
a) Prey-Predators
b) Herbivore
c) Primary Carnivore-Secondary Carnivore
d) Host-Parasite

300. Which of the following requires silica for survival?
a) Coral reefs b) Cyanobacteria
c) Diatoms d) Molluscs
[CSIR (NET/JRF) Exam. June 2007]

301. Which of the following show predator-prey
a) 0 - b) - -
c) + - d) + +

302. Which of the following show protocooperation?
a) + - b) + 0
c) + + d) 0 0

303. Which of the following show unlimited and catastrophic environment?
a) Logistic growth and J-shaped growth curve in a population
b) Geometric growth and S-shaped growth curve in a population
c) Logistic growth and S-shaped growth curve in a population
d) Exponential growth and J-shaped growth curve in a population.

304. Which of the following shows degree of change in species composition between sites or communities or along gradients?
   a) α-diversity b) β-diversity
   c) γ-diversity d) Epsilon diversity

305. Which of the following statement is NOT correct for deep sea vent communities?
   a) They are islands of warmth in oceans.
   b) they support unique communities, rich in endemic species.
   c) they may have been the birth place of all life on earth.
   d) These are the only communities of deep ocean which can trap solar radiation.

306. Which of the following statements is not correct for coral reefs?
   a) They are the oldest community on Earth
   b) They are rich in diversity
   c) They are most productive
   d) Their contribution in global production is highest

307. Which of the following statements is not correct?
   a) Biodiversity is maximum in those ecosystems which face intermediate disturbance.
   b) Island populations are more prone to extinction.
   c) Nutrient cycling is very fast in coral reefs.
   d) Open ocean has very poor productivity because of "fertilization effect".

308. Which of the following statements is not correct?
   a) Bottlenecked populations are more prone to extinction
   b) Species exhibiting allozyme variation are more threatened
   c) The highest species extinction occurs on Islands
   d) Bottlenecked populations are poor in genetic diversity

309. Which of the following statements is not correct?
   a) organisms showing pattern I survivourship curve are K-selected.
   b) organisms showing pattern III survivourship curve are less prone to extinction.
   c) organisms showing J-shaped growth curve are opportunistic.
   d) organisms showing S-shaped growth curve are less prone to extinction.

310. Which of the following statements is not correct?
   a) r-selected species follows pattern-I survivorship curve
   b) k-selected species have narrow niche range
   c) r-selected species are semelparous
   d) k-selected species are more prone to extinction

311. Which of the following statements is not correct?
   a) r-selected species are poor competitors
   b) K-selected species are vegetatively very strong
   c) r-selected species tend to disperse well
   d) K-selected species produce more offsprings

312. Which of the following statements is not correct?
   a) r-strategist exceeds carrying capacity of an ecosystem.
   b) Savanna is a grassland with scattered trees.
   c) Desert ecosystems are fragile.
   d) A species is said to be iteroparous if individuals reproduce only one in their lives.

313. Which of the following statements is not correct?
   a) The biodiversity of coral reefs is extraordinary
   b) The tight recycling of nutrients provides coral reefs so biologically diverse
   c) The greatest abundance of corals located closest to the equator
   d) Coral bleaching occurs when corals rapidly increase their numbers

314. Which of the following statements is not correct?
   a) When two species with similar requirement coexist each typically occupies its fundamental niche
   b) Resource partitioning is the outcome of the coevolution of species with extensive but not total-niche overlap
   c) The net transfer of energy between trophic levels is roughly 10%
   d) Ocean is the major sink of CO2

315. Which of the following states of India is richest in rhinoceros population?
   a) Assam   b) Kerala
   c) Madhya Pradesh   d) Uttarakhand

316. Which of the following types of biomes is found in California and in the coastal lands of Mediterranean sea?
   a) Taiga   b) Savanna
   c) Chapparal   d) Temperate deciduous forest

317. Which of the following will be more important ecologically?
   a) + -   b) 0 -
   c) + 0   d) + +

318. Which of the following will not favour extinction of a species?
   a) Trophic specialization   b) High rate of reproduction
   c) K-selection   d) Narrow niche range

319. Which one of the following biogeochemical cycles has both atmospheric

phase and a lithospheric phase

a) Carbon cycle b) Nitrogen cycle
c) Phosphorus cycle d) Sulphur cycle

320. Which one of the following can NOT form coral reef?
a) Cnidaria
b) Coralline red algae and green calcerous algae
c) Foraminifera and mollusks. .
d) Brown algae

321. Which one of the following characters make a species more prone to extinction?
a) High fecundity b) Trophic specialization
c) r-selection d) High dispersal ability

322. Which one of the following factors does not make any contribution to make tropical rain forest most productive of the Earth's biomes?
a) High solar radiation received throughout the year.
b) regular and reliable rainfall.
c) Nutrient rich soil.
d) High rate of decomposition of detritous.

323. Wild Ass are found in
a) Assam b) Gujarat
c) Kerala d) Meghalaya

[CSIR (NET/JRF) Exam. Dec. 2004]

324. Which one of the following has status of a National Park, Biosphere Reserve and a World Heritage site?
a) Nilgiri b) Sundarbans
c) Banarghatta d) Kaziranga **(ICMR 2007)**

325. Which one of the following is NOT a character of healthy population?
a) Maximum number of juveniles
b) High reproductive rates
c) Urn shaped age structure pyramid
d) Early stage maturity

326. _____________ survivorship curves are usually associated with organisms that have high mortality rates in the early stages of life.
a) Type I b) Type III
c) Type II and III d) Type I and II

327. What is the minimum condition needed to prevent a continuously breeding

population from going extinct?

a) r > 0
b) r < 0
c) r = 1
d) r > 1

328. In the Lotka-Voltera competition models, if K2/β < K1 and K1/α > K2, then

a) N1 is eliminated
b) N_2 is eliminated
c) Both species co exist
d) Either species may be eliminated depending on starting conditions

329. Which of the following relationships is not a type of commensalism

a) Phorey
b) Inquilinism
c) Metabiosis
d) VAM

330. Mutual interference between predators tends to

a) Bend the predator isocline to the right
b) Bend the predator isocline to the left
c) Bend the prey isocline to the right
d) Bend the prey isocline to the left

331. Which is a characteristic of species during the later seral stages of succession?

a) Low plant efficiency at low light
b) Small biomass
c) Low species richness
d) Short seed longevity

332. On which type of island would you expect species richness to be greatest?

a) Small, near mainland
b) Small, distant from mainland
c) Large, near mainland
d) Large, distant from mainland

333. The most highly productive terrestrial communities are

a) Forests
b) Grasslands
c) Deserts
d) Tundra

334. In unpolluted areas of tropical oceans, primary productivity is limited most often by

a) N
b) P
c) Fe
d) N, Fe and P

335. A measure of eutrophication is

a) BOD
b) COD
c) DO
d) All of the above

336. Altruism

a) is only possible with reciprocity.
b) is only possible with kin selection.

c) cannot be explained given the way natural selection operates.
d) will only occur when the fitness benefit of a given act is greater than the fitness cost.

337. Which of the following ecosystems has the highest consumption efficiency?
a) Forest
b) Grassland
c) Aquatic ecosystems
d) Deserts

338. The total biomass in an ecosystem at any one point in time is called
a) Gross production
b) Production efficiency
c) Standing crop
d) Net production

339. Which of the following will decompose rapidly?
a) Pine branch (high lignin+ high nitrogen)
b) Pine needle (low nitrogen)
c) Pin-cherry leaf (high nitrogen)
d) Both (a) and (b)

340. The existing average temperature of Earth is
a) + 17ºC +29ºC
b) + 25ºC
c) + 200ºC
d) + 15ºC

341. Which of the following is the least disturbed biome in the world?
a) Tundra
b) Savanna
c) Tropical wet forests
d) Deserts

342. Which of the following can cause the realized niche of a species to be smaller than its fundamental niche?
a) Predation
b) Competition
c) Commensalism
d) Both (a) and (b)

343. When a predator preferentially eats the superior competitor in a pair of competing species
a) the inferior competitor is more likely to go extinct.
b) the superior competitor is more likely to persist.
c) coexistence of the competing species is more likely.
d) None of the above

344. What two factors are most important in biome distribution?
a) Temperature and latitude
b) Rainfall and temperature
c) Latitude and rainfall
d) Temperature and soil type

345. Carrying capacity of a forest is 40 tonnes with 20% in its biomass annually.

For sustainable forestery how much trees can be harvested for timber so that it has minimum effect on forest and can be harvested annually.
a) 8 tonnes
b) 4 tonnes
c) 6 tonnes
d) 20 tonnes

346. Which of the following is characteristic feature of climax community.
a) Simple food chain
b) High resilence
c) High productivity
d) Narrow niche specialization

347. During winters in Tundra when the lake freezes into ice, the temperature of water just beneath the ice would be
a) 0°C
b) -4°C
c) -10°C
d) 4°C

348. From the perspective of females, extra-pair copulations (EPCs)
a) are always disadvantageous to females
b) can be associated with receiving male aid
c) are too rare to affect female fitness
d) can only be of benefit if the EPC male has elaborate secondary sexual traits

349. In a population in which individuals are uniformly distributed
a) The population is probably well below its carrying capacity
b) Natural selection should favor traits that maximize the ability to compete for resources
c) Immigration from the other population is probably keeping the population from going extinct
d) None of the above

350. In which of the following ecosystems, the maximum of primary productivity is consumed by animals?
a) Forests and deserts
b) Freshwater ecosystems
c) Oceanic ecosystems
d) Tundra

351. Selection that lowers an individual's own fitness but enhances that of a relative is known as
a) Altruism
b) Kin selection
c) Inclusive fitness
d) Hamilton's rule

352. In which of the following species interactions realized niche would be greater than fundamental niche?
a) Parasitism
b) Commensalism

c) Amensalism d) Mutualism

353. Which of the following does not follow the theory of natural selection
a) Neutral evolution
b) Genetic drift
c) Hardy-Weinberg population
d) All of the above

354. Which of the following is not applicable for Darwin's finches?
a) Character displacements b) Niche diversion
c) Resource partitioning d) Competitive exclusion

355. Evolutionarily, with which of the following could parental care in animals be associated?
a) Semalparity b) Greater longevity
c) Polygamy d) Smaller clutch size

356. When species have a strong effect on community structure not because of their abundance, but because of the roles they play in their communities, are called
a) Dominant species b) Pioneer species
c) Relic species d) Keystone species

357. Genes that are found in two different species and have arisen from a common ancestral gene are known as
a) Orthologous b) Paralogous
c) Homeologous d) Neologous

358. Competition coefficients describe
a) The effect of one species on the other
b) The predator-prey relationship
c) Effect of competition on natural selection
d) Effect of resources on logistic growth

359. Which of the following contributes maximum to the earth's primary productivity?
a) C_3 plants b) C_4 plants
c) CAM plants d) Both (b) and (c)

360. To measure the dominant species in an ecosystem, preferentially used
a) Simpson index b) Shanon's index
c) Hardy-Weinberg equation d) Lotka-Voltera equation

361. If two species coexist in a stable environment then which of the following does not well define its state

a) Niche complementarity b) Resource partitioning
c) Character displacement d) Ecological release

362. Most fragile community on Earth is
a) Tropical rain forests b) Estuaries
c) Cold-seep communities d) Mangroves

363. Upwelling zone of ocean is present in between the latitude of
a) 10^0 North to 10^0 South
b) $23\frac{1}{2}^0$ North to $23\frac{1}{2}^0$ South
c) 40^0 to 60^0 North and South
d) 0 to 30^0 North and South

364. Marine snow is
a) Dead organic matter in benthic region of ocean.
b) Iceberg in ocean.
c) Chilling of water at night.
d) Ice precipitation at high latitudes.

365. Ecological foot printing is
a) Study of extinct organisms
b) Adverse effects due to consumption of resources
c) Decrease in atmospheric radioactive CO_2
d) Study of fossils

366. Demography is
a) Study of climatic condition of desert.
b) Quantitative study of population.
c) Qualitative study of population.
d) Study of ocean currents.

367. The highest rates of decomposition are under
a) Cold and wet conditions. b) Cold and dry conditions.
c) Warm and wet conditions. d) Warm and dry conditions.

368. Temperature increases with increasing hight in
a) Troposphere b) Stratosphere
c) Mesophere d) None of the above

369. Lotka-Voltera model is based on
a) Interspecific competition
b) Logistic growth equation
c) Explain prey-predatory dynamics
d) All of the above

370. Shannon index is measure of

a) Species richness b) Population
c) Species abundance d) Speciation

371. Which is not the characteristic feature of a species, which are more prone to extinction
a) have high degree of specialization
b) have low reproductive capability
c) have genetic variability
d) have high trophic status

372. Which is the hottest biodiversity hotspots on the earth
a) Himalaya b) Philippines
c) Atlantic forest d) New Zealand

373. Leaf nodules are formed by
a) *Klebsiella* b) *Azorhizobium*
c) *Mesorhizobium loti* d) *Sinorhizobium fredii*

374. Global warming is due to
a) Absorption of UV light by ozone
b) Absorption of IR light by CO_2
c) Absorption of IR light by ozone
d) Absorption of UV light by CO_2

375. Stabilizing selection differs from directional selection because
a) In the former, phenotypic variation is reduced but the average phenotype stays the same, whereas in the latter both the variation and the mean phenotype change.
b) The former requires genetic variation but the latter does not.
c) Intermediate phenotypes are favoured in directional selections.
d) None of the above.

376. During the history of life on Earth
a) There have been major extinction events.
b) Species diversity has steadily increased.
c) Species diversity has stayed relatively constant.
d) Extinction rates have been completely offset by speciation rates.

377. Character displacement
a) Arises through competition and natural selection, favouring divergence in resource use.
b) Arises through competition and natural selection, favouring convergence in resource use.
c) Does not promote speciation.
d) All of the above.

378. Asian brown haze located in the
   a) Troposphere b) Thermosphere
   c) Stratosphere d) Mesosphere

379. Alfalfa is used as biofertilizer due to presence of
   a) *Rhizobium* b) *Sinorhizobium*
   c) *Mesorhizobium* d) *Azorhizobium*

380. CO_2 absorbs
   a) Red light b) Far-red light
   c) Infrared light d) UV light

381. The overall process of nitrogen fixation in bacteria involves
   a) Oxidation of NO_2 b) Reduction of NO_2
   c) Oxidation of NH_3 d) Reduction of N_2

382. Biodegradable plastics are made using which of the following compounds?
   a) Proteins b) Lipids
   c) Poly β-hydroxy alconates d) Alkaloids

[CSIR (NET/JRF) Exam. June 2001]

383. DMSO is a frequently used cryoprotectant. It is obtained from
   a) Marine Fish b) Marine Algae
   c) Chemosynthesis d) Gymnosperms

384. Methemoglobinema in infants is caused by
   a) Nitrate b) Nitrite
   c) Ammonium d) Urea

385. Aquatic primary production was measured using Light-and-Dark Bottle technique. If the initial oxygen concentration was I and the final oxygen concentration in the light bottle was L and that in the dark bottle D, the gross productivity (in terms of oxygen released) is given as
   a) L-I b) I-D
   c) I-L d) L-D

[CSIR (NET/JRF) Exam. Dec. 2011]

386. Which of the following groups of species are typical of grassland habitats in India
   a) Black buck, wolf, great Indian bustard, lesser florican
   b) Spotted deer, dhole, peacock, finch-lark
   c) Sambar, tiger, paradise fly catcher
   d) Otter, cormorant, darter, pelican **[CSIR (NET/JRF) Exam. Dec. 2011]**

387. The Hutchinsonian concept of ecological niche is based on
   a) microhabitat occupied
   b) multidimensional hypervolume

c) role played in the ecosystem
d) a combination of role played and microhabitat occupied

[CSIR (NET/JRF) Exam. Dec. 2011]

388. A specialist species has a
a) wider niche and high efficiency of niche utilization
b) narrower niche and high efficiency of niche utilization
c) wider niche and low efficiency of niche utilization
d) narrower niche and low efficiency of niche utilization

[CSIR (NET/JRF) Exam. Dec. 2011]

389. Which of the following is NOT a physiological characteristic of early successional plants?
a) High respiration rate b) Inhibition by far-red light
c) High transpiration rate d) Low photosynthetic rate

[CSIR (NET/JRF) Exam. Dec. 2011]

390. Wetlands are conserved internationally through an effort called as
a) Basel Convention b) Rio Convention
c) Montreal Convention d) Ramsar Convention

[CSIR (NET/JRF) Exam. Dec. 2011]

391. A much greater proportion of energy fixed by autotrophs is transferred to the herbivore level in the open ocean ecosystem than in a forest ecosystem because
a) aquatic autoptrophs are small.
b) aquatic herbivores are more efficient feeders.
c) terrestrial autotrophs are less efficient feeders.
d) terrestrial autotrophs have more indigestible tissues.

[CSIR (NET/JRF) Exam. June 2011]

392. Which of the following is a characteristic of an early seral community?
a) Narrow niche specialization.
b) High species diversity.
c) Low community production.
d) Open mineral cycling. **[CSIR (NET/JRF) Exam. June 2011]**

393. Following figure shows McArthur and Wilson's equilibrium model of biota on a single island. In this figure, terms A, B, C and D in order are
a) extinction, immigration, equilibrium number of species, size of species pool.
b) immigration, extinction, equilibrium number of species, size of species pool.
c) extinction, immigration, size of species pool, equilibrium number of species.

d) immigration, extinction, size of species pool, equilibrium number of species. **[CSIR (NET/JRF) Exam. June 2011]**

394. In an altruistic act, if a donor sacrifices 'C' offspring which helps the recipient to gain 'B' offspring and the donor is related to the recipient by a coefficient, under which condition would kin selection favour this altruistic trait?

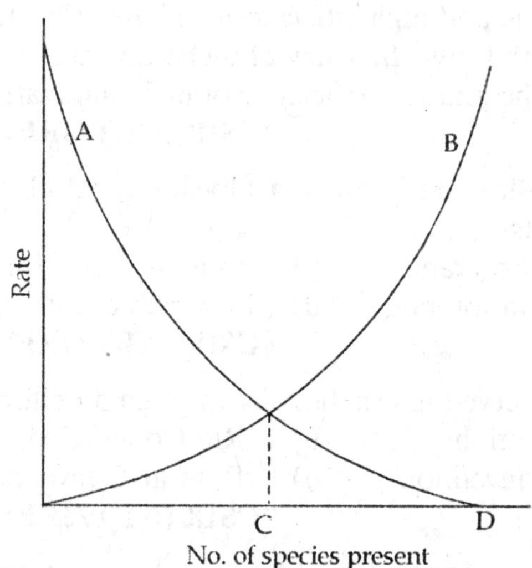

a) B > C.
b) B > γC.
c) γB - C = 0.
d) B - C > 0.

[CSIR (NET/JRF) Exam. June 2011]

395. The most commonly used method of estimating primary productivity of a pond involves measurement of the amount of
a) CO_2 utilized.
b) autotroph biomass.
c) oxygen released
d) organic carbon.

[CSIR (NET/JRF) Exam. June 2011]

396. One life history trait that is not characteristic of very small sized organisms is
a) delayed age at first reproduction.
b) earlier age at first reproduction.
c) high population growth rate.
d) short lifespan. **[CSIR Model Paper 2011]**

397. Which of the following statement is the most appropriate example of character displacement?
a) Two related species depending on the same prey species avoid competition by feeding at different times of the day.
b) The body sizes of two related species are very similar when they are

allopatric, but in geographical areas of sympatry, one species is significantly smaller than the other.

c) The food niche of a species is generally wider in the absence of competing species than in their presence.

d) Closely related species can coexist if their densities are regulated by a predator. **[CSIR Model Paper 2011]**

398. In a population growing logistically and approaching Carrying Capacity (K), the change in density (N) per unit time (dN/dt) is maximum when N equals to

a) K2 b) K/2.

c) K. d) K. **[CSIR Model Paper 2011]**

399. The losses of ozone over Arctic are significantly lower than that over Antarctica because

a) polar vortex over Arctic is not as tight as over Antarctic.

b) Arctic stratosphere warms slower in the spring.

c) concentration of chlorine in the atmosphere over Arctic is less than over Antarctic.

d) freezing of NO_2 and CH_4 are slower over Arctic than over Antarctic. **[CSIR Model Paper 2011]**

400. Which of the following species replacement sequence depicts tolerance model of community succession?

[CSIR Model Paper 2011]

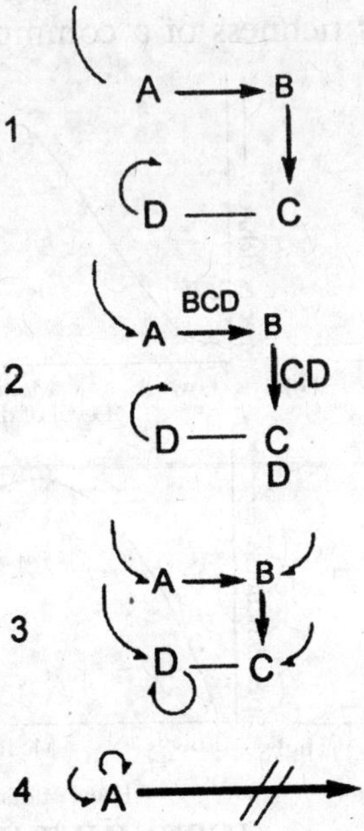

Part C

1. The genetic relatedness (r) of an individual to his nephew is 0.25. The alleles that cause uncles to care for nephews will spread, according to Hamilton's Rule, only if the fitness benefit is
   a) equal to the cost of care
   b) more than the cost of care by 25%
   c) double the cost of care
   d) four times the cost of care **[CSIR (NET/JRF) Exam. Dec. 2011]**
2. Which of the following is NOT true for a critically endangered species?
   a) Reduction of population breeding ability due to increased relatedness through the action of incompatibility mechanisms in plants or behavioural difficulties in animals.
   b) The individuals of the species which have declined to low numbers are still a genetically open system.
   c) Loss of some alleles from the species causing loss of genetic diversity with consequent inability to respond rapidly to selection.
   d) Expression of deleterious alleles and increased homozygosity increases mortality of young, and inbreeding depression leads to reduced offspring fitness. **[CSIR (NET/JRF) Exam. Dec. 2011]**
3. Which of the following graphs illustrates the current consensus on the role of disturbance on the species richness of a community?

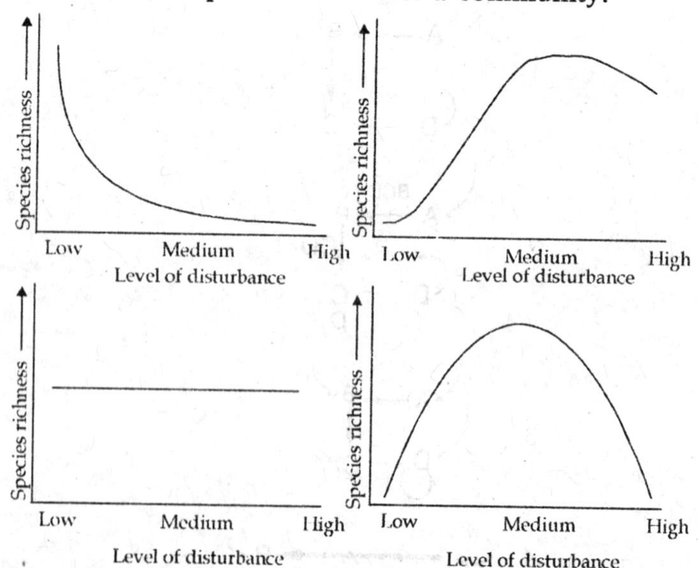

[CSIR (NET/JRF) Exam. Dec. 2011]

4. Suppose you discovered a new species about which you know only two facts: it is small-sized (<10cm) and short-lived (<20d). Which of the following reproductive strategies is most likely to be true for this species?
   a) Breeds early and more than once in life and produces large number of small-sized offspring
   b) Breeds late and only once in life and produces large number of small-sized offspring
   c) Breeds early and only once in life and produces large number of small-sized offspring
   d) Breeds early and only once in life and produces a small number of large-sized offspring **[CSIR (NET/JRF) Exam. Dec. 2011]**

5. Autotrophs in the aquatic ecosystem, unlike their counterparts in the terrestrial ecosystem, are mostly microscopic and very low in indigestible (to the herbivores) matter. This explains the fact that compared to the terrestrial ecosystem, in the aquatic ecosystem
   a) Productivity/Biomass ratios are higher and energy transfer rates to higher trophic levels are faster.
   b) Productivity/Biomass ratios are lower and the energy transfer rates to higher trophic level are slower.
   c) Productivity/Biomass ratios are lower and the energy transfer rate to higher trophic levels are faster
   d) Productivity/Biomass ratios are higher and the energy transfer rate to higher trophic levels are slower **[CSIR (NET/JRF) Exam. Dec. 2011]**

6. Ecological compression differs from character displacement in that it operates on a
   a) shorter timescale and does not involve heritable change.
   b) longer timescale and does not involve heritable change.
   c) shorter timescale and involves heritable change.
   d) longer timescale and involves heritable change.
   [CSIR (NET-JRF) Exam. Dec. 2011]

7. Gause's 'Competitive exclusion' principle states that two species with identical niches cannot coexist indefinitely. Which of the following statements is the most appropriate regarding the validity of the principle?
   a) It depends on how one defines niche.
   b) There are in nature many instances of continued coexistence of closely related species.
   c) The principle is universally true.
   d) It does not predict the outcome where both the species are equally strong competitors. **[CSIR (NET/JRF) Exam. June 2011]**

8. According to MacArthur and Wilson's equilibrium theory, which of the following is true?
   a) Larger islands and islands closer to continent are expected to have more species than smaller and isolated islands.
   b) Smaller islands and islands far from the continent are expected to have more species than larger and isolated islands.
   c) Smaller islands and islands closer to the continent are expected to have more species than far away smaller and isolated islands.
   d) More species are expected on all islands irrespective of their size and distance from the continent. **[CSIR (NET/JRF) Exam. June 2011]**

9. The graph below shows the relationships of per capita population growth rate (r). fecundity (b) and age at first reproduction (a) in an animal species.

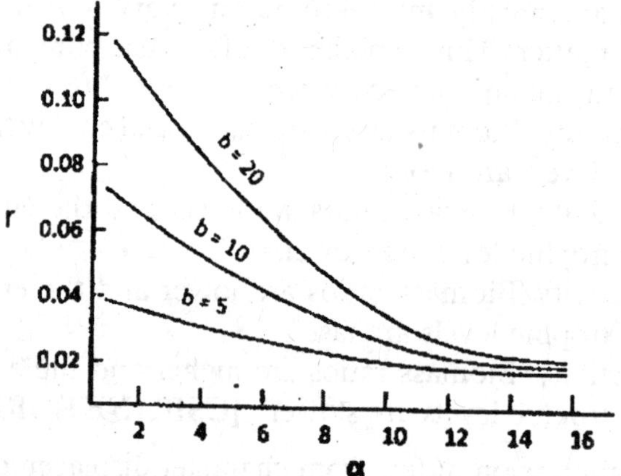

What is the most important conclusion to be drawn from the graph?
   a) The later the age of first reproduction, the lower is the population growth rate achieved.
   b) The population growth rate decreases as first reproduction is postponed to a later stagsssse, regardless of the fecundity.
   c) At any, the higher the fecundity, the higher is the population growth rate achieved.
   d) As the age at first reproduction is postponed further, the benefits of increasing fecundity on the population growth rate become progressively negligible. **[CSIR (NET/JRF) Exam. June 2011]**

10. Primary production in aquatic ecosystem is measured using Light-and-Dark-Bottle technique. In this method, as an indirect measure of photosynthetic production, dissolved oxygen concentration of the pond water enclosed in a BOD bottle is measured initially (I) and after a fixed duration of incubation in a light bottle (L) and a dark bottle (D). Then, the gross and net primary

productions are estimated as

a) (L-D) and (L-I), respectively.
b) (L-I) and (L-D), respectively.
c) (L-I) and (I-D), respectively.
d) (L-D) and (I-D), respectively. **[CSIR (NET/JRF) Exam. June 2011]**

11. In a lake ecosystem, bottom-up effects (B) refer to control of a lower trophic levelby the higher trophic levels and top-down effects (T) refer to the opposite. In a lake with three trophic levels-Phytoplankton (P), Zooplankton (Z) and primary Carnivore (C),
a) P and C are controlled by B, and Z is controlled by T.
b) P, Z and C are all controlled by T.
c) P is controlled by B, Z is controlled by T and C is controlled by B.
d) P is controlled by T, Z is controlled by B and C is controlled by T.

[CSIR (NET/JRF) Exam. June 2011]

12. In Galapagos Islands study of Darwins finches, different species seem to segregate based on resource factors, such as location of prey items. This differentiation among the niches of these finches is known as
a) Competitive exclusion b) Resource partitioning
c) Character displacement d) Proportional similarity

13. Which of the following is the correct order of mass extinctions according to percent of species extinct?
a) Permian > Devonian > Ordovician
b) Ordovician > Permian > Devonian
c) Devonian > Ordovician > Permian
d) Permian > Ordovician > Devonian

14. Which of the following statements is NOT correct?
a) Assimilation efficiency depends on the quality of food eaten and the physiological efficiency of the consumer
b) Carnivores assimilation efficiencies are higher than herbivores
c) Aquatic herbivores have higher assimilation efficiencies than terrestrial herbivores
d) Trophic-level transfer efficiencies appears to average around 30%

15. Which of the following is the correct order of green house gases according to their contribution in global warming?
a) Water vapor > CO_2 > N_2O > CH_4 > CFCs
b) CO_2 > water vapor > CH_4 > N_2O > CFCs
c) CH_4 > N_2O > CO_2 > CFCs > water vapor
d) CO_2 > CH_4 > water vapor > N_2O > CFCs

16. Which of the following is NOT true for the equilibrium model of island biogeography?
    a) Larger islands have more species than smaller islands.
    b) The species richness of an island is determined by colonization and extinction.
    c) Smaller islands have lower rates of extinction.
    d) Islands closer to the mainland will have higher colonization rates.
17. Which of the following statement is incorrect?
    a) Logistic growth is density dependent growth.
    b) Population will experience a positive growth rate when the population size exceeds the carrying capacity.
    c) Growth rate approaches zero if population approaches K.
    d) In logistic growth, the rate of population growth is slowed as population size increases.
18. In the evolution of life histories of populations living in uncertain and catastrophic environments, natural selection should favour
    a) Earlier age at maturity and low fecundity
    b) Earlier age at maturity and high fecundity
    c) Later age at maturity and high fecundity
    d) Later age at maturity and low fecundity

[CSIR (NET/JRF) Exam. June 2001]

19. Tropical semievergreen forests are found in the region having rainfall
    1. > 3000 mm. 2. 2000 - 2500 mm.
    3. 1200-2500 mm. 4. 800-1200 mm.

[CSIR Model Paper 2011]

20. Complete the following sentence using options given below the sentence as a, b, c, d and e.
    "Species are critically endangered when it is not endangered but is facing ___c___ risk of extinction in the wild in the ____d____ future".
    (a) high
    (b) very high
    (c) extremely high
    (d) near
    (e) immediate
    a) a, a b) b, c
    c) c, e d) c, d

[CSIR Model Paper 2011]

21. Which one of the following trait set characterizes best a r selected species?
 a) Usually a type III survivorship curve, short life span and density dependent mortality
 b) Usually a type I survivorship curve, short life span and density dependent mortality
 c) Usually a type I survivorship curve, long life span and density independent mortality
 d) Usually a type III survivorship curve, short life span and density independent mortality **[CSIR Model Paper 2011]**

22. The following graphs show the population growth of two species P and Q, each growing either alone (a) or in the presence of other species (b).

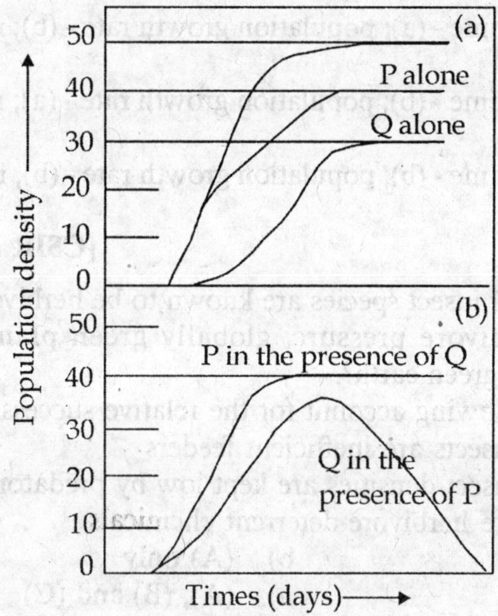

The most important conclusion to be drawn from the graph is
 a) P and Q are equally competitive.
 b) In competition, the growth of both species is adversely affected.
 c) In competition, species P remains unaffected while Q suffers.
 d) There is no evidence of competitive exclusion.

[CSIR Model Paper 2011]

23. Three important biological parameters - generation time, population growth rate (r) and metabolic rate per gram body weight are a function of the organism?s body size. Which of the curves (a) or (b) represents the correct relation of each of the parameters to body size?

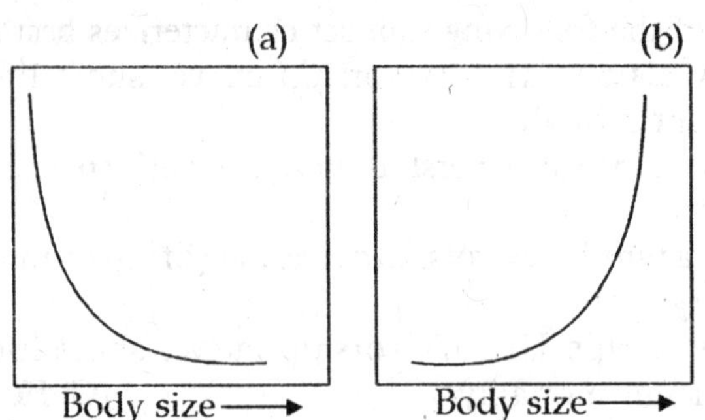

a) Generation time - (a); population growth rate - (b); metabolic rate/g bw- (a)
b) Generation time - (a); population growth rate - (b); metabolic rate/g bw - (b)
c) Generation time - (b); population growth rate - (a); metabolic rate/g bw - (a)
d) Generation time - (b); population growth rate - (b), metabolic rate rate/ g bw - (a)

[CSIR Model Paper 2011]

24. Nearly 25% of all insect species are known to be herbivores. Yet, in spite of such heavy herbivore pressure, globally green plants tend to persist, contributing to a green earth?.
Which of the following account for the relative success of green plants?
(A) Herbivore insects are inefficient feeders
(B) Herbivore insect densities are kept low by predators
(C) Plants secrete herbivore-deterrent chemicals
a) (B) and (C) b) (A) only
c) (B) and (C) d) (A), (B) and (C)

[CSIR Model Paper 2011]

25. In the process of nitrification by organisms, the respective bacteria A and B in the following reaction are:

$$NH_4 + \frac{1}{2}O_2 \xrightarrow{A} NO_2^- + 2H^+ + H_2O$$

$$NO_2^- + \frac{1}{2}O_2 \xrightarrow{B} NO_3^-$$

a) Azotobacter, Nitrobacter b) Nitrobacter, Azotobacter
c) Nitrosomonas, Nitrobacter d) Nitrobacter, Nitrosomonas

[CSIR Model Paper 2011]

26. In column I are given equations and in column II what the equations represent. Column I and II are incorrectly matched.

I	II
$\frac{dN_1}{dt} = r_1N_1\left(\frac{K_1 - N_1}{K_1}\right)$	(a) Population growth of species1 in the presence of competing species 2
$\frac{dN_1}{dt} = r_1N_1$	(b) Logistic population growth of species 1
$\frac{dN_1}{dt} = r_1N_1\left(\frac{K_1 - N_1 - \alpha N_2}{K_1}\right)$	(c) Population growth of prey species 1 in the presence of predator species 2.
$\frac{dN_1}{dt} = N_1b_1 - d_1N_1N_2$	(d) Exponential population growth of species 1.

The correct match in sequence of the four equations from column II is

a) b, d, a and c
b) d, b, c and d
c) b, d, c and a
d) d, b, a and c

[CSIR Model Paper 2011]

27. Following are some statements about tolerance model of succession

(A) Early colonists modify the environment so that it becomes suitable for subsequent colonization by early successional species but more suitable for colonization by late successional species.

(B) Early colonists modify the environment so that it becomes less suitable for subsequent colonization by both early and late successional species.

(C) Juveniles of later successional species that colonize or are already present grow to maturity despite the continued presence of healthy individuals of early successional species. In time, earlier species are eliminated.

(D) As long as individual of the early successful species persist, they exclude or suppress subsequent colonists of all species.

Which one of the following combination of above statements is true?

a) A and D
b) B and C
c) Only C
d) Only B

28. Which of the following graph shows correct correlation between population size and their extinctions?

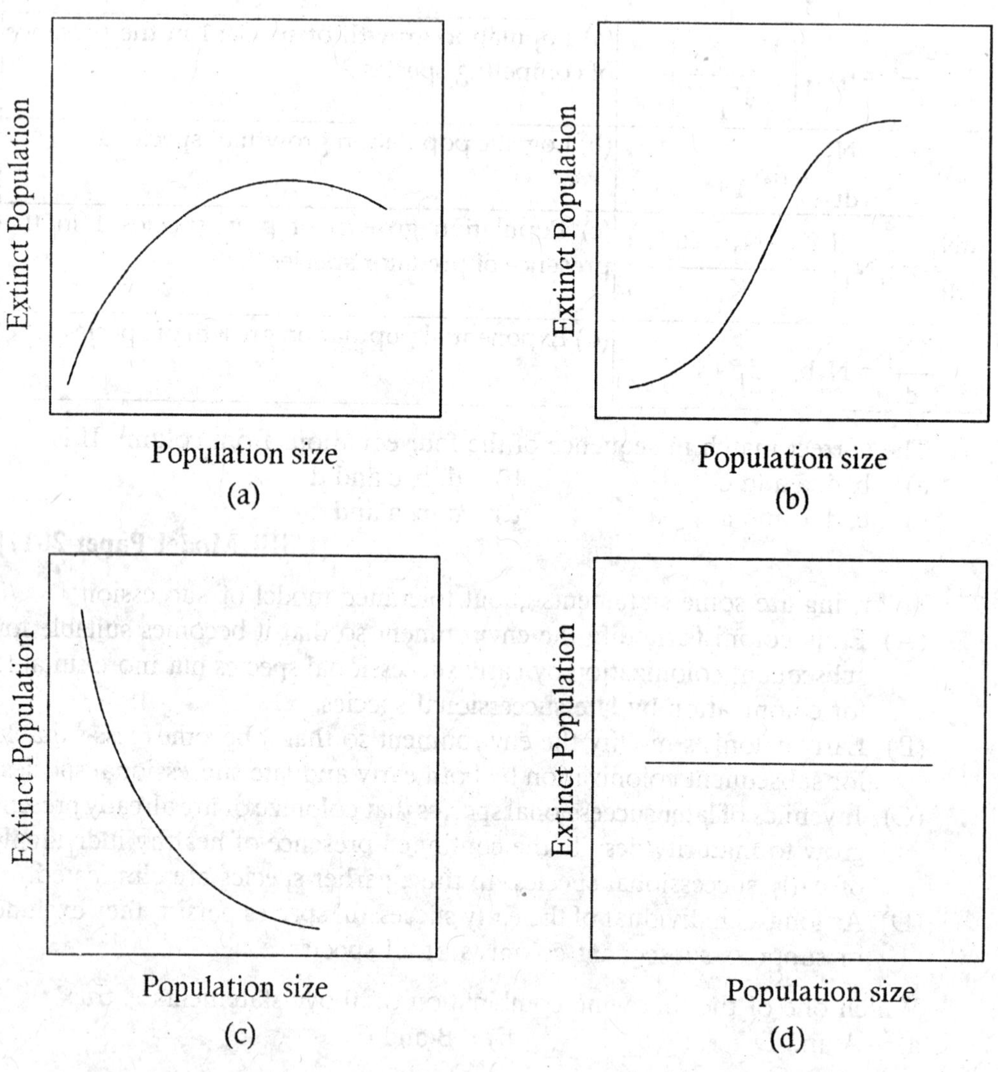

29. Which of the following graph of the Lotka-Voltera model of competion between two species represents coexistence

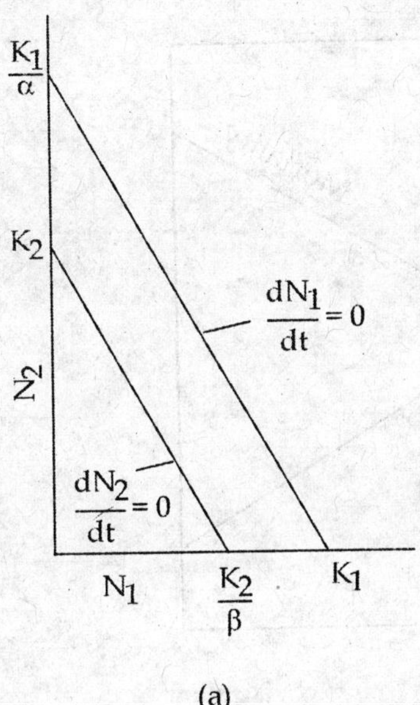

(a)

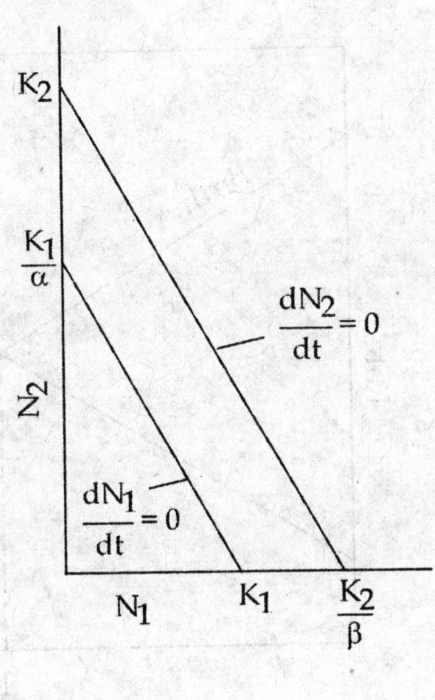

(b)

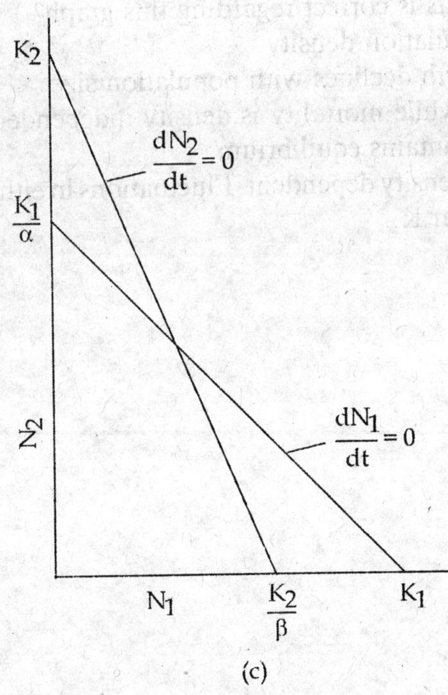

(c)

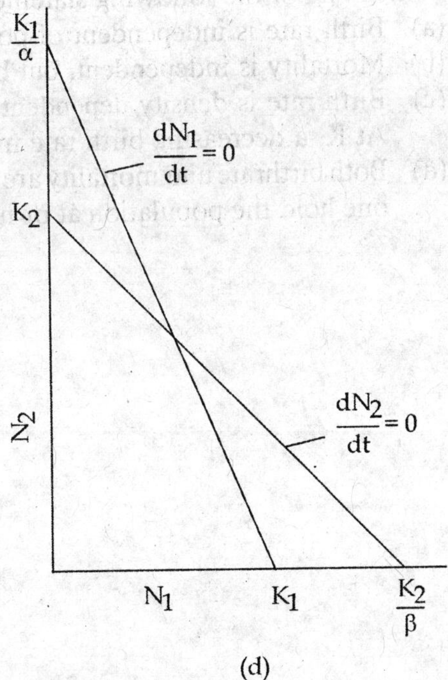

(d)

30. Following graph represents regulation of population size.

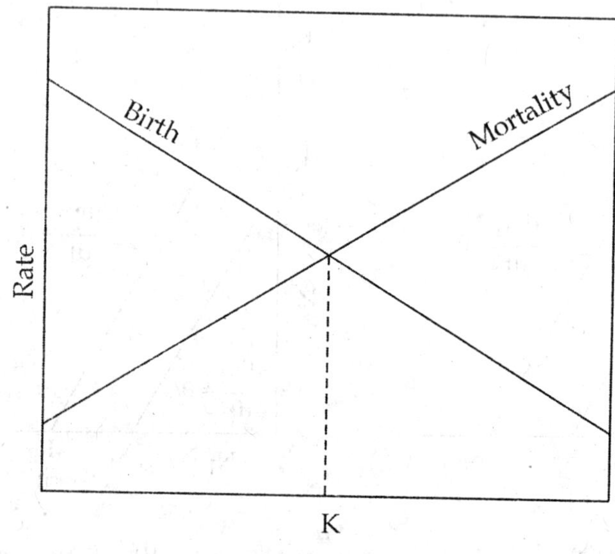

Which one of the following statements is correct regarding this graph?

(a) Birth rate is independent of population density

(b) Mortality is independent, but birth declines with population size.

(c) Birth rate is density dependent while mortality is density independent. At K, a decreasing birth rate maintains equilibrium.

(d) Both birthrate and mortality are density dependent. Fluctuations in either one hold the population at or near K.

Answer Sheet

Part – B

1.	b	2.	c	3.	a	4.	c	5.	d	6.	b
7.	a	8.	c	9.	a	10.	d	11.	b	12.	c
13.	b	14.	b	15.	d	16.	a	17.	a	18.	a
19.	b	20.	d	21.	c	22.	c	23.	a	24.	d
25.	a	26.	a	27.	d	28.	b	29.	b	30.	b
31.	a	32.	b	33.	a	34.	b	35.	c	36.	d
37.	d	38.	b	39.	a	40.	c	41.	a	42.	b
43.	a	44.	d	45.	b	46.	c	47.	d	48.	c
49.	b	50.	d	51.	b	52.	c	53.	b	54.	d
55.	c	56.	d	57.	c	58.	b	59.	a	60.	c
61.	d	62.	b	63.	a	64.	a	65.	a	66.	a
67.	b	68.	d	69.	c	70.	b	71.	c	72.	d
73.	a	74.	a	75.	b	76.	b	77.	d	78.	b
79.	c	80.	d	81.	b	82.	d	83.	b	84.	c
85.	a	86.	b	87.	b	88.	c	89.	d	90.	a
91.	c	92.	d	93.	a	94.	a	95.	b	96.	a
97.	b	98.	c	99.	d	100.	a	101.	b	102.	c
103.	a	104.	d	105.	d	106.	d	107.	a	108.	c
109.	c	110.	a	111.	d	112.	b	113.	c	114.	b
115.	c	116.	b	117.	a	118.	c	119.	c	120.	c
121.	b	122.	c	123.	d	124.	b	125.	d	126.	b
127.	c	128.	a	129.	b	130.	c	131.	c	132.	d
133.	d	134.	b	135.	a	136.	c	137.	b	138.	c
139.	d	140.	d	141.	a	142.	d	143.	a	144.	b
145.	b	146.	b	147.	b	148.	c	149.	b	150.	b
151.	b	152.	b	153.	c	154.	d	155.	b	156.	c
157.	c	158.	a	159.	d	160.	c	161.	c	162.	b
163.	d	164.	d	165.	c	166.	c	167.	b	168.	d
169.	a	170.	d	171.	b	172.	d	173.	d	174.	a
175.	d	176.	c	177.	b	178.	a	179.	c	180.	a
181.	d	182.	b	183.	d	184.	d	185.	c	186.	c
187.	d	188.	c	189.	b	190.	d	191.	d	192.	c
193.	a	194.	c	195.	b	196.	a	197.	a	198.	c
199.	c	200.	c	201.	a	202.	d	203.	a	204.	b
205.	c	206.	c	207.	a	208.	d	209.	c	210.	b

211.	b	212.	d	213.	c	214.	b	215.	c	216.	c
217.	b	218.	c	219.	c	220.	c	221.	b	222.	b
223.	d	224.	b	225.	a	226.	a	227.	d	228.	b
229.	c	230.	d	231.	c	232.	c	233.	a	234.	b
235.	b	236.	c	237.	d	238.	b	239.	c	240.	b
241.	b	242.	b	243.	a	244.	d	245.	b	246.	d
247.	c	248.	c	249.	b	250.	a	251.	a	252.	a
253.	c	254.	c	255.	d	256.	c	257.	d	258.	d
259.	d	260.	d	261.	a	262.	b	263.	b	264.	b
265.	d	266.	c	267.	c	268.	a	269.	d	270.	d
271.	c	272.	b	273.	b	274.	b	275.	a	276.	c
277.	c	278.	d	279.	d	280.	d	281.	a	282.	d
283.	b	284.	d	285.	d	286.	d	287.	d	288.	d
289.	d	290.	c	291.	c	292.	c	293.	b	294.	c
295.	d	296.	c	297.	d	298.	b	299.	d	300.	c
301.	c	302.	c	303.	c	304.	d	305.	b	306.	d
307.	d	308.	d	309.	b	310.	d	311.	a	312.	d
313.	d	314.	d	315.	a	316.	a	317.	c	318.	d
319.	b	320.	d	321.	d	322.	b	323.	c	324.	b
325.	b	326.	c	327.	b	328.	a	329.	b	330.	d
331.	a	332.	d	333.	c	334.	a	335.	d	336.	a
337.	d	338.	c	339.	c	340.	c	341.	d	342.	a
343.	d	344.	c	345.	b	346.	b	347.	d	348.	d
349.	d	350.	b	351.	c	352.	b	353.	b	354.	d
355.	d	356.	d	357.	d	358.	a	359.	a	360.	a
361.	a	362.	d	363.	a	364.	c	365.	a	366.	b
367.	b	368.	c	369.	a	370.	d	371.	a	372.	c
373.	b	374.	a	375.	b	376.	a	377.	c	378.	a
379.	a	380.	b	381.	c	382.	d	383.	c	384.	b
385.	a	386.	d	387.	b	388.	b	389.	b	390.	d
391.	d	392.	d	393.	d	394.	b	395.	d	396.	c
397.	a	398.	b	399.	b	400.	c				

Part – C

1.	b	2.	a	3.	b	4.	c	5.	a	6.	a
7.	d	8.	a	9.	c	10.	a	11.	c	12.	b
13.	d	14.	d	15.	a	16.	c	17.	b	18.	b
19.	b	20.	d	21.	d	22.	c	23.	c	24.	c
25.	d	26.	a	27.	c	28.	c	29.	d	30.	d

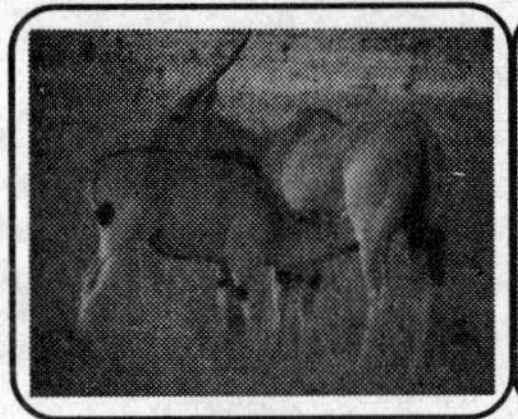

Chapter 10

Evolution & Behaviour

Part B

1. Fossils are abundantly found in
   a) Igneous Rocks b) Sedimentary Rocks
   c) Metamorphic Rocks d) All of these
   [CSIR (NET/JRF] Exam. June 2005]

2. Classification of amino acids into two groups : functional and non functional was proposed by
   a) Pauling b) Woese
   c) Berzilius d) Kimura

3. "Industrial Melanism" can not explain
   a) Natural Selection b) Speciation
   c) Adaptation d) Migration

4. "Species are groups of interbreeding natural populations that are reproductively isolated from other such groups" It is true for
   a) Taxonomic species concept b) Evolutionary species concept
   c) Genetic species concept d) Biological species concept

5. ____________operates to eliminate intermediate phenotypes
   a) Directional selection b) Stabilizing selection
   c) Disruptive selection d) Random chance

6. A Mendelian population represents a population showing
   a) Extensive migration b) Active speciation
   c) Selective mating d) Hardy-Weinberg equilibrium

7. A mode of speciation that is both sympatric and instantaneous is -
   a) Ecological speciation b) Allopatric speciation
   c) Polyploidy d) Parapatric speciation

8. A non harmful species copies a harmful and tasteless form, the type of mimicry shown is
   a) Batesian b) Mullerian
   c) Darwinian d) Morganian

9. A population is said to be polymorphic for a locus if it has at least
   a) Two genotypes for the locus
   b) Two different alleles at that locus
   c) Three genotypes for that locus
   d) Three different alleles at that locus

10. A population mating at non-random in the absence of evolutionary forces.
    a) Allele frequencies will remain constant.
    b). Genotype frequencies will remain constant.
    c) Both allele and genotype frequencies will remain constant.
    d) Zygote frequencies will remain constant.

11. A strategy which, when adapted by most members of the population, cannot be beaten by any other strategy is known as
    a) An evolutionary stable strategy
    b) A functional response
    c) A life history strategy
    d) An adaptive strategy

12. A type of selection which favours an optimal phenotype and works against the extremes is called
    a) Directional selection b) Mass selection
    c) Disruptive selection d) Stabilising selection
    [CSIR (NET/JRF) Exam. June 2003]

13. Abrupt change in gene frequency of small population is termed as
    a) Genetic loss b) Genetic erosion
    c) Genetic drift d) Genetic load

14. African cheetah population has lost nearly all its genetic variation due to the
    a) Founder effect b) Bottleneck effect
    c) Baldwin effect d) Rescue effect

15. Albinism, an autosomal recessive trait, has an incidence of about 1/10,000 in some population. Calculate the frequency of the allele
    a) 0.001 b) 0.01
    c) 1.00 d) 0.02

16. All genes of Mendelian population makes
    a) Genome b) Genotype
    c) Alleles d) Gene pool

17. All of the following are believed to contribute to genomic diversity among various species except
    a) Gene duplication
    b) Gene transcription

c) Chromosomal rearrangements
d) Lateral gene transfer

18. All proteins are polymer of -L-amino acids. What can you assume from this fact?
   a) α-L-amino acids are more stable than α-D-amino acids
   b) α-L-amino acids are naturally selected due to some other selective advantages
   c) all living organisms are derived from one cell line
   d) α-L-amino acids were formed before α-D-amino acids during course of evolution

19. Altruistic behaviour between relatives is explained by
   a) Clinal selection
   b) Cyclic selection
   c) Kin selection
   d) Balancing selection

20. A balanced polymorphism can be maintained by the following mechanisms except
   a) Disruptive selection
   b) Frequency-dependent selection
   c) Directional selection
   d) Heterozygote advantage

21. Among the following which would lead into new species formation
   a) Increased resources
   b) Niche overlapping tolerance
   c) Niche specialization
   d) Lack of competition

22. An animal is said of the eusocial if
   a) Group members interact very intensively.
   b) A dominance hierarchy exists among group members.
   c) Young individuals remain in the group to help their parents rear other offspring.
   d) The social group contains sterile individuals.

23. An evolutionary bottleneck is best described as
   a) Loss of genetic variability in a population during a period of reduced population size
   b) Permanent loss of genetic information by natural selection
   c) The rate-limiting step in evolutionary change, such as mutation rate
   d) Very slow phenotypic change within a population over time.

24. At present, the relationship between human and monkey can be stated as
   a) They both have common ancestors
   b) Human have evolved from monkey
   c) Both have very distinct phylogeny
   d) Relationship can not be established

[CSIR (NET/JRF) Exam. June 2007]

25. Who said "Evolution is irreversible"?
    a) Jordan b) Cope
    c) Williston d) Dolo
26. A common means of sympatric speciation is
    a) Polyploidy b) Disruptive selection
    c) Hybrid infertility d) Polymorphism in population
27. Classification of organisms based on rRNA type was propounded by
    a) Haldane b) Mayr
    c) Woese d) Racker

[CSIR (NET/JRF) Exam. June 2002]

28. Concept of neutral evolution is based on
    a) Natural selection b) Genetic drift.
    c) Founder effect. d) Hardy-Weinberg principle.
29. Dendrogram is
    a) Family tree b) Phylogenetic relationship
    c) Matching species similarity d) Evolutionary relationship

[CSIR (NET/JRF] Exam. June/ Dec. 2005]

30. Disaster such as earthquake or fire may reduce the size of population drastically and the genetic make up of the small surviving population is unlikely to be representative of make up of original population. The situation is termed as
    a) Adaptive radiation b) Founder effect
    c) Bottle neck effect d) Gene migration

[CSIR (NET/JRF) Exam. June 2007]

31. Division of sympatric isolation into two isolating mechanism was given by
    a) Fox b) Mayr
    c) Woese d) Newman
32. Which type of speciation occur among very sedentary species?
    a) Allopatric b) Parapatric
    c) Peripatric d) Sympatric
33. Which of the following, when acting alone, does not have any significant effect of the allele frequency in a population?
    a) Selection and Mutation b) Mutation
    c) Inbreeding d) Migration
34. During evolution the limbs of snakes were lost. The explanation for this is
    a) Limbs were not desirable
    b) This was more adapted
    c) Limbs degenerated due to disuse

d) None of the above

35. During the process of natural selection environment acts upon
   a) Phenotypic variations b) Genotypic variations
   c) Physiological variations d) New alleles

36. Ernst Mayer gave the concept of
   a) Biological species b) Ecological species
   c) Evolution species d) Phylogenetic species

[CSIR (NET/JRF) Exam. Dec. 2005]

37. Evolutionary radiations
   a) Often happen on continents, but rarely on island archipelagos
   b) Never happen in species-poor environments
   c) Characterize birds and plants, but not other taxonomic groups
   d) Have happened on continents as well as on islands

38. Finches speciated in the Galapogos Islands because
   a) The Galapagos Islands are not far from the main land.
   b) The Galapogos Islands are small.
   c) The Islands of Galapagos archipelago are close enough to one another that there is considerable migration among them.
   d) The Islands of Galapagos archipelago are sufficiently isolated from one another that there is little migration among them.

39. First mammals appeared in
   a) Devonian b) Cretaceous
   c) Triassic d) Jurassic

40. First multicellular organisms appeared in
   a) Precambrian b) Cambrian
   c) Permian d) Silurian

41. Formation of various species from one common ancestor is termed as
   a) Natural selection b) Phylogeny
   c) Cladistics d) Adaptive radiation

42. From Galapages Islands Darwin has had collected specimens of
   a) Mocking birds b) Humming birds
   c) Game birds d) Flightless birds

43. Genes in different species that are sufficiently similar in their nucleotide sequences to suggest that they have orginated from a common ancestral gene are
   a) Duplicate b) Paralogous
   c) Orthologous d) Microevolutionary

[CSIR (NET/JRF) Exam. June 2006]

44. Genes that are passed in a straight line from one generation to the next but have ended up in different gene pools because of speciation are called
    a) Orthologous b) Paralogous
    c) Homologous d) Neologous

45. Genetic drift can not occur via
    a) Large scale migration b) Bottle neck effect
    c) Founder effect d) Sampling error

46. Genetic drift is the result of
    a) Sampling error leading to random fixation of alleles
    b) Positive assortative mating
    c) Inbreeding
    d) Out breeding **[CSIR (NET/JRF) Exam. June 2001]**

47. Genetic variation that decreases the average fitness of a population is referred to as
    a) Genomic abnormality b) Genetic load
    c) Junk genetic variation d) None of the above

48. Genotype frequency remains constant from generation to generation in a population, under following conditions except
    a) Random mating b) Large populaltion
    c) Absence of natural selction d) Assortative mating

49. Geographically Isolated local population will be
    a) Coenospecies b) Ecospecies
    c) Demes d) Evolved species

50. Germplasm theory of organic evolution was given by
    a) Weisman b) Lamark
    c) de Varies d) Morgan
    [CSIR (NET/JRF) Exam. Dec. 2005]

51. Which of the following will not change genotype frequency in a population?
    a) Assortative mating b) Inbreeding
    c) Random mating d) Consanguineous marriages

52. Hardy-Weinberg equilibrium is true for
    a) Large and random mating population having individuals with selective advantage
    b) Large and non-random mating population
    c) Large population in which selection and random mating occurs rarely
    d) Large and random mating population which has no selective advantage among individuals

53. Hardy-Weinberg law in a population represents
   a) Allele frequency b) Genotype frequency
   c) Homozygote frequency d) Heterozygote frequency
   [CSIR (NET/JRF) Exam. June 2006]

54. Hardy-Weinberg law is thought to be a null hypothesis because
   a) It is true for a very large population
   b) It is against evolution
   c) It disfavors theory of natural selection
   d) It is true only when certain assumptions are met.

55. Hardy-Weinberg population is
   a) Non-evolving b) Gradually evolving
   c) Spontaneously evolving d) Differential evolving
   [CSIR (NET/JRF) Exam. June 2005]

56. Horizontal gene transfer is common in
   a) Only eukaryotes b) Prokaryotes
   c) Mesokaryotes d) None of these

57. Identify the correct statement-
   a) In Hardy-Weinberg equilibrium generations are overlapping
   b) In Hardy-Weinberg equilibrium the proportion of heterozygotes is minimum when allele frequency are equal.
   c) Hardy-Weinberg population is non-evolutionary
   d) Hardy-Weinberg equilibrium is applicable to calculating the frequency of genotype but not allele.

58. If a certain parasitic bacteria on insect prevents cross breeding among them. It well lead into
   a) Rapid speciation b) Divergence of insects
   c) Extinction of insects d) No effect
   [CSIR (NET/JRF) Exam. Dec 2006]

59. If a gene have three alleles namely p, q and r. The Hardy-Weinberg law can be represented as
   a) (p+q+r)2 b) (p+q+r)3
   c) (p+q+r) d) (p+q)2
   [CSIR (NET/JRF) Exam. Dec 2007]

60. If a gene product in species A is 90% similar to gene product of species B. Such genes are termed as
   a) Homologous b) Paralogous
   c) Orthologous d) Allologous

61. If gene and genotype frequencies remain constant generation after generation in natural populations, the populations would have constant genetic composition and there would be
a) Fast evolution
b) No evolution
c) Slow evolution
d) Sympatric speciation

62. If genes move between species the phenomenon is called
a) Vertical gene transfer
b) Lateral gene transfer
c) Genetic recombination
d) Migration

63. If the two or more morphological forms are favoured against heterozygotes, such a selection is termed as
a) Stabilizing
b) Cyclic
c) Directional
d) Disruptive

64. If there are 3 alleles for a genetic locus in a population, phenotypic proportion will be
a) $(P+q)^2$
b) $(p+q)^3$
c) $(P+q+r)^2$
d) $(P+q+r)^3$

[CSIR (NET/JRF) Exam. June 2005]

65. In a diploid organism, what is the maximum number of alleles that can exist in a population for any given gene?
a) 1
b) 2
c) 4
d) Unlimited

66. In a genotype, frequency of recessive allele 'a' is 0.12 and dominant allele 'A' is 0.88. Frequency of carrier heterozygote will be
a) 21.1
b) 10.5
c) 17.4
d) 0.21

[CSIR (NET/JRF) Exam. Dec. 2005]

67. In a habitat where environment is stable which type of selection will probably operate there?
a) Stabilising selction
b) Directional selection
c) Disruptive selection
d) Oscillating selection

68. In a population at Hardy-Weinberg equilibrium in which the frequency of A allele (p) is 0.3, the expected frequency of Aa individual is
a) 0.42
b) 0.18
c) 0.36
d) 0.63

[CSIR (NET/JRF) Exam. Dec 2005]

69. In a population frequency of a homozygous recessive disease is 16% then the frequency of dominant allele would be
a) 0.4
b) 0.16
c) 0.84
d) 0.6

70. In a population obeying Hardy-Weinberg equillibrium, the frequency of recessive allele is 0.88, while of dominant allele is 0.12, The frequency of heterozygotes in population will be
a) 14.4% b) 10.56%
c) 21.1% d) 11.1%

71. In evolution adaptation of two or more species occur in this way that each one has strong selective force on the other. It is an example of
a) Complementation b) Coevolution
c) Cooperation d) Convergent evolution
[CSIR (NET/JRF) Exam. Dec 2005]

72. In peppered moths, the black colouration is selected when soot covers tree bark, this phenomenon is called
a) Oscillating selection b) Convergent evolution
c) Industrial melanism d) Transient polymorphism

73. In present condition origin of life from inorganic molecules is not possible because of
a) Absence of raw material b) Presence of oxygen
c) Low enthalpy d) Presence of ozone layer
[CSIR (NET/JRF) Exam. June 2007]

74. Which of the following was not used by Miller in his experiment?
a) Methane b) Ammonia
c) Water d) Nitrogen

75. In their early embryonic stages, fish, turtles, chickens, mice and humans all develop tails and gill slits. But only fish retain gills as adults, and only fish, turtles and mice retain substantial tails. It indicates that
a) Fish are more advanced than others.
b) They have originated from different parental stock.
c) They have common origin.
d) Mice are more close to fish than turtles.

76. In which of the following diseases the heterozygotes are resistant to tuberculosis?
a) Sickle-cell anemia b) Cystic fibrosis
c) PKU d) Tay-sachs disease

77. In which of the following situations the frequency of an allele changes significantly but the changes is not the result of selection are called
a) Assoratative mating b) Random mating
c) Genetic drift d) None of the above

78. Independently evolved traits subjects to similar selective pressures may become superficially similar as a result of
    a) Mega evolution
    b) Divergent evolution
    c) Convergent evolution
    d) Evolutionary reversad

79. Kin selection favours
    a) Direct fitness
    b) Indirect fitness
    c) Inclusive fitness
    d) Selfishness

80. Life is believed to have originated on earth
    a) 3.6 billion years ago
    b) 3.6 million years ago
    c) 4.5 billion years ago
    d) 4.5 million years ago

[CSIR (NET/JRF) Exam. Dec 2001]

81. Locally adapted and genetically distinctive populations within a species are called
    a) Cline
    b) Ecads
    c) Ecotype
    d) Race

82. Which of the following statements is not true?
    a) Natural selection always operates in nature.
    b) Arrival of fittest was the greatest finding of Darwin's theory of evolution.
    c) Genetic drift operates in small populations.
    d) Cladogenesis means true speciation.

83. Loss of genetic information from a small population is called
    a) Genetic drift
    b) Bottleneck effect
    c) Founder effect
    d) Inbreeding depression

[CSIR (NET/JRF) Exam. June 2005]

84. Mitochondria and chloroplasts are suggested to have evolved from symbiotic prokaryotes present in primitive eukaryotic cells. One evidence for this is that
    a) These organelles contain cristae and thylakoids
    b) These organelles contain electron transport chain
    c) The ribosomes in these organelles share properties with those of prokaryotes
    d) The genetic code in these organelles is same as in all organisms

85. Mitochondrial DNA sequences are useful in studying the recent evolution of closely related species because
    a) They evolve only in a neutral fashion
    b) Some mitochondrial genes accumulate mutations very rapidly
    c) They are highly constrained in function
    d) They recombine every generation

86. Modern humans are closely related to
    a) Cro-Magnons b) Neanderthals
    c) Java d) Australopithecus

87. Molecular phylogenetics is based on
    a) Natural selection b) Neutral evolution
    c) Parallel evolution d) Coevolution

88. Molecular polymorphism can be explained by
    a) Darwinism b) Lamarkism
    c) Neutral theory d) All of the above

89. Molecular systematics deals commonly exclusively with the utilization of
    a) Nucleic acids b) Proteins
    c) Flavonoids d) Phenolics

90. Morphologically similar but reproductively isolated species are called
    a) Sibling species b) Compilo species
    c) Parapatric species d) Sympatric species

91. Morphologicaly distinct but not reproductively-isolated species are
    a) Subspecies b) Cryptic species
    c) Compilo species d) Sibling species

92. Most of new species are formed by the process of
    a) Anagenesis b) Cladogenesis
    c) Sympatric speciation d) Phylogenetic evolution
    [CSIR (NET/JRF) Exam. Dec 2002]

93. Natural selection that favours values of trait at one end of its distribution is
    a) Disruptive selection b) Stabilizing selection
    c) Directional selection d) Oscillating selection
    [CSIR (NET/JRF) Exam. Dec 2005]

94. Natural selection that preserves existing allele frequencies is called
    a) Stabilizing selection b) Directional selection
    c) Preserving selection d) Oscillating selection

95. Natural selection usually reduces variations in a population but sometimes it increases variations such as
    a) Directional selection.
    b) Kin selection.
    c) Frequency dependent selection.
    d) Sexual selection.

96. Niche differentiation is the basis of
   a) Sympatric speciation b) Allopatric speciation
   c) Peripatric speciation d) Parapatric speciation

97. Once they evolved,________forever changed the atmosphere on earth
   a) Bacteria b) Archaebacteria
   c) Cyanobacteria d) Eukaryotes

98. One of the practical applications of the Hardy-Weinberg law is the estimation of
   a) Gamete frequency in a population
   b) Zygote frequency in a population
   c) Heterozygote frequency in a population
   d) Allele frequency in a population

99. Overtime, the same bones in different vertebrates were put to different uses. This falls under the category of
   a) Missing links b) Vestigial structures
   c) Analogous structures d) Homologous structures

100. Pelvic girdle and hind limbs in python are example of
   a) Homologous organ b) Analogous organ
   c) Vestigial organ d) Orthologous organ

101. Phenomenon of "industrial melanism" demonstrates
   a) Reproductive isolation b) Induced mutation
   c) Natural selection d) Geographical isolation

102. Phenotypic extremes are selected in
   a) Stabilizing selection b) Directional selection
   c) Disruptive selection d) Balancing selection

[CSIR (NET/JRF) Exam. June 2004]

103. Philopatry defines
   a) Mating behavior in peacocks.
   b) Parental care in birds.
   c) The tendency of some organisms to remain in the same area throughout their lives.
   d) The tendency of some organisms to change the area after each generation.

104. Phylogenetic relationship cannot be established on the basis of
   a) 5S r-RNA b) 16S r-RNA
   c) Ribosomal DNA d) Mitochondrial genes

105. Prezygotic isolating mechanisms include all of the following except-
   a) Courtship rituals b) Habitat separation
   c) Hybrid sterility d) Seasonal reproduction

106. Reinforcement is necessary requirement for
   a) Allopatric speciation   b) Parapatric speciation
   c) Allopatric and parapatric   d) Sympatric and parapatric

107. Reinforcement means that
   a) Natural selection acts to increase the prezygotic isolation between two populations
   b) Speciation is proceeding either sympatrically or parapatrically, rather than allopatrically
   c) Hybrids have lower fitness than either of the two parental forms
   d) All of these

108. Reproductive isolation and the evolution of species could occur through which of the following?
   a) Founder effect   b) Reinforcement
   c) Adaptation   d) All of these

109. Reproductive isolation is essential for
   a) Typological species concept
   b) Biological species concept
   c) Evolutionary species concept
   d) Genetic species concept

110. Resistance to insecticides in natural populations of insects is an example of
   a) Directional selection
   b) Stabilizing selection
   c) Disruptive selection
   d) Frequency-dependent selection

[CSIR (NET/JRF) Exam. June 2006]

111. Ribosomal RNA are better molecules for phylogenetic studies because
   a) They are present in 70s and 80s ribosomes
   b) They can easily be sequenced
   c) Antiquity of protein synthesizing process
   d) None of these

112. Ribosomal RNA sequences are useful addressing the evolutionary relationships of lineages that diverged in ancient times because they
   a) Evolve at rapid rate
   b) Are molecules that all organisms have
   c) Consist of mainly neutral characters
   d) Have undergone convergent evolution many lineages

113. Selection that favours the survival of organisms in a population that is at an intermediate phenotypic value for a particular character is called
   a) Directional selection b) Balancing selection
   c) Stabilizing selection d) Diversifying selection

114. Selection which operates against any direction and do not allow to disrupt the present mean is termed as
   a) Balancing b) Disruptive
   c) Directional d) Stabilizing
   [CSIR (NET/JRF) Exam. June 2002]

115. Selection, in which allelic frequency changes as altitude and latitude changes, is
   a) Stabilising selection b) Clinal selection
   c) Directional selection d) Genotypic selection

116. Similarities in organisms with different genotypes indicates
   a) Microevolution b) Macroevolution
   c) Convergent evolution d) Divergent evolution

117. Slow-moving organisms show
   a) Sympatric speciation b) Peripatric speciation
   c) Parapatric speciation d) Gradual speciation
   [CSIR (NET/JRF) Exam. Dec. 2004]

118. Small populations give rise to new species through
   a) Bottleneck effect b) Founder effect
   c) Assortative mating d) Genetic drift

119. Some insects have wings shaped and sculptured like leaves, such wings are examples of
   a) Homologous structures b) Analogous structures
   c) Homoplastic structures d) None of the above

120. Sometimes blind luck can cause a population to evolve unpredictably. This mechanism of evolution can be explained in the light of
   a) Assortative mating b) Genetic drift
   c) Anagenesis d) Adaptive radiation

121. Speciation occurs most frequently in populations that are-
   a) Sympatric b) Undergoing disruptive selection
   c) Allopatric d) Parapatric

122. Speciation occurs when
   a) Niches of two closely-related individuals get overlapped
   b) Competition occurs between members of two populations for resources

c) Nutrients limit gene flow between individuals
d) Gene flow within the common pool is interrupted by an isolating mechanism

123. Species A changes into B in due course of time, the phenomenon is called as
a) Cladogenesis b) Stasigenesis
c) Anagenesis d) Punctuated equilibrium

124. Species X has few genes very much similar to that of species Y. These are called
a) Paralogous b) Homologous
c) Orthologous d) Homeologous

125. Taxonomists strive to include taxa in biological classifications that are
a) Monophyletic b) Paraphyletic
c) Polyphyletic d) Homoplastic

126. Tay-Sach's disease is related to
a) Genetic drift b) Polymorphism
c) Mutation d) Heterosis

127. The appropriate unit for defining and measuring genetic variation is the
a) Individual b) Population
c) Community d) Ecosystem

128. Which one of the following classes of compounds is most useful in comparative studies for determining the ancestral relationships ?
a) Nucleic acid b) Proteins
c) Amino acids d) Nucleotide sequences

129. The change of prey brings changes in predator and vice-versa. Such an evolution due to competition for existence is termed as
a) Diverging evolution b) Converging evolution
c) Parallel evolution d) Coevolution

130. The chemical evolution of biomolecules has been taken place from
a) Amino acids b) HCN
c) Purine and Pyrimidines d) HCHO

[CSIR (NET/JRF) Exam. Dec. 2002]

131. The choice of mating partner may be based on
a) The inherent qualities of a potential mate.
b) The resources held by a potential mate.
c) Both (a) and (b)
d) The courtship display of a potential mate.

132. The combination of closely-linked genetic markers which tend to be transmitted as a unit to the next generation is called
   a) Allotype b) Haplotype
   c) Karyotype d) Isotype

133. The concept of a "molecular clock" implies that
   a) Organisms evolve at a constant rate
   b) All molecules change at the same rate in evolution
   c) Many proteins show a constancy in rate of change with time
   d) One can date evolutionary events with molecules alone

[CSIR (NET/JRF) Exam. Dec. 2001]

134. The concept of Genetic drift was given by
   a) Sewall Wright b) Mayr
   c) Stebbins d) Dobzhansky

135. The evolution of antibiotic resistance in bacteria is an example of
   a) Stabilizing selection b) Directional selection
   c) Disruptive selection d) Balancing selection

[CSIR (NET/JRF) Exam. Dec 2006]

136. The evolutionary divergence of higher taxonomic groups is due to
   a) Adaptive radiation b) Anagenesis
   c) Cladogenesis d) Stasigenesis

[CSIR (NET/JRF) Exam. June 2005]

137. The finch species of the Galapagos islands are grouped according to their food sources. Which of the following is not a finch food source?
   a) Seeds b) Insects
   c) Carrion d) Tree buds

138. The first animals to move onto land were
   a) Arthropods b) Amphibians
   c) Reptiles d) Mammals

139. The first living cells are
   a) Anaerobic heterotrophs b) Aerobic heterotrophs
   c) Aerobic autotrophs d) Anaerobic autotrophs

140. The frequency of an allele in a large random mating population is 0.2. What is the frequency of the heterozygous carriers ?
   a) 0.08 b) 0.16
   c) 0.32 d) 0.64

141. The frequency of cystic fibrosis in North America Caucasians is approximately 1 in 2000, what will be the frequency of heterozygous carriers of the gene?
a) 0.2
b) 0.98
c) 0.42
d) 0.02

142. The genes that are most extensively used to determine evolutionary relationships among plants are
a) Genes of flowers
b) Mitochondrial genes
c) Chloroplast genes
d) Nuclear genes

143. The gradual mode of speciation in single lineage in which species diverge in spurts of relatively rapid change which result in increase in species is termed is
a) Cladogenesis
b) Adaptive radiation
c) Anagenesis
d) Punctuated equilibrium

[CSIR (NET/JRF) Exam. Dec 2001]

144. The high altitude variety of a plant species 'A' differs morphologically from the same species growing in the valley. The high altitude plant should be categorised as a
a) Subspecies
b) Ecotype
c) Race
d) Different species

145. The hypothesis of "molecular clock" of evolution considers
a) Analysis of 16 SrRNA
b) DNA-DNA hybridization
c) Molecular profiling
d) Rate of amino acid change in a protein

146. The hypothesis that evolution occurs in spurts, with great amounts of evolutionary change followed by periods of stasis, is
a) Gradualism
b) Stasigenesis
c) Punctuated equilibrium
d) Hardy-Weinberg equilibrium

[CSIR (NET/JRF) Exam. June 2000]

147. The large number of Hawaiian Drosophila species has likely resulted from
a) Adaptive radiation
b) A single common ancestor
c) Geographic isolation
d) All of these

148. The largest unit in which gene flow is possible is a
a) Species
b) Phylum
c) Subspecies
d) Population

[CSIR (NET/JRF) Exam. Dec. 2001]

149. The maintenance of the sickle cell allele in human population in Central Africa is an example of
a) Gene flow
b) Genetic drift
c) Balancing selection
d) Non-random mating

[CSIR (NET/JRF) Exam. June 2002]

150. The maternal progenitors of plant species are assessed by the analysis of variation in
   a) Chloroplast DNA alone
   b) Both chloroplast and mitochondrial DNA
   c) Nuclear DNA
   d) Mitochondrial DNA alone

151. The mitochondria of eukaryotic cells most likely arose as a result of endosymbiosis between a eukaryotic cell and a
   a) Red alga b) Purple sulfur bacteria
   c) Non-sulfur purple bacteria d) Cyanobacterium

152. The modern single toed horse has evolved from a
   a) Four toed horse b) Five toed horse
   c) Three toed horse d) Single toed horse

153. The natural selection which maintains balanced polymorphism is called
   a) Stabilizing selection b) Balancing selection
   c) Directional selection d) Disruptive selection

154. Which of the following statements is not true for Hardy-Weinberg theorem?
   a) It describes a hypothetical population that is not evolving
   b) It is a null hypothesis
   c) It describes a hypothetical large, random mating population that is evolving
   d) It describes a population where mutation, migration and natural selection is not operating

155. The phenomenon wherein organisms change the relative time of appearance and rate of development of characters is called
   a) Adaptation
   b) Developmental plasticity
   c) Modularity
   d) Heterochrony

156. The phenomenon which can fix rare allele is called
   a) Genetic drift b) Mutation
   c) Natural selection d) Recombination

157. The pre-biotic environment on Earth was
   a) Reducing b) Oxidising
   c) Nitrifying d) Rich in ozone

[CSIR (NET/JRF) Exam. Dec 2003]

158. The present concept for origin of life is
   a) At hydrothermal vents b) In mid oceans
   c) Pangenesis d) On land

159. The process of evolving reproductive isolation between subpopulation that exists in the same territory is called
   a) Allopatric speciation b) Sympatric speciation
   c) Anagenesis d) Peripatric speciation

160. The rate of fixation of neutral mutations is
   a) Higher in small populations than in large populations.
   b) Higher in larger populations than in small populations
   c) Independent of population size..
   d) Slower than the rate of fixation of deleterious mutations.

161. The RNA moleule often used to determine evolutionary relatedness is
   a) mRNA b) rRNA
   c) tRNA d) SnRNA

162. Which of these is not a requirement for maintaining the Hardy-Weinberg equilibrium?
   a) Random mating
   b) Infinite population size
   c) Absence of gene flow between populations
   d) Selection

163. The shape of the beaks of Darwin's finches, industrial melanism, and the changes in horse teeth are examples of
   a) Individual selection b) Natural selection
   c) Convergent evolution d) Homologous structures

164. The smallest biological unit evolved over time is
   a) Species b) Population
   c) Individual d) Cell

[CSIR (NET/JRF) Exam. June 2005]

165. Which of these is not a condition for natural selection?
   a) Variation in fitness b) Excess fecundity
   c) Reproduction d) None of these

166. The term "molecular clock" refers to
   a) An RNA or protein molecule that is expressed in rhythmic manner
   b) A molecule involved in the aging process
   c) The concept that macromolecules like nucleic acids and proteins evolve

at a constant rate

d) A molecule that controls circadian rhythms

167. The theory of special creation was given by

a) Cuvire b) Haeckel

c) Father Suez d) Arrhenius and Ritcher

168. Two alleles in a population are in Hardy-Weinberg equilibrium. This means that

a) Neither of the alleles is being selected

b) Neither of the alleles contribute to the fitness of the population

c) Both the alleles are being selected

d) Selection is ineffective

169. Two populations, A and B, can be designated as two distinct species if they are

a) Morphologically dissmiliar

b) Geographically isolated

c) Reproductively isolated

d) Morphologically and anatomically dissimilar

170. Under what type of speciation might we expect evolution to be faster during speciation than between speciating events ?

a) Sympatric speciation b) Hybridization

c) Peripheral speciation d) Parapatric speciation

171. Variations are produced by

a) Mutation b) Random fertilization

c) Recombination d) All of the above

172. What is not true about mutation?

a) It is non-random event b) It produces new alleles.

c) It is generally recessive d) It causes polymorphism

173. What is the fundamental unit on which natural selection acts

a) Gene b) Individual

c) Species d) Population

[CSIR (NET/JRF) Exam. June 2001]

174. What type of selection could lead to a population splitting into two ?

a) Stabilizing selection b) Directional selection

c) Disruptive selection d) Group selection

175. Which of the following statement is not correct?

a) Natural selection acts on individuals, but it is populations that are changed by evolution.

b) Natural selection acts only on existing variation among phenotypes
c) Natural selection can act directly on the genotypes of individual organsims
d) Natural selection with exceptions removes variations from the populations

176. When a colony derived from a more wide spread 'parent population' diverges and acquires reproductive isolation, it is known as
a) Vicariant speciation b) Peripheral speciation
c) Parapatric speciation d) Sympatric speciation

177. When a single or small group of ancestral species rapidly diversifies into a large number of descendant species that occupy a wide variety of ecological niches the event is called
a) Allopatric speciation b) Cladogenesis
c) Adaptive radiation d) Convergent evolution

178. When an individual prefers a phenotypically or genotypically similar individual for mating it is called
a) Random mating b) Non-assortative mating
c) Assortative mating d) None of these

179. When an organ develops for a function but it also perform another function, it is called
a) Adaptive radiation b) Adaptation
c) Conversion d) Co-evolution

180. When different species formed are touching a boundary, such a speciation is termed as
a) Parapatric b) Allopatric
c) Sympatric d) Allo-Sympatric

181. When dissimilar phenotypes mate preferentially, the phenomenon is called
a) Random mating b) Assortative mating
c) Disassortative mating d) Inbreeding

182. When larva attains sexual maturity and starts reproduction, it is called
a) Abnormality b) Neoteny
c) Compatibity d) Promorphogenesis

183. When natural selection causes non-homologous structures serve similar functions to resemble one another, the phenomenon is called
a) Divergent evolution. b) Convergent evolution
c) Mega evolution d) Adaptive radiation.

184. Which insect suddenly disappeared from London after clean Air Act 1959

a) *Drosophilla melanogaster* b) *Biston betularia*
c) *Biston betularia carbonaria* d) *Periplanata*

[CSIR (NET/JRF) Exam. Dec. 2005]

185. Which is not prezygotic isolating mechanism?
a) Habitat isolation b) Ecological isolation
c) Temporal isolation d) Hybrid inviability

186. Which of the following appears to play a role in the evolution of eusociality?
a) Clinal selection. b) Reciprocal altruism.
c) Kin selection. d) Sexual selection.

187. Which of the following can not be used in evolutionary studies?
a) Allozymes b) Cytochrome
c) Restriction enzymes d) Myoglobin

188. Which of the following can not be used in establishing phylogenetic relationship ?
a) Cytochrome-c b) Allozymes
c) Allelozymes d) Abzymes

189. Which of the following conditions is not needed for natural selection to occur in a population ?
a) Individuals must be able to move between populations
b) Variations must be genetically inherited
c) Certain variations allow an individual to produce more offspring that survive in the next generation
d) There must be variations in the phenotypes of individuals

190. Which of the following did Darwin regard as a major challenge to the theory of evolution by natural selection?
a) The occurrence of marine mammals with fish-like morphology
b) The fact that several species have persistent unchanged over millions of years
c) The fact that some insect taxa are more specific than others
d) The occurrence of sterile workers individuals in colonies of social insects.

191. Which of the following does not cause evolution?
a) Mutation b) Selection
c) Genetic drift d) Random mating

192. Which of the following elements is very reactive element commonly found in volcanic rocks such as granite and basalt and is used in radiometric dating

of rocks.
a) Ag^{40} b) K^{40}
c) C^{14} d) U^{235}

193. Which of the following groups of Darwin's finches show character displacement?
a) Tree finches b) Warbler finches
c) Ground finches d) All of these

194. Which of the following is a major force in changing allelic frequencies?
a) Mutation b) Genetic drift
c) Migration d) Natural selection

195. Which of the following is also considered as 'founder effect speciation'?
a) Allopatric speciation b) Peripatric speciation
c) Parapatric speciation d) Sympatric speciation

196. Which of the following is commonly called as "spice of life"?
a) Speciation b) Variation
c) Mutation d) Natural selection

197. Which of the following is considered as the "chemical fingerprints" of evolutionary history?
a) Nucleic acid b) Proteins
c) Amino acid d) Ribosomes

198. Which of the following is important for evolution
a) Mutation b) Recombination
c) Isolation d) All of these

[CSIR (NET/JRF) Exam. June 2005]

199. Which of the following is not an assumption of the Hardy-Weinberg equilibrium?
a) The size of the population is large
b) There is no migration
c) Mating occurs preferentially
d) There is no mutaion

200. Which of the following is not an implication of the Hardy-Weinberg law?
a) a population can not evolve if it meets the Hardy-Weinberg assumptions
b) When a population is in Hardy-Weinberg equilibrium, the genotypic frequencies are determined by the allelic frequencies
c) a single generation of random mating produces the equilibrium of p2,2pq and q2
d) None of the above

201. Which of the following statement is not correct?
   a) The composition of gene pool can not change from generation to generation in some population
   b) Allele frequency is the proportion of all alleles of a particular gene
   c) The haplotype contains a minimum of two loci on the same chromosome
   d) In the Hardy-Weinberg principle, the population should be mendelian.

202. Which of the following is not essential for evolution ?
   a) Mutations b) Variations
   c) Natural selection d) Migration

203. Which of the following is not essential for speciation ?
   a) Reproductive isolation b) Fitness
   c) Preferential Mating d) Variations and Natural selection

204. Which of the following is not thought to be one of the primary causes of genome evolution?
   a) Exon shuffling b) Gene duplication
   c) Horizontal gene transfer d) Vertical gene transfer

205. Which of the following is not true for a species?
   a) Members of a species can interbreed
   b) Variations occur among members of a species
   c) Each species is reproductively-isolated from every other species
   d) Gene flow does not occur between the populations of a species

206. Which of the following is not true for Darwin's theory of evolution?
   a) This theory is a variational theory of change
   b) It holds that all species have descended from one or a few original forms of life
   c) It supports natural selection
   d) It suggests that common ancestry plays almost no role in evolution

207. Which of the following is related to the molecular systematics?
   a) Holotype b) Syntype
   c) Haplotype d) Paratype

208. Which of the following is responsible for formation of new taxa?
   a) Stasigenesis b) Punctuated equilibrium
   c) Cladogenesis d) Anagenesis

[CSIR (NET/JRF) Exam. June 2005]

209. Which of the following is the exception of Hardy-Weinberg equillibrium
   a) Non-preferential fusion of gametes

b) Size of population infinite
c) No equal fitness of genotype
d) Sexually reproducing population

210. Which of the following is the form of selection that operates in most natural population ?
a) Disruptive selection
b) Directional selection
c) Oscillation selection
d) Stabilizing selection

211. Which of the following is the most common mode of speciation?
a) Sympatric speciation
b) Parapatric speciation
c) Allopatric speciation
d) Hybrid speciation

212. Which of the following is the most primitive molecule?
a) DNA
b) RNA
c) HCN
d) Amino Acids

213. Which of the following is the ultimate source of genetic variation in a population?
a) Gene flow
b) Assortative mating
c) Selection
d) Mutation

214. Which of the following is true speciation ?
a) Anagenesis
b) Cladogenesis
c) Stasigenesis
d) Anagiogenesis

[CSIR (NET/JRF) Exam. Dec. 2003]

215. Which of the following macromolecules are called "documents of evolutionary history"?
a) Protein
b) DNA
c) Amino acids
d) RNA

216. Which of the following statements is not correct ?
a) PAM is percentage of accepted point mutations
b) PAM is the proteins evolved at highly different rates
c) PAM is percentage of average mutations
d) PAM values are used to estimate evolutionary distance between two homologous proteins

217. Which of the following statements is not correct?
a) Mitochondrial DNA is used in molecular systematics
b) In Protein-coding sequences the third position is more prone to mutation
c) Codons within the middle of a pyrimidine generally specify for a hydrophobic amino acid
d) The concept of "molecular clock" is against Kimura's neutral theory of evolution

218. The first living beings on earth were anaerobic because
   a) there was no oxygen in air
   b) oxygen damages proteins
   c) oxygen interferes with the action of ribozymes
   d) they evolved in deep sea [CSIR (NET/JRF) Exam. Dec. 2011]

219. Which of the following processes interferes in sequence-based phylogeny?
   a) Horizontal gene transfer b) Adaptive mutations
   c) DNA repair d) Reverse transcription
   [CSIR (NET/JRF) Exam. Dec. 2011]

220. The peacock's tail is an example of
   a) natural selection b) diversifying selection
   c) sexual selection d) group selection
   [CSIR (NET/JRF) Exam. Dec. 2011]

221. Which one of the following is often used to establish family trees for organisms because it is present in all organisms and does not accumulate mutations quickly?
   a) rRNA b) Fibrinopeptides
   c) Mitochondrial DNA d) All of the above

222. Recent studies on Archaea suggest that life could have originated
   a) extraterrestrially and seeded through meteorite impacts.
   b) in shallow coastal areas.
   c) in deep hydrothermal vents.
   d) in hot, terrestrial habitats. [CSIR (NET/JRF) Exam. June 2011]

223. The frequencies of alleles 'A' and 'a' in a population at Hardy-Weinburg equilibrium are 0.7 and 0.3, respectively. In a random sample of 250 individuals taken from the population, how many are expected to be heterozygous?
   a) 112 b) 81
   c) 105 d) 145
   [CSIR (NET/JRF) Exam. June 2011]

224. A trait determined by an X-linked dominant allele shows 100% penetrance and is expressed in 36% of the females in a population. Assuming that the population is in HWE, what proportion of the males in this population express the trait?
   a) 0.2 b) 0.8
   b) 0.16 d) 0.32

225. During chemical evolution of life, purine is evolved from
   a) Cyanoacetylene b) Nitriles
   c) Cyanamide d) None of the above

226. Stromatolites are
   a) Rock like structures formed by cyanobacteria
   b) Asteroids like particles
   c) Ocean of storms on Moon's surface
   d) Cupier objects of our solar system

227. Which of the following statement is incorrect?
   a) Natural selection acts at population level
   b) Disruptive selection is the rarest form of selection
   c) Positive frequency dependent selection maintains variation
   d) Disruptive selection maintains balanced polymorphism

228. In geological time scale, the era of reptiles is
   a) Paleozoic   b) Mesozoic
   c) Holozoic   d) Proterozoic

229. Age of fossils is usually determined by
   a) Sediment deposition
   b) Mineral deposition
   c) Radioactive decay of isotopes
   d) Age of surrounding rocks

230. Clads are evolutionary units and refers to
   a) A common ancestor and all of its descendents.
   b) A common ancestor and not include their descendents.
   c) Only their descendents.
   d) Most common ancestor of all members of the group.

231. Which of the following is/are the example of the directional selection?
   a) Industrial melanism.
   b) Resistance of insects of DDT.
   c) Resistance of bacteria to drugs or antibiotics.
   d) All of the above.

232. Which of the following selection maintains the variation in the nature?
   a) Negative frequency dependent solution.
   b) Positive frequency dependent solution.
   c) Directional selection.
   d) Disruptive selection.

233. The most abundant element in living organisms, in terms of percentage of total number of atoms is
   a) Hydrogen   b) Nitrogen
   c) Oxygen   d) Carbon

234. Evolutionary conservation occurs when a characteristic is
   a) Important to the life of the organism.

b) Not influenced by evolution.
c) Reduced to its least complex form.
d) Found in more primitive organism.

235. How does the field of molecular genetics helps support the concept of evolution?
a) Comparisons of genes demonstrate a relationship between all living things.
b) Different organisms have different genomes.
c) Sequencing allows for the identification of unique genes.
d) The number of genes in an organism increase with the complexity of organism.

236. Assortative mating
a) Affects genotype frequencies expected under Hardy-Weinberg equilibrium.
b) Affects allele frequencies expected under Hardy-Weinberg equilibrium.
c) Has no effect as the genotypic frequencies expected under Hardy-Weinberg equilibrium because it does not affect the relative proportion of alleles in a population.
d) Increases the frequency of heterozygous individuals above Hardy-Weinberg expectations.

237. Which of the following is most primitive molecule?
a) HCN
b) Cyanoacetate
c) Nitriles
d) Cyanamide

238. Evolutionarily, with which of the following could parental care in animals be associated?
a)

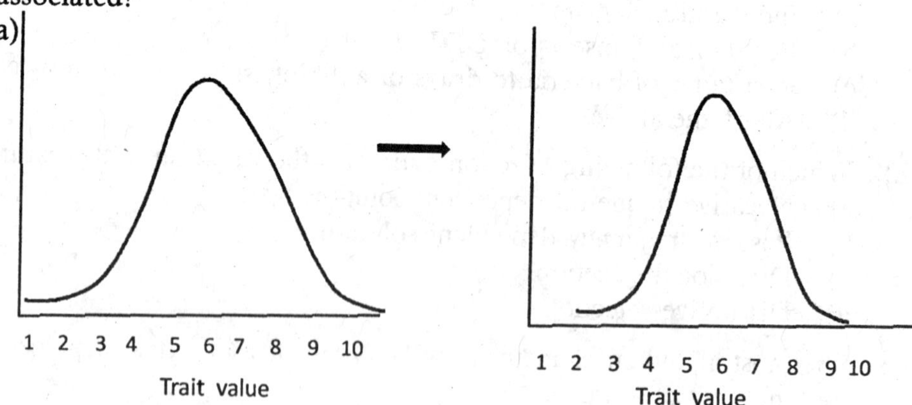

c) Greater longevity.
d) Semelparity.

[CSIR Model Paper 2011]

239.

The change in a trait with time as a result of natural selection is shown above. This type of natural selection is

a) directional. b) disruptive.
c) stabilizing. d) random. **[CSIR Model Paper 2011]**

240. During which geological period did the greatest diversification of life on earth occur?

a) Permian b) Jurassic
c) Cambrian d) Ordovician

[CSIR Model Paper 2011]

241. Which of the following plant groups evolved during the Silurian period?

a) Bryophyta b) Psilophyta
c) Lycophyta d) Spherrophyta

[CSIR Model Paper 2011]

242. Similarities in sequence and function of two proteins indicate that they are members of a family that share a common ancestor. If they are from different species, they are called

a) homologs. b) orthologs.

c) paralogs. d) proteologs. **[CSIR Model Paper 2011]**

Part C

Experimental Conditions	Observations
A. Light : light dark cycle-12h : 12h	N-trials
B. Bright light – 24h	Significantly more trials than 'N'
C. Bright light -24 h + continuous physical disturbance	Significantly more trials than 'N'
D. Dark light – 24h + continuous physical disturbance	Significantly more trials than 'N'

1. Number of trials required for rats to learn a task when they were exposed to various conditions were as follows:
Which of the following inferences is most appropriate?
   a) Continuous light enhanced learning
   b) Continuous darkness inhibited learning
   c) Physical activity inhibited learning
   d) Learning was reduced by sleep loss

[CSIR (NET-JRF) Exam. Dec. 2011]

2. Assume a male sparrow (species X) is hatched and reared in isolation and allowed a critical imprinting period to hear the song of a male of another sparrow (species Y). Now after the isolation, what kind of behaviour will species X show?
   a) It will sing the song of species Y that it had heard in the critical period.
   b) It will sing the song of its own species X.
   c) It will not sing at all.
   d) It will sing a song not sung by either X or Y.

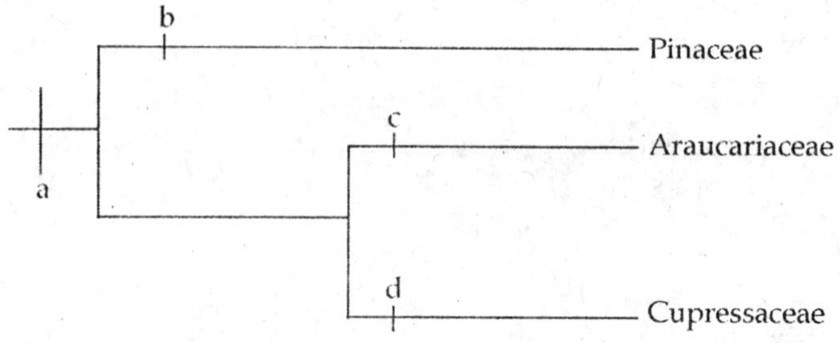

[CSIR (NET-JRF) Exam. Dec. 2011]

3. Identify the synapomorphies in the following cladogram:
   a) (a) seeds with long terminal wing; (b) ovules 1-20 per scale; (c) resin canals; (d) 1 ovule per scale
   b) (a) resin canals; (b) seeds with long terminal wing; (c) 1 ovule per scale; (d) ovules 1-20 per scale
   c) (a) resin canals; (b) ovules 1-20 per scale; (c) seeds with long terminal wing; (d)1 ovule per scale
   d) (a) seeds with long terminal wing; (b) ovules1-20 per scale; (c) 1 ovule per scale; (d) resin canals **[CSIR (NET/JRF) Exam. Dec. 2011]**

4. Several distinct time periods and different routes might explain the entrance of marsupials into Australia.
   A. Late Jurassic - early therians arrived in Antarctica - Australia where the marsupials subsequently evolved.
   B. Early to middle Cretaceous - early marsupials arrived in Australia from northern regions and then radiated in isolation.
   C. Paleocene - marsupials entered Australia from South-East Asia.
   D. Eocene - chance dispersal of marsupials into Australia.
   Which of the following is the correct combination?
   a) (A) (B) (C) b) (A) (C) (D)
   c) (B) (C) (D) d) (A) (B) (D)
   [CSIR (NET/JRF) Exam. Dec. 2011]

5. Which of the following behavioural changes are expected in a rat when its

	1	2	3	4	5
A	0	0	0	0	0
B	0	1	1	0	0
C	0	1	0	0	0
D	0	1	1	0	1

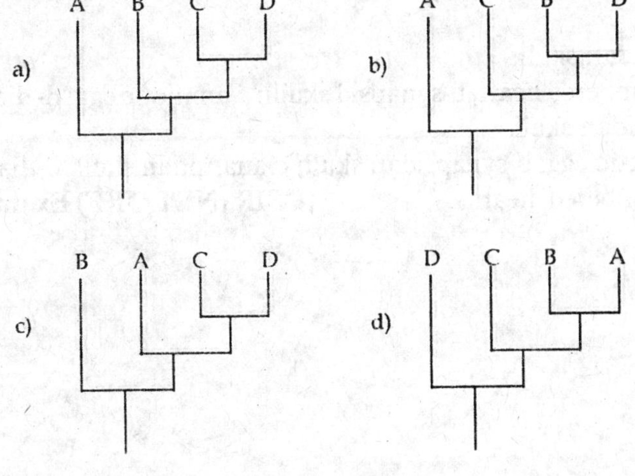

nucleus accumbens is experimentally ablated?

a) Aggressive behaviour increases
b) Exploratory behaviour decreases
c) Nest-building activity increases
d) Level of parental care drops **[CSIR (NET-JRF) Exam. Dec. 2011]**

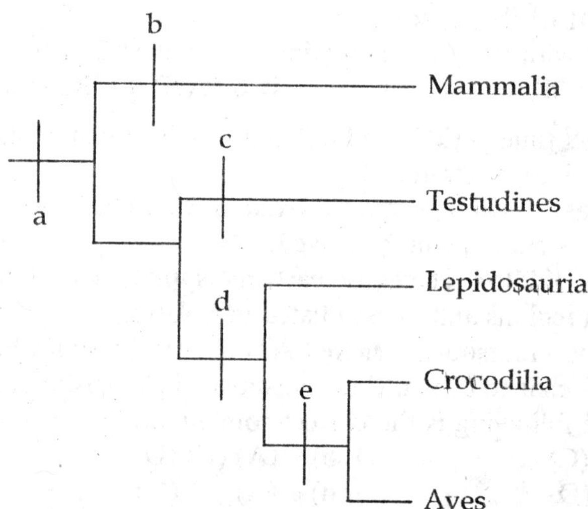

6. Identify the most appropriate cladogram that can be constructed using the data matrix given below, assuming '0's are plesiomorphic and '1's are apomorphic characters.

[CSIR (NET/JRF) Exam. June 2011]

7. Identify the apomorphic characters marked in the cladogram:
   a) a-amniotic egg; b-4-chambered heart; c-anapsidan skull; d-diapsidan skull; e-synapsid skull.
   b) a-amniotic egg; b-synapsidan skull; c-4-chambered heart; d-anapsidan skull;
   e-diapsidan skull.
   c) a-4-chambered heart; b-synapsid skulll; c-amniotic egg; d- diapsidan skull; e-anapsidan skull.
   d) a-aminotic egg; b-synapsidan skull; c-anapsidan skull; d-diapsidan skull; c-4-chambered heart. **[CSIR (NET/JRF) Exam. June 2011]**

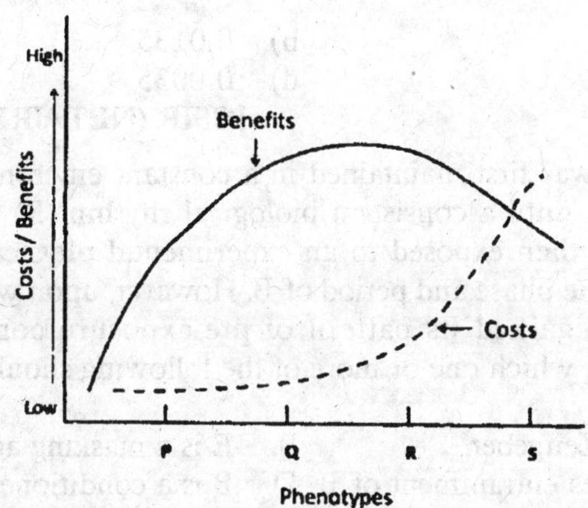

8. Shown in the graph below are the fitness costs and benefits of four alternative behavioural phenotypes (P,Q,R,S). Given sufficient evolutionary time, which phenotype(s) is likely to evolve as an adaptation?
   a) Q and R
   b) Q only
   c) P, Q and R
   d) S only

[CSIR (NET/JRF) Exam. June 2011]

9. The following geological eras mark the advent of important events in the history of earth-origin of terrestrial plants, origin of mammals, and break up of the land mass Pangaea:
   A. Early Cambrian
   B. Late Devonian
   C. Late Cretaceous
   D. Late Jurassic.

   Identify the correct match of the events with the geological era.
   a) Origin of terrestrial plants-(c); Origin of mammals-(d); Break-up of Pangaea-(a)
   b) Origin of terrestrial plants-(b); Origin of mammals-(d); Break-up of Pangaea-(c)
   c) Origin of terrestrial plants-(d); Origin of mammals-(c); Break-up of Pangaea-(b)
   d) Origin of terrestrial plants-(b);Origin of mammals-(c); Break-up of Pangaea-(d)

[CSIR (NET/JRF) Exam. June 2011]

10. Using molecular clock, it was estimated that two species A and B must have diverged from their common ancestor about 9 × 106 years ago. If the rate of divergence per base pair is estimated to be 0.0015 per million years, what is the proportion of base pairs that differ between the two species now?

a) 0.0270 b) 0.0135
c) 0.00017 d) 0.0035

[CSIR (NET/JRF) Exam. June 2011]

11. An animal was first maintained in a constant environmental condition for several days until a consistent biological rhythm (B) was established. The animal was then exposed to an experimental physical rhythm (E) which modulates the phase and period of B. However, upon withdrawal of E, the B gradually regained its pattern of pre-exposure condition. From these observations which one or more of the following should be the most logical inference?
A. E is a Zeitgeber. B. E is a masking agent.
C. E causes entrainment of B. D. B is a conditioned to E.
The correct answer is
a) A and C b) B and D
c) B only d) D only

[CSIR (NET/JRF) Exam. June 2011]

12. Which of the following statement is incorrect?
 a) Synteny refers to the conserved arrangements of segments of DNA in related genomes.
 b) The field of comparative genomics studies the variable regions of genomes among organisms.
 c) DNA microarray allow the expression of all of the genes in a cell to be monitored at once.
 d) Genomic haplotypes are regions of chromosomes that are not exchanged by recombnination.

13. Genetic drift and natural selection can both lead to rapid rates of evolution. However,
 a) Genetic drift works fastest in large populations.
 b) Only genetic drift leads to adaptation.
 c) Natural selection requires genetic drift to produce new variation in populations.
 d) Both processes of evolution can be slowed by gene flow.

14. When the environment changes from year to year and different phenotypes have different fitness in different environments.
 a) Natural selection will operate in a frequency dependent manner.
 b) The effect of natural selection may oscillate from year to year, favouring alternative phenotypes in different years.

c) Genetic variation is not required to get evolutionary change by natural selection.
d) None of the above.

15. In a given population, the allele 'a' at a specific locus confers reduced fitness compared to the normal allele 'A'. However, the allele frequencies of 'a' and 'A' remain constant over a long period of time. It is because -
a) The population size is too small
b) F1 alleles has no effect on allele frequency
c) The population size is too large
d) Selection may be balanced by mutation

16. Which statement is correct if we compare a protein and its DNA for phylogenetic studies
a) Differences in DNA and protein do not have any similarity
b) DNA is more similar than the protein sequences
c) DNA and protein have similar differences
d) Proteins are more similar than DNA

17. Speciation is often rapid within groups whose species have complex behavior because
a) Such species have complex relationship with their environments.
b) Such species have high reproductive rates.
c) Such species have short generation time.
d) Individuals of such species make fine discriminations among potential mating partners.

18. Which of the following statement is not correct?
a) Natural selection acts on individuals, but its consequences occur in populations.
b) Natural selection acts on phenotypes, but evolution consists of changes in allele frequencies.
c) New traits can evolve, even though natural selection acts on existing traits.
d) None of the above.

19. When a population rapidly declines to a few surviving individuals and remains so for sometime, one time we find
a) No change in heterozygosity or proportion of polymorphic loci
b) A major increase in the number of heterozygous loci
c) Decreased levels of genetic heterozygosity and many loci fixed for one allele
d) Increased level of genetic diversity

20. Which of the following statement is not correct about speciation?
    a) Speciation always requires isolation followed by divergence
    b) True speciation occurs through cladogenesis
    c) Allopatric speciation is not very common
    d) Genetic drift causes speciation without natural selection

21. The flightless birds ostrich, rhea and emu are distributed on different continents. What is the most plausible explanation that is given by an evolutionary biologist for this discontinuous observation?
    a) The birds were able to fly earlier, but lost their flight ability later
    b) Prehistoric humans transported these birds to different continents
    c) The birds, although flightless, may have used drifting logs to cross the ocean and reach other continents
    d) All the continents used to be one single supercontinent earlier and the flightless birds were isolated after the break up of the landmass.

[CSIR Model Paper 2011]

22. Inspite of its two-fold cost, sexual reproduction is the most dominant mode of reproduction among the living organisms. Which of the following reasons might account for this?
    (A) Sexual reproduction generates genetic heterogeneity through recombination
    (B) Sexual reproduction helps in purging deleterious mutations
    (C) Sexual reproduction evolved to stay evolutionarily ahead of fast evolving internal parasites.

    a) (A) only
    b) (A) and (B)
    c) (C) only
    d) (A), (B) and (C)

[CSIR Model Paper 2011]

23. A moth species occurs as two distinct morphs based on wing colour - pale and dark. In the forest there are trees with dark coloured trunks as well as those with light coloured trunks and the moths can rest on either tree. Birds capture the resting moths and eat. In a field experiment, the proportion (%) of dark and pale morphs captured from dark and light trunk trees was recorded.

	Moth morph	
Tree Trunk Colour	Dark	Pale
Dark	45	55
Light	48	52

The most plausible conclusion to be drawn from the results is
    a) Natural selection favours dark morphs in forests where trees with dark trunks are dominant.
    b) Birds can detect dark morphs better than light morphs.

c) Pale morphs prefer to rest on light coloured trunks
d) Birds detect the moths by cues other than their wing colour.

[CSIR Model Paper 2011]

24. It is found that people with the genetic disease called sickle cell anaemia are resistant to malaria. Which of the following best describes the underlying mechanism?
a) Frequency-dependent selection
b) Superiority of heterozygotes
c) Transient polymorphism
d) Balanced polymorphism **[CSIR Model Paper 2011]**

25. In a bird species A, the male alone builds the nest, incubates the eggs and feeds the nestling. In bird species B, it is the female that does all that. In bird species C, both sexes contribute equally to the above activities. In species A and B, the uninvolved partner may fly away and mate again. Which sex among A, B and C is most likely to develop colourful plumage during breeding season?
a) Male in species A and B, both sexes in species C.
b) Female in species A, male in species B and C.
c) Female in species A and B, neither in species C.
d) Female in species A, male in species B, neither in species C.

[CSIR Model Paper 2011]

Answer Sheet

Part – B

1.	b	2.	b	3.	d	4.	d	5.	c	6.	b
7.	c	8.	a	9.	a	10.	a	11.	d	12.	d
13.	c	14.	b	15.	b	16.	d	17.	b	18.	c
19.	c	20.	c	21.	c	22.	d	23.	a	24.	a
25.	d	26.	a	27.	c	28.	b	29.	a	30.	c
31.	b	32.	b	33.	b	34.	b	35.	a	36.	a
37.	d	38.	c	39.	c	40.	a	41.	d	42.	a
43.	c	44.	b	45.	a	46.	a	47.	b	48.	d
49.	b	50.	a	51.	c	52.	d	53.	a	54.	d
55.	a	56.	b	57.	d	58.	a	59.	a	60.	c
61.	b	62.	b	63.	d	64.	c	65.	b	66.	d
67.	a	68.	a	69.	d	70.	c	71.	b	72.	c
73.	b	74.	d	75.	c	76.	d	77.	c	78.	c
79.	c	80.	a	81.	c	82.	b	83.	a	84.	c
85.	a	86.	a	87.	b	88.	c	89.	a	90.	a
91.	c	92.	b	93.	c	94.	a	95.	c	96.	d
97.	c	98.	d	99.	d	100.	c	101.	c	102.	c
103.	c	104.	c	105.	c	106.	d	107.	d	108.	d
109.	b	110.	a	111.	c	112.	b	113.	c	114.	d
115.	b	116.	c	117.	c	118.	d	119.	c	120.	b
121.	c	122.	d	123.	c	124.	c	125.	a	126.	c
127.	b	128.	d	129.	d	130.	b	131.	c	132.	b
133.	c	134.	a	135.	b	136.	c	137.	c	138.	a
139.	a	140.	c	141.	c	142.	c	143.	d	144.	a
145.	d	146.	c	147.	d	148.	d	149.	c	150.	b
151.	b	152.	b	153.	d	154.	c	155.	d	156.	a
157.	a	158.	a	159.	b	160.	a	161.	b	162.	d
163.	b	164.	a	165.	d	166.	c	167.	c	168.	a
169.	c	170.	b	171.	d	172.	a	173.	d	174.	c
175.	c	176.	b	177.	c	178.	c	179.	b	180.	a
181.	c	182.	b	183.	b	184.	c	185.	d	186.	c
187.	c	188.	d	189.	a	190.	d	191.	d	192.	b
193.	d	194.	d	195.	b	196.	b	197.	b	198.	d
199.	c	200.	d	201.	a	202.	d	203.	c	204.	d
205.	d	206.	d	207.	c	208.	c	209.	c	210.	d

211.	c	212.	c	213.	d	214.	b	215.	b	216.	c
217.	d	218.	d	219.	a	220.	c	221.	a	222.	c
223.	c	224.	a	225.	c	226.	a	227.	c	228.	b
229.	c	230.	a	231.	d	232.	a	233.	a	234.	d
235.	d	236.	a	237.	a	238.	a	239.	c	240.	c
241.	b	242.	b								

Part – C

1.	b	2.	a	3.	b	4.	b	5.	b	6.	b
7.	d	8.	a	9.	d	10.	b	11.	a	12.	b
13.	d	14.	b	15.	c	16.	d	17.	d	18.	d
19.	a	20.	c	21.	d	22.	a	23.	b	24.	d
25.	d										

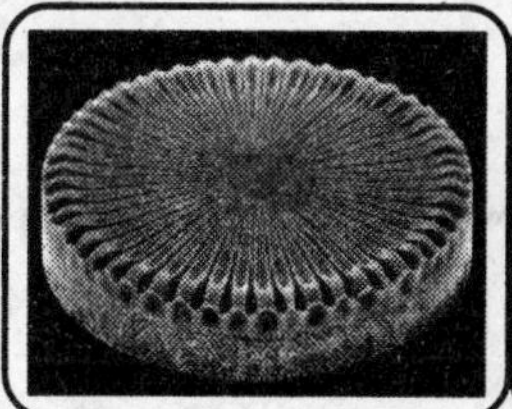

Chapter 11
Life Forms & Applied Biology

Part B

1. Which element is present in Diatoms?
   a) Si b) C
   c) Mg d) Al
   [CSIR (NET/JRF] Exam. June 2005]
2. Which of the following grouping list only domains?
   a) Eukarya, bacteria and animalia
   b) Plantae, protista and archaea
   c) Archaea, bacteria and ciliates
   d) Archaea, bacteria and eukarya
3. Which of the following is pathogenic yeast?
   a) Saccharomyces cerevisiae b) Saccharomyces apiculatus
   c) Saccharomyces fructuum d) *Candida albicans*
   [CSIR (NET/JRF] Exam. Dec. 2006]
4. Chordates are most closely related to
   a) Cnidarians b) Molluscs
   c) Echinoderms d) Arthropods
5. Water is made purified by adding
   a) NaCl b) NaOCl
   c) $CaCl_2$ d) $BaCl_2$
6. "Chagas disease" in man is caused by
   a) *Trypanosoma gambiense* b) *T. cruzi*
   c) *T. equinum* d) *T. brueci*
7. Commercial production of fumeric acid is produced by
   a) *Aspergilus* species b) *Acetobactor* species
   c) *Penicillum* species d) *Lactobacillus* species

8. Horse shoe crabs belong to the group
   a) Onychophora
   b) Chelicerata
   c) Uniramia
   d) Crustacea

[CSIR (NET/JRF) Exam. Dec. 2011]

9. The atmosphere in a sealed space craft contains
   a) pure oxygen
   b) a mix of oxygen and nitrogen
   c) a mix of oxygen and carbon dioxide
   d) pressurized atmospheric air available normally on earth

[CSIR (NET/JRF) Exam. Dec. 2011]

10. The presence of *Salmonella* in tap water is indicative of contamination with
    a) industrial effluents
    b) human excreta
    c) agriculture waste
    d) kitchen waste

[CSIR (NET/JRF) Exam. Dec. 2011]

11. In transverse sections of a young stem, if vallecular canals and carinal canals are present, then the plant belongs to
    a) Lycopodiales
    b) Isoetales
    c) Selaginellales
    d) Equisetales

[CSIR (NET/JRF) Exam. Dec. 2011]

12. Batrachochytrium dendrobatidis, a fungus, has been implicated in the decline of populations of
    a) fish
    b) frogs
    c) pelicans
    d) bats

[CSIR (NET/JRF) Exam. Dec. 2011]

13. The rattans and canes that we use in furniture belong to
    a) bamboos
    b) palms
    c) arborescent lilies
    d) legumes

[CSIR (NET/JRF) Exam. Dec. 2011]

14. The whole original individual which is selected for nonanclature by author is known as
    a) Holotype
    b) Isotype
    c) Paratype
    d) Syntype

15. The duplicate of holotype is
    a) Paratype
    b) Isotype
    c) Lectotype
    d) Syntype

16. If all the material is missing on which the description of a new species was based then a new specimen is selected which is known as
    a) Neotype
    b) Lectotyoe
    c) Isotype
    d) None of the above

17. The phylogenetic relationship among species can be predicted by which of the following?
    a) Tistogram b) Cladogram
    c) Dendogram d) Pie chart

18. Which system of classification is based on phylogenetic relationship
    a) Classification proposed by Linnaeus
    b) Classification proposed by Benthom and Hooker
    c) Classification proposed by Hutchinson
    d) Both (b) & (c)

19. The relationship between comparable structure is called
    a) Homology b) Analogy
    c) Ontogeny d) Phylogeny

20. A species is taxonomically:
    a) A fundamental unit in the phylogenetic history of organism
    b) A group of evolutionary related population
    c) A base category to which most taxonomic information is attached
    d) A population with common characteristics as evolutionary base of variation

21 It is possible to imagine the various level of taxonomic classification as a kind of "family tree" for an organism. If the kingdom is analogous to the trunk of the tree, what taxonomic category would be analogous to large limbs coming of that trunk?
    a) Class b) Genus
    c) Family d) Division or phylum

22. Two or more species occupying identical or overlapping areas are known as?
    a) Sympatric b) Subspecies
    c) Allopatric d) Sibling species

23. The different form of interbreeding species that live in different geographical region are called
    a) Sibling species b) Allopatric species
    c) Sympatric species d) Polytypic species

24. An artificial classification was given by
    a) Linnaeus b) Darwin
    c) Lamark d) Wallce

25. Four kingdom classification was proposed by
    a) Hackel b) Whittaker
    c) Copeland d) Carl woese

26. Kingdom Monera comprises:-
    a) All eukaryotes
    b) All prokaryotes
    c) Both prokaryotes and emparyotes
    d) Viruses

27. Plant decomposers are
    a) Monera and fungi
    b) Fungi and plantae
    c) Protista and animalia
    d) Animalia and monera

28. In five kingdom classification, the bluegreen alage, nitrogen fixing bacteria and methanogenic archaebacteria are included is
    a) Fungi
    b) Plantae
    c) Monera
    d) Protist

29. Biological species concept emphasizes on?
    a) Geographical isolation
    b) Reproductive isolation
    c) Physiological isolation
    d) All of above

30. The closely related morphologically similar sympatric population but reproductively isolated are designated as
    a) Clines
    b) Demes
    c) Clones
    d) Sibling species

31. Match the following

A) Porifera	p) Cell-tissue
B) Protozoa	q) Protoplasmic
C) Cnidaria	r) Organ specific
D) Chordata	s) Cellular

    a) A = s, B = q, C = p, D = r
    b) A = q, B = r, C = s, D = p
    c) A = s, B = r, C = q, D = p
    d) A = r, B = q, C = 5, D = p

32. Radial symmetry occurs in
    a) Porifera and coelentrata
    b) Cnidaria and ctenophora
    c) Mollusca and coelentrata
    d) Mollusca and echinodermata

33. Bilateral symmetry is absent in
    a) Obelia
    b) Frog
    c) Octopus
    d) Mammal

34. Match the following

A) Playhelminthes	p) Enterocoel
B) Nematoda	q) No body cavity
C) Annelida	r) Pseudocoel
D) Echinodermata	s) Schizocoel

a) A = s, B = q, C = r, D = p
b) A = q, B = r, C = s, D = p
c) A = s, B = r, C = q, D = p
d) A = r, B = q, C = s, D = p

35. Which of the following group is deuterosome?
a) Annelida, Mollusca, chordata
b) Annelida , Arthropoda, Mollusca
c) Arthropoda, Mollusca, Echinodermata
d) Echinodermata, Hemichordata, Chordata

36. Match the following

A) Polycheata	p) Scorpion
B) Trematoda	q) Pila
C) Arachnida	r) Liver fluke
D) Gastropoda	s) Neris
	t) Starfish

a) A = s, B = r, C = p, D = q
b) A = r, B = s, C = p, D = t
c) A = q, B = s, C = t, D = p
d) A = t, B = d, C = s, D = r

37. Which one of the following is correctly matched with its own characteristics and taxon.

	Animal	Characteristic	Taxon
a)	Millipede	Ventral nerve cord	Arachnida
b)	Duck bill platypus	Oviparous	Mammalian
c)	Silver fish	Pactoral and Pelvic fins	Chordate
d)	Sea anemone	Triploblastic	Cnidaria

38. A plant which produces seeds but lacks the flowers will be placed in the group
a) Fungi b) Bryophyta
c) Pteridophyta d) Gymnosperm

39 Which plant group is known as vascular cryptopams?
a) Thallophyta b) Phanerogams
c) Pteridophyta d) Gymnosperm

40. Sex organs are multicellular and jacketed in
a) Algae b) Fungi
c) Mossess d) All of the above

41. A plant having thallose plant body, developing embryo and reproducing by means of spores will be placed is?
    a) Algae b) Fungi
    c) Ferns d) Liver worts

42. The main plant body is always gametophytic (haploid) in
    a) Bryophyta b) Pteridophyta
    c) Gymnosperm d) Angiosperm

43. Whittaker's classification is not based on
    a) Complexity of body structure
    b) Complexity of cell structure
    c) Presence or absence of vascular tissue
    d) Trophic structure

44. The ancient form from which archaebacteria and eubacteria arósem is
    a) Viruses b) Cyanobacteria
    c) Progenote d) None of these

45 Reserve food in the form of glycogen and cell wall made of chitin is characteristics of the kingdom
    a) Protista b) Fungi
    c) Monera d) All of these

46. Which of the following plants show independent "alternation of generations"?
    a) Angiosperm b) Gymnosperm
    c) Pleridophyta d) Bryophyta

47. In which group would you place a plant which produces spores, has vascular tissue and lacks seeds
    a) Gymnosperm b) Algae
    c) Pteridophytes d) Bryophytes

48. Archegoniate include
    a) Algae, fungi and virus
    b) Algae, lichens and bryophytes
    c) Algae, lichens and fungi
    d) Bryophytes, pteridophytes and gymnosperm

49. Important evolutionary feature of alternation of generation from algae to flowering plant is
    a) Gradual elaboration of gametophyte
    b) Gradual elaboration sporophyte
    c) Elimination of sporophyte
    d) Gradual elaboration of both gametophyte and sporophyte

50. In which group of plants the gametophytic phase is embedded in sporophyte?
    a) Bryophytes b) Pteridophytes
    c) Gymnosperms d) Angiosperms

51. Decomposers are
    a) Autotrophs b) Heterotrophs
    c) Autoheterotrophs d) Organotrophs

52. If decomposers on the earth are totally extinct, the most seven effect would be that
    a) Carnivores will not get food
    b) Biomagnification
    c) Minerals will not get recyeled
    d) Nitrogen fixation will suffer

53. An American plant which is a troublesome terrestrial weed in India is?
    a) Eichhornia b) Argemone
    c) Parthenium d) Chenopodium

54. Which one of the following gene is defective in patients suffering from severe combined immuno deficiency syndrome (SCID)
    a) CFTR b) Adenosine deaminase
    c) Ribonucleotide reductase d) 2-microglobulin

55. Genetically engineered male sterile crop plants may be produced by inserting
    a) BT toxin gene b) Barnase gene
    c) Lectine gene d) Chitinase gene

56. What role do opines play in crown gall diseases?
    a) Source of carbon , nitrogen , and energy for Agrobacterium.
    b) Transfer of T-DNA to plant cells
    c) Attachment of Agrobacterium to plants
    d) Induction of the expression of the vir genes.

57. Identify the incorrect statement for the model plant Arabdopsis thaliana.
    a) Its mutants can be easily produced and characterized
    b) Its genome sequence is known
    c) All the genes encompassing its genome have already been identified.
    d) The molecular genetics of its flowering has been extensively studied.

58. For a plasmid to become a cloning vector the minimum elements required are?
    a) Origin of replication, multiple cloning site, selection marker.
    b) Origin of replication, multiple cloning site, selection marker, promoter
    c) Origin of replication, multiple cloning site, selection marker, translation start site
    d) Origin of replication, multiple cloning site, promoter

59. Terminator seeds produced by seed companies using techniques of genetic engineering are infact
    a) Hybrid seeds which germinate in farmer's field but do not produce seed in next generation
    b) Hybrid seed which give a very high yeild
    c) Seeds which germinates and produce incompatible gametes.
    d) Seeds that develop into fertile plants which produce non germinable seeds

60. Yeast artificial chromosome is used for cloning
    a) Large segment of DNA   b) Yeast DNA
    c) Bacterial DNA.   d) mRNA

61. The product commercially produced by animal cell culture is:
    a) Insulin   b) Tissue plasminogen activator
    c) Interferon   d) Heptitis B vaccine

62. Hydrated synthetic seeds which are produced by ion exchange reaction involve mixing the somatic embryo in a solution of
    a) Sodium alginate and dropping it in a solution of calcium nitrate
    b) Calcium alginate and dropping it in solution of ammonium nitrate.
    c) Calcium alginate and dropping it in a solution of ammonium nitrate.
    d) Mannitol and dropping it in a solution of sodium nitrate

63. Shoot organogenesis by tissue culture results into :-
    a) A bipolar structure that has no vascular connection with explant
    b) A monopolar structure that has a strong connection with the pre-existing vascular tissue of explant.
    c) Monopolar structure that has no vascular connection with explant
    d) A bipolar structure that has a strong connection with pre existing vascular tissue of explant.

64. Proteinase K enzyme which is used in DNA isolation, is obtained from
    a) Fungus   b) Algae
    c) Bacteria   d) All of the aove

65. Phenol is used as
    a) Antiseptic   b) Disinfectant
    c) Insecticide   d) None of the above

66. Cancer drug Vinblastin is obtained from
    a) *Catharanthus roseus*   b) *Taxus baccata*
    c) *Podophyllum*   d) *Digitalis perpurea*

[CSIR (NET/JRF] Exam. June 2005]

67. Vincristine is an anticancerous drug. It is obtained from
   a) *Taxus baccata* b) *Catharanthus roseus*
   c) *Atropa* d) *Colchicum*

68. Caffeine and nicotine are
   a) Steroids b) Cortisones
   c) Alkaloids d) Terpenes

69. Which of the following is correct for biosensor?
   a) It should be highly specific for the analyte.
   b) The response should be linear over a useful range of analyte concentrations.
   c) The device should be tiny and biocompatible.
   d) All of the above.

70. Which of the following biosensor is used for the detection of lipid breakdown in to fatty acids?
   a) Calorimetric b) Potentiometric
   c) Conductimetric d) Amperometric

71. Bioremediation reduces or eliminates toxic pollutants from contaminated sites by
   a) Degradation b) Assimilation
   c) Transpiration d) All of the above

72. Bioremediation process is mediated by
   a) Bacteria b) Fungi
   c) Plants d) All of the above

73. Which is incorrect for the xenobiotic compounds?
   a) Man-made chemicals that is present in the environment at unnaturally high concentrations.
   b) Their small molecular size facilitates entry in to microbial cells.
   c) Chemically and biologically inert due to the presence of substitution groups (like halogen groups).
   d) They are not recognized by the existing degradative enzymes.

74. Phytoremediation may occur due to
   a) Accumulation of the organics in plant tissues.
   b) Translocation of the organics to leaf and volatilization from the leaf surface.
   c) The organics may be metabolized in plant tissues.
   d) All of the above.

75. In which of the following marker will you prefer to check the expression of resistance to a toxin?
a) GFP
b) Scorable reporter gene
c) Selectable reporter gene
d) All of the above

76. Most common method used for the transformation of DNA into plant cell is
a) *Agrobacterium* mediated gene transfer
b) Chemical method
c) Electroporation
d) Particle gun method

77. Wheat is non native crop in India, It is originally came from
a) Iraq
b) Iran
c) Egypt
d) Saudi Arabia

78. The typical growth curve of bacteria is observed by
a) Solid state fermentation
b) Submerged fermentation
c) Aerobic fermentation
d) Immobilized cell bioreactors

79. Which of the following is incorrect?
a) Fruit ripening in tomato is controlled by the gene addition method.
b) Major GM crops developed by terminator technology.
c) The tac promoter is a hybrid between trp and lac promoters.
d) Archaegenetics is the study of DNA based human prehistory.

80. The horizontal transfer of DNA using a plasmid is an example of
a) Transduction
b) Transformation
c) Conjugation
d) Transfaction

81. If you want to design an artificial cell that can safely carry drugs inside the body. Which of the following molecule would need to mimic to deter the immune system?
a) MHC I
b) Interleukin I
c) Antigen
d) Complement

82. If you are asked how would clean up a trichloroethylene (TCE) spill without having to resort to burning or other chemical methods, how would you do it?
a) Plant popular trees to phytoremediate the soil.
b) Plant bean plants to replace the TCE with fixed nitrogen.
c) Plant Brassica plants to phytoaccumulate the TCE.
d) Plant Indian pipe because it is not adversely affected by TCE in the soil.

83. What is a Ti plasmid?
a) A vector that can transfer recombinant genes in to plant genomes.
b) A vector that can be used to produce recombinant proteins in yeast.
c) A vector is that is specific to ceral plants like rice and corn.
d) A vector that is specific to embryonic stem cells.

84. What is proteome?
    a) The collection of all genes encoding proteins.
    b) The collection of all proteins encoded by the genome.
    c) The collection of all proteins present in a cell.
    d) The amino acid sequence of a protein.

85. Which of the following statement is incorrect?
    a) Synteny refers to the conserved arrangements of segments of DNA in related genomes.
    b) The field of comparative genomics studies the variable regions of genomes among organisms.
    c) DNA microarray allow the expression of all of the genes in a cell to be monitored at once.
    d) Genomic haplotypes are regions of chromosomes that are not exchanged by recombnination.

86. For the selection of hybrid cell we use
    a) Broth medium
    b) HAT medium
    c) ME medium
    d) ITES-ERDF medium

87. Which of the following is most appropriate for cybrids?
    a) Containing cytoplasm from both the parental species.
    b) Containing cytoplasm of one species but nucleus from both the parental species.
    c) Containing nucleus of one species but cytoplasm from both the parental species.
    d) Enucleate protoplast of one species.

88. Which of the following species is exported for the fixation of heavy metals present in the polluted lakes and rivers?
    a) *Lantana camara*
    b) *Agrotemma githogo*
    c) *Casuraina*
    d) *Eichornia*

89. Which of the following would be an example of biomarker?
    a) A microfossil found in a meteorite.
    b) A hydrocarbon found in an ancient rock layer.
    c) An area that is high in Carbon 12 concentration in a rock layer.
    d) A newly discovered formation of the stromatolites.

90. Phycobilins are the signature pigment of
    a) Red algae
    b) Green algae
    c) Brown algae
    d) All algae

91. Which group has the greatest number of species?
   a) Crustaceans
   b) Mollusks
   c) Insects
   d) Round worms

92. Phytoremediation may occur due to
   a) Accumulation of the organics in plant tissues.
   b) Translocation of the organics to leaf and volatilization from the leaf surface.
   c) The organics may be metabolized in plant tissues.
   d) All of the above.

93. Which of the following is the most popular approach to deliver genes?
   a) Bacterial vectors
   b) Liposomes
   c) Viral vectors
   d) Gene gun

94. How are pathogens detected by using biosensors?
   a) By antibodies that are connected to components to give electrical signals or trigger light emission.
   b) Biosensors detect antibodies against specific pathogens, similar to a western blot.
   c) By isolating the pathogen directly from the sample.
   d) None of the above

95. In India, brown antlered deer (sangai) is found only in the floating landmasses of
   a) Wular lake.
   b) Sasthamkotta lake.
   c) Dal lake.
   d) Lok Tak lake.

[CSIR (NET/JRF) Exam. June 2011]

96. Which of the following is not a characteristic of phylum Chordata?
   a) Pharyngeal slits
   b) Amniotic egg
   c) Postanal tail
   d) Notochord

[CSIR (NET/JRF) Exam. June 2011]

97. 'Imperfect fungi' is a group represented by fungal species which have
   a) simple mycelia.
   b) no known mechanisms of sexual reproduction.
   c) unknown phylogenetic relationship.
   d) lost its survival mechanism against harsh environments.

[CSIR (NET/JRF) Exam. June 2011]

98. Which of the following food crops has recently been genetically engineered to obtain edible vaccine to develop immunity against hepatitis B?
   a) Banana
   b) Maize
   c) Potato
   d) Tomato

[CSIR (NET/JRF) Exam. June 2011]

99. Routinely used glucose biosensor estimates blood glucose level by sensing the concentration of
    a) glucose. b) oxygen.
    c) δ-gluconolactone. d) H_2O_2

[CSIR (NET/JRF) Exam. June 2011]

100. Release of nutrients, oxidants or electron donors into the environment to stimulate naturally occurring microorganisms to degrade a contaminant, is referred to as
    a) biostimulation b) phytoremediation
    c) bioaugmentation d) bioremediation.

[CSIR (NET/JRF) Exam. June 2011]

101. Bergad is
    a) *Ficus religiosa* b) *Ficus bengalensis*
    c) *Ficus elastica* d) None of these

[CSIR. (NET/JRF] Exam. June 2005]

102. Cataloging and classification of plant species in India is maintained by
    a) Forest Survey of India b) National Botanical Research Institute
    c) Botanical Survey of India d) Forest Research Institute

103. Which of the following shows bioluminescence
    a) Copepod b) Dinoflagellates
    c) Brown algae d) Red algae

[CSIR (NET-J.R.F) Exam Dec. 2005]

104. Which of the following was previously a fossil but now become living
    a) *Ginkgo biloba* b) *Pteris*
    c) *Sequoia* d) *Welwitschia*

105. Which of the following plants can be used to remove arsenic and uranium from the soil?
    a) Helianthus annuus
    b) Thalsphi caenilescens
    c) Brassica juncea
    d) Transgenic plants containing genes for bacterial enzymes

106. There is neither a single-drug nor any vaccine against AIDS virus because
    a) It contains DNA as genetic material
    b) It contains RNA as genetic material
    c) Proof reading machinery for repairing genetic material is very weak
    d) It contains two sets of genetic material

[CSIR (NET/JRF) Exam. June 2007]

107. 'I.C.B.N.' stands for
   a) International Council for Botanical Nomenclature
   b) International Code for Botanical Nomenclature
   c) International Code for Biological Nomenclature
   d) International Council for Nomenclature

[CSIR. (NET/JRF] Exam. June 2005]

108. A set of virulence genes (vir genes), located in the Agrobacterium Ti-plasmid, is activated by
   a) octopine.
   b) nopaline.
   c) acetosyringone.
   d) auxin. **[CSIR Model Paper 2011]**

109. The reptilian order Squamata includes
   a) crocodiles and alligators.
   b) the living fossil 'tuatara'.
   c) turtles and tortoises.
   d) snakes and lizards.

[CSIR Model Paper 2011]

110. Cultivated bananas are sterile because
   a) male flower-bearing plants are very rare.
   b) they lack natural pollinators in the crop plants.
   c) they are triploid and therefore seeds are not set.
   d) they are a cross of two unrelated species. **[CSIR Model Paper 2011]**

111. Which of the following GM crops is the most widely cultivated globally?
   a) Herbicide resistant soybean.
   b) Insect resistant cotton.
   c) Insect resistant brinjal.
   d) delayed ripening tomato. **[CSIR Model Paper 2011]**

112. The genes whose promoters are extensively used for production of pharmaceutical proteins in transgenic dairy cattles are
   a) lactalbumin and ovalbumin.
   b) lactoglobulin and casein.
   c) lactoferrin and transferrin.
   d) casein and ovalbumin. **[CSIR Model Paper 2011]**

113. Adenoviral vector system is a very common vector system for human gene therapy because it
   a) Can infact most of the non dividing human cells
   b) Has a RNA genome, which can integrate easily after reverse transcription through homologous recombination
   c) Has an DNA genome which can integrate easily through homologous recombination
   d) Small vector size

114. Which of the following is a suicide gene, and is used for the treatment of certain cancers?
   a) Thymidine kinase
   b) Thymidine reductase
   c) Adenine kinase
   d) Adenine reductase

115. Which of the following two genes are used by researchers in gene therapy of cancer.
   a) *gag*, and *pol*
   b) *gag*, and *rev*
   c) *rev*, and *euv*
   d) *rev* and *pol*

116. What process is used to produce transgenic animals?
   a) Particle bombardment
   b) Nuclear microinjection
   c) Nuclear fusion
   d) Germ line transformation

117. What is used by targeting vectors to insert transgenes at specific locations within the host genome?
   a) Homologous recombination
   b) Transfection
   c) Transduction
   d) All of the above

118. Why are Cre/loxp or flp/FRT used in transgenic animals?
   a) Activation of transgene by removing blocking sequences flanked by this loxp or FRT sites
   b) Creation of conditional knockout mutants
   c) Removal of selectable markers that are no longer needed
   d) All of these

119. Which of the following is a predominant microorganism for bioremediation?
   a) *Pseudomonas*
   b) *Bacillus sp.*
   c) *Xanthomonas sp.*
   d) *Nocardia sp.*

120. Which of the following statement is correct?
   a) The Ti plasmid has been used by genetic engineers to transfer gene into plants to confer a particular trait.
   b) The Ti plasmid produces tumors on plant roots.
   c) The Ti plasmid carries genes for opine uptake and metabolism, as well as genes for virulence.
   d) All of the above

121. What is the significance of using the Cre/loxp system in plant biotechnology
   a) This system promotes the transgene from recombining into the plant genome
   b) This system creates a mare efficient way to integrate useful genes into the plant chromosome

c) This system provide a way to remove selectable marker gene or reporter gene from the plants
d) All of these

122. Which of the following about Bt toxin is true?
a) Bt toxin kills insect like cotton bollworms and corn borers
b) Bt toxin is released by Cry proteins of bacillus spores that are ingested by insects
c) Bt toxin is produced by *Bacillus thurigiensis*
d) All of the above

123. What can be produced upon chemical modification of β-lactams?
a) β-lactum antibioties that are resistant to β-lactamases
b) Antibiotics that are easily absorbed in the intestines
c) Antibiocties that can penetrate bacterial cell wall more efficiently
d) All of these

124. Which of the following degrades aromatic compounds by specially adding a single oxygen atom
a) Monooxygenase
b) Oxygenase
c) Dioxygenase
d) All of these

Part C

1. Enzymes are nowadays used extensively in bioprocessing industries. Enzyme 1 is used for treatment of hides to provide a finer texture , in leather processing and manufacture of glue. Enzyme 2 is used for clarification of fruit juices. Identify Enzymes 1 and 2

Enzyme1	Enzyme 2
a) Amylase	Pectinase
b) Protease	Amylase
c) Protease	Pectinase
d) Pectinase	Amylase

[CSIR (NET/JRF) Exam. Dec. 2011]

2. Chlorophyll pigment composition and carbohydrate food reserves of some algal groups are given below:
Pigments : (i) Chlorophyta a and b; (ii) Chlorophyll a and c.
Carbohydrate food reserve : (a) Paramylon; (b) Starch; (c) Laminarin; (d) Leucosin.
Identify the correct combination of the characters for the given groups.
a) Euglenophyta - (i and a); Bacillariophyta - (ii and d); Phaeophyta - (ii and c); Chlorophyta - (i and b)
b) Euglenophyta - (ii and a); Bacillariophyta - (ii and d); Phaeophyta - (i and c); Chlorophyta - (i and b)
c) Euglenophyta - (i and a); Bacillariophyta - (ii and b); Phaeophyta - (i and c); Chlorophyta - (ii and d)
d) Euglenophyta - (i and d); Bacillariophyta - (ii and a); Phaeophyta - (ii and c); Chlorophyta - (i and b)

[CSIR (NET/JRF) Exam. Dec. 2011]

3. During a field study, three insects with the following characteristics were observed:
A. elongate, membranous wings with netlike venation, long and slender abdomen, large compound eyes
B. small bodied, sucking mouth parts, narrow wings fringed with setae
C. sclerotized forewings, membranous hindwings, chewing mouth parts
They can be identified to their respective orders as
a) A-Orthoptera; B-Hemiptera; C-Coleoptera
b) A- Odonata; B-Coleoptera; C-Hemiptera
c) A-Orthoptera; B-Odonata; C-Coleoptera
d) A-Odonata; B-Thysanoptera; C-Coleoptera

[CSIR (NET/JRF) Exam. Dec. 2011]

4. Aspirin is commonly used as analgesic, antipyretic and anti-inflamatory agents in daily routine life. What is the mode of action of this drug to our immune system.
   A. Inhibition of prostaglandin and prosacyclin synthesis
   B. Activation of prostaglandin and prostacyclin
   C. It irreversively inhibits the cyclooxygenases
   D. It activates cyclooxygenases
   Which of the following combination is correct
   a) A and D b) B and D
   c) A and C d) B and C

5. Hairy roots induced in vitro by infection of Agrobacterium rhizogenes are characterized by
   A. A high degree of lateral branching
   B. Genetic instability of culture
   C. An absence of geotropism
   D. Poor biomass production
   Which of the following combination is true?
   a) A and C b) A and B
   c) B and C d) C and D

6. Macth the following

A.	Hepetitis A virus	1.	Heparan sulphate
B.	Human immuno deficiency virus	2.	Acetylcholine receptor
C.	Rabies virus	3.	CD_4 region
D.	Herpes simplex virus type-1	4.	α-2 Macroglobulin

   a) A-1, B-3, C-2, D-4 b) A-3, B-4, C-1, D-2
   c) A-4, B-3, C-2, D-1 d) A-2, B-3, C-1, D-4

7. Match items in group I with group II

Group I		Group II	
A.	Alzheimer's disease	1.	H_1N_1
B.	Mad cow disease	2.	Hemoglobin
C.	Sickle cell anemia	3.	Prion
D.	Swine flue	4.	Amyloid

   a) A-4, B-3, C-2, D-1 b) A-3, B-4, C-1, D-2
   c) A-2, B-1, C-4, D-3 d) A-1, B-2, C-3, D-4

8. Retroviruses and adenoviruses are extensively used in gene therapy. They transfer the genes to eukaryotic system successfully.
   The following statements are correlated with these viruses
   (A) Retroviruses are class of enveloped virus containing single stranded RNA molecule as genome.

(B) Adenoviruses are viruses that carry their genetic material in the form of double stranded DNA.
(C) The genetic material of the adenoviruses is not incorporated into host cells genetic material.
(D) The retroviral genome is reverse transcribed into double stranded DNA which integrates into host genome.

Which of the following combination is true?

a) A and B b) A and D
c) B and C d) A, B, C and D

9. A panel of cell lines was created from mouse-human somatic cell fusion. Each line was examined for presence of human chromosome and for the production of an enzyme. The following results were obtained:

Cell line	Enzyme	Human chromosome											
		1	2	3	4	5	6	7	8	9	10	17	22
A	-	+	-	-	-	+	-	-	-	-	-	+	-
B	+	+	+	-	-	-	-	-	+	-	-	+	+
C	-	+	-	-	-	+	-	-	-	-	-	-	+
D	-	-	-	-	+	-	-	-	-	-	-	-	
E	+	+	-	-	-	-	-	-	+	-	+	+	-

On the basis of these results the following chromosome could possibly contain the genes encoding the enzyme

(A) Chromosome 17 (B) Chromosome 1
(C) Chromosome 22 (D) Chromosome 2

Which of the following is correct?

a) Only A b) A and B
c) A and C d) B and C

10. Assume a new subspecies Ficus callosa subsp. *microcarpa* has been published by Jacobs. The nomenclature of the resulting entities would be

a) *F. callosa* and *F. callosa* subsp. *microcarpa Jacobs*
b) *F. callosa* subsp. *microcarpa* Jacobs and other yet to be named subspecies of *F. callosa*
c) *F. callosa* subsp. *callosa Jacobs* and *F. callosa* subsp. *microcarpa* Jacobs.
d) *F. callosa* subsp. *callosa* and *F. callosa* subsp. *microcarpa* Jacobs.

[CSIR (NET/JRF) Exam. June 2011]

11. Two new plant species, A and B, were described in 1872. Subsequently it was found that the type for species A was never designated and for species B there was one specimen designated as type but missing. As per International Code of Botanical Nomenclature (ICBN), typification should be

a) neotype for A only.
b) neotypes for both A and B.
c) neotype for A and lectotype for B.
d) lectotypes for both A and B. **[CSIR (NET/JRF) Exam. June 2011]**

12. An organism has the following architectural pattern :
i. multicellular with germ layers
ii. a coelom derived from the mesoderm
iii. primary bilateral symmetry with secondary radial symmetry
iv. presence of endoskeletal plates
Such an organism is most likely to
A. have mesohyl as its connective tissue.
B. undergo torsion, whereby the mouth and anus are properly oriented.
C. be devoid of a brain but have calcareous spicules.
D. have comb plates to help in locomotion.
Which of the following is true?
a) A and C
b) C only
c) D only
d) B and C
[CSIR (NET/JRF) Exam. June 2011]

13. Industrial products in which bacteria are employed for production are shown in the following table:

I List of products	II Microorganism
A. 2,3-Butane diol	i) *Leuconostoc*
B. Dextran	ii) *Brevibacterium*
C. Glutamic acid	iii) *Bacillus polymyxa*
D. Cobalamine	iv) *Propionibacterium*

The correct combination is
a) A - iii; B - i; C-ii, D-iv
b) A-i; B-ii; C-iii; D-iv
c) A-iii; B-ii; C-iv; D-i
d) A-ii; B-iii; C-iv; D-i **[CSIR (NET/JRF) Exam. June 2011]**

14. Which of the following characteristic differentiate Eubacteria from Archaebacteria?
a) Circular nature of chromosome.
b) Absence of nuclear membrane.
c) Presence of 70S ribosomes.
d) Presence of murein in cell wall. **[CSIR Model Paper 2011]**

15. The following table lists some of the enzymes of fungi and bacteria having wide variety of industrial applications, including alcoholic beverages, food, detergents and pharmaceuticals, along with their microbial original

Enzyme	Microorganism
A. Amylase	E. *Azotobacter vinelandii*
B. Asparginase	F. *Serratia marcescens*
C. Lipase	G. *Aspergillus aureus*
D. Pectinase	H. *Aspergillus oryzae*

The correct combinations are

a) A and H b) B and G
c) C and E d) D and F **[CSIR Model Paper 2011]**

16. The common name of animals and their groups are shown in the following table

Animal	**Group**
(A) Sea lemon	(i) Annelida
(B) Coconut crab	(ii) Mollusca
(C) Sea mouse	(iii) Crustacea
(D) Mud puppy	(iv) Amphibia

The correct combination is

a) A-(ii), B-(iii), C-(i), D-(iv)
b) A-(iv), B-(ii), C-(iv), D-(i)
c) A-(iii), B-(i), C-(ii), D-(iv)
d) A-(i), B-(ii), C-(iii), D-(iv)

17. On the basis of human gene therapy trials various diseases causing genes are modified now a days. Match the following dieseases with their respective defective gene

Diseases	**Gene**
(A) Hemophilia B	(i) p53
(B) Thalassemia	(ii) β globin
(C) Sickle cell anemia	(iii) Factor IX
(D) Head and neck cancer	(iv) α or β globin

a) A- (iii), B-(iv), C-(ii), D-(i)
b) A- (iv), B-(ii), C-(i), D-(iii)
c) A- (iv), B-(iii), C-(ii), D-(i)
d) A- (i), B-(ii), C-(iii), D-(iv)

Answer Sheet

Part – B

1.	a	2.	d	3.	d	4.	c	5.	b	6.	b
7.	c	8.	b	9.	b	10.	b	11.	d	12.	b
13.	b	14.	a	15.	b	16.	a	17.	b	18.	c
19.	a	20.	d	21.	d	22.	a	23.	b	24.	a
25.	c	26.	b	27.	a	28.	c	29.	b	30.	a
31.	a	32.	c	33.	a	34.	b	35.	d	36.	a
37.	b	38.	d	39.	c	40.	c	41.	d	42.	a
43.	c	44.	c	45.	b	46.	d	47.	c	48.	d
49.	b	50.	c	51.	b	52.	c	53.	c	54.	b
55.	b	56.	a	57.	c	58.	a	59.	d	60.	a
61.	b	62.	a	63.	b	64.	a	65.	b	66.	a
67.	b	68.	c	69.	d	70.	d	71.	d	72.	d
73.	c	74.	d	75.	c	76.	a	77.	a	78.	b
79.	a	80.	b	81.	a	82.	a	83.	a	84.	b
85.	b	86.	b	87.	c	88.	d	89.	d	90.	a
91.	c	92.	d	93.	c	94.	a	95.	d	96.	b
97.	b	98.	c	99.	d	100.	a	101.	b	102.	c
103.	b	104.	c	105.	c	106.	b	107.	b	108.	c
109.	d	110.	c	111.	b	112.	b	113.	a	114.	a
115.	c	116.	b	117.	a	118.	d	119.	a	120.	d
121.	c	122.	d	123.	d	124.	a				

Part – C

1.	c	2.	a	3.	d	4.	c	5.	a	6.	c
7.	a	8.	d	9.	a	10.	b	11.	c	12.	b
13.	a	14.	d	15.	d	16.	a	17.	a		

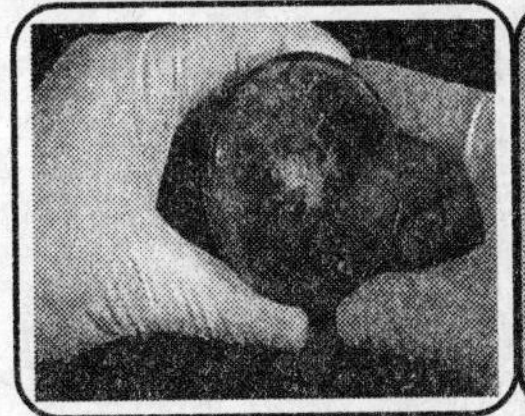

Chapter 12 Biological Techniques

Part B

1. 3-D structure can be seen under
   a) Light microscope
   b) Phse-contrast microscope
   c) SEM
   d) TEM

2. Restriction endonucleases hydrolyze a polynucleotide from
   a) Only the 5' end
   b) From either terminal
   c) At an internal phosphodiester bond
   d) A phosphodiester bond within a specific sequence

3. Several staining techniques yield characteristic patterns of alternating light and dark chromosome bands which results from the preferential binding of stains to
   a) AT-rich versus GC-rich DNA
   b) AG-rich versus CT-rich DNA
   c) Exon-rich versus intron-rich DNA
   d) Histone rich versus non-histone rich DNA

4. Which of the following is not used in somatic cell fusion?
   a) PEG
   b) Sendi virus
   c) $CaCl_2$
   d) $NaNO_3$

5. A liver cell is gently ruptured and the components of cell lysate is subjected for density gradient centrifugation. Arrange the following orgenelles in order to form the top to bottom in centrifuge tube.
   (A) Nuclei (B) Mitochondria (C) Lysosomes (D) ribosomal subunit
   a) CBAD
   b) ADCB
   c) ABCD
   d) DCBA

6. If you have a fragment of DNA of 50 kb and you want to digest it by the EcoRI approximately how many fragment you will get?
   a) 12
   b) 11
   c) 15
   d) 14

7. A piece of DNA of 7 kb is digested with EcoRI then we get the fragment of 4 kb and 3 kb, when this fragment is digested with Hind III then we get fragment of 4.5 kb and 2.5 kb. If we digest this fragment with both enzyme simultaneously fragment will be of
   a) 4 kb, .5 kb, 2.5 kb
   b) 3.5kb, .5 kb, 3 kb
   c) 4 kb, 2 kb, 1 kb
   d) None of the above

8. There are 6 variables in a data and their standard deviation is 5. If one is added to all the variable, the standard deviation of new series will be
   a) 4
   b) 5
   c) 6
   d) 7

9. The test for testing the significance of difference between the means of two different samples of small size is
   a) t - test
   b) standard deviation
   c) chi square test
   d) ANOVA

10. The best technique for analyzing total mRNA in cytoplasm of oocyte is
    a) Northern analysis
    b) Southern analysis
    c) DNA hybridization
    d) RNA in situ hybridization

11. The most common method for purifying proteins is
    a) Column chromatography
    b) HPLC
    c) TLC
    d) SDS-PAGE

12. You mix 100 ml of solution of pH1 with 100 ml of solution of pH3. The pH of the new 200 ml solution will be
    a) 1.0
    b) 2.0
    c) Between pH 1.0 and pH 2.0
    d) Between pH 2.0 and pH 3.0

13. Renaturation of human genome has revealed that it contains both repetitive and non-repetitive sequences. Which of the following statement is correct?
    a) Unique sequences renature fast
    b) Repetitive sequences are located only to the centromere
    c) Humans have more unique sequences
    d) Repetitive sequences renature fast

14. The somatic cell hybridization of human and mouse cell can effectively carried out by using
    a) Dextron
    b) PEG
    c) Enzymatic treatment
    d) Inactivated sendai virus

15. Which of the following methods is commonly used to demonstrate the association between proteins and DNA in vivo?
   a) Electrophoretic mobility shift assay (EMSA)
   b) DNAase I foot printing
   c) Chromatin immunoprecipitation
   d) Pull-down assay

16. The interaction between the protein with a DNA binding domain and the protein containing an activation domain can be studied by which of the following methods?
   a) Fluorescence resonance energy transfer (FRET)
   b) Coimmunoprecipitation assay
   c) Yeast two-hybrid assay
   d) Cryoelectron microscopy

17. Which of the following techniques cannot be used to examine chromosomal rearrangements?
   a) Chromosome painting b) Spectral karyotyping
   c) aCGH d) DNA profiling

18. Which of the following techniques is used to determine genome-wide expression patterns?
   a) qRT-PCR b) Northern blot analysis
   c) DNA microarray analysis d) RNase protection assay

19. The topography of membranes and membrane bound proteins can be characterized and analyzed by
   a) TEM b) SEM
   c) Atomic Force Microscopy d) Confocal microscopy

20. Which of the following techniques has NOT been devised to locate transcription initiation sites?
   a) S1 mapping
   b) Primer extension
   c) Run-Off transcription method
   d) Foot printing

21. For the selection of hybrid cell we use
   a) Broth medium b) HAT medium
   c) ME medium d) ITES-ERDF medium

22. Which of the following techniques is used for the physical mapping of the genome?
   a) RFLPs b) STRs
   c) SNPs d) FISH

23. Which of the following markers fail to distinguish AA from Aa genotypes in the given population?
    a) RFLP b) Microsatellite
    c) RAPD d) Expressed sequence tag

24. In a population of human, characters are regulated by more than one gene and inherited vertically. If you want to observe their genomic similarity or dissimilarity, which technique will you prefer
    a) SNPs b) Microsatellite
    c) RFLPs d) QTL

25. Suppose you have a managed sequences, which database you will prefer to submit your sequences?
    a) Gene Bank b) DDBJ
    c) Prosite d) PDB

26. For determining structure and function of similar query cDNA sequences which of the following will you prefer?
    a) Blast-P b) Blast-N
    c) Blast-X d) T Blast-X

27. Numerical aperture of compound microscope is
    a) A measure of the ability of a lens to collect light from the specimen.
    b) A measure of ability of a lens to collect light from light source.
    c) The resolution of the lens measures the ability to distinguish between two objects in the specimen.
    d) The resolving power of the microscope

28. Which of the following will be used for viewing unstained cell growing in tissue culture?
    a) Bright field microscopy b) Phase contrast microscopy
    c) Fluorescence microscopy d) All of the above

29. Resolution power of confocal/ multiple photon microscopy is
    a) 0.5 μm b) 0.25 μm
    c) 0.05 μm d) 0.3 μm

30. Which of the following DNA polymerase is used in the RT-PCR?
    a) T4 DNA pol. b) Taq DNA pol.
    c) Tth DNA pol. d) T7 DNA pol.

31. Ligase chain reaction technique is used for
    a) Viral detection b) Mutation detection
    c) Gene transfer detection d) All of the above

32. The enzymatic method of DNA sequencing is
    a) Sanger sequencing
    b) Maxum and Gilbert sequencing
    c) Direct PCR pyrosequencing
    d) Automated fluorescent DNA sequencing

33. Denaturing gradient gel electrophoresis (DGGE) detects
    a) Conformation difference of DNA strands.
    b) Melting temperature of DNA strands.
    c) Labeled probe hybridization to DNA.
    d) oligonucleotide matching to DNA sample.

34. HPLC/FPLC separates the molecules on the basis of their
    a) Size
    b) Surface charge
    c) Specificity
    d) All of the above

35. Primary structure determination of protein in a Edman degradation proceeds removal of amino acid from
    a) - N terminus of a protein
    b) - C terminus of protein
    c) Either side of the protein
    d) Breaks disulphide bond

36. Which of the following electromagnetic radiation is used in resonance phenomenon of nuclear magnetic resonance spectroscopy?
    a) X-rays
    b) Infrared
    c) Radiofrequency waves
    d) Microwaves

37. In a sequencing reaction, the dATP was left out of the tube to which ddATP was added, what would be the consequence?
    a) No DNA synthesis will occur.
    b) Synthesis would always stop at the position at which the first A was incorporated.
    c) Synthesis would terminate randomly regardless of the nucleotide incorporated.
    d) Normal DNA synthesis would occur.

38. The presence of metal ions in a protein solution can be found by
    a) Atomic absorption spectroscopy.
    b) Infrared spectroscopy.
    c) Thin layer chromatography.
    d) Fluorescence spectroscopy.

39. Optical density of 1 means
    a) 1% of the incident light is absorbed.
    b) 10% of the incident light is transmitted.
    c) 10% of the incident light is absorbed.
    d) 90% of the incident light is transmitted.

40. Which of the following antigen-antibody interactions does not involve in precipitation reaction?
    a) Radial immunodiffusion
    b) Ouchterlany
    c) ELISA
    d) Immunoelectrophoresis
41. Which of the following is correct for shuttle vector?
    a) It can replicate in the cells of more than one organism.
    b) It is a λ vector constructed by deleting segment of non-essential DNA.
    c) It is a cloning vector and expressed in the host genome.
    d) It is a cloning vector consisting of the λ cos site.
42. Protein binding sites on a DNA molecule is identified by
    a) RACE
    b) Foot printing
    c) SAGE
    d) OFAGE
43. To know the native protein after post transcriptional modification, researcher use
    a) Eastern blotting
    b) Western blotting
    c) NMR spectroscopy
    d) OFAGE
44. Biochips are
    a) DNA chips
    b) RNA chips
    c) Protein chips
    d) All of the above
45. DNA foot printing is a method to study
    a) DNA-protein interaction
    b) DNA-RNA interaction
    c) mRNA-protein interaction
    d) DNA-cDNA interaction
46. If we increase the concentration of any solution, then what would happen
    a) Decrease in freezing point
    b) Increase in freezing point
    c) Initially increases and then decreases
    d) No relation between freezing point and solute concentration
47. Which of the following vectors holds the largest pieces of DNA?
    a) Plasmids
    b) Bacteriophage
    c) Cosmids
    d) YACs
48. Light waves projected on oil surface show seven colors due to
    a) Polarization
    b) Diffraction
    c) Refraction
    d) Interference
49. During *in vitro* DNA replication, which of the following components is not required?
    a) Single stranded-DNA
    b) A primer containing a 3'-OH
    c) DNA helicase to separate the strands
    d) DNA polymerase to catalyze the reaction

50. Which of the following techniques would allow a researcher to determine the genetic relatedness between two samples of DNA?
   a) Inverse PCR
   b) RT-PCR
   c) Overlap PCR
   d) Randomly amplified polymorphic DNA

51. Why would a researcher want to use RT-PCR?
   a) RT-PCR is used to compare two different samples of DNA for relatedness
   b) RT-PCR creates an mRNA molecule from a known DNA sequence
   c) RT-PCR generates a DNA molecule without the noncoding introns from eukaryotic mRNA
   d) All of the above are applications for RT-PCR

52. Which method was used to sequence the human genome?
   a) Cytogenetic mapping   b) Shotgun sequencing
   c) Chromosome walking   d) Radiation hybrid mapping

53. Which of the following is used to quantify proteins with mass spectroscopy?
   a) ^{2}H b) ^{33}P
   c) ^{35}S d) ^{32}P

54. What is a bacmid?
   a) A virus used to infect bacterial cells
   b) A recombinant protein from bacteria that is expressed in insect cells
   c) A shuttle vector that replicates as a plasmid in E. coli and a virus in insect cells
   d) A general term for bacterial expression vectors

55. To detect the HIV infection by ELISA, detection occurs through
   a) Serum antigen   b) Serum antibody against antigen of HIV
   c) Both   d) None

56. Which of the following techniques can be used to measure the level of gene expression in mutant cells compared to wild-type cells growing under different growth conditions?
   a) Microarrays   b) quantitativePCR
   c) In situ DNA hybridization   d) Northern blotting

57. Which of the following has become an important enzyme in DNA biotechnology?
   a) β-galactosidase   b) Transacetylase
   c) β-galactoside permease   d) IPTG

58. Why is the lac operon of E. coli is important to biotechnology research?
   a) IPTG is a cheaper additive than lactose to growing cultures
   b) The lac operon controls the amount of lactose that E. coli metabolizes
   c) The inducers and regulators of the lac operon are used to control the expression of genes in model organisms
   d) All of the above

59. Which one of the following fusion proteins does not require some kind of chemical substrate to observe activity?
   a) Luciferase b) Alkaline phosphatase
   c) Green fluorescent protein d) β-galactosidase

60. One of the methods for finding common regulatory motifs present in a set of co-regulated gene is
   a) Prosite b) MEME
   c) Mat Inspector d) PSSM

[CSIR (NET/JRF) Exam. Dec. 2011]

61. A sample counted for one minute shows a count rate of 752 cpm. For how many minutes should it be counted to have 1% probable error?
   a) 13 b) 5
   c) 2 d) 75

[CSIR (NET/JRF) Exam. Dec. 2011]

62. An averge molecular weight of amino acid is 110 dalton. Suppose that a polypeptide has 120 amino acids, calculate the molecular weight of the polypeptide
   a) 13200 dalton b) 11040 dalton
   c) 11058 dalton d) None of these

63. The most popular tool to conduct phylogenetic analysis is
   a) BLAST b) Phylip
   c) Array express d) PDB

64. Array express is a computational tool, it is used for
   a) Sequence analysis b) Homology modeling
   c) Microarray d) Phylogenetic analysis

65. Which of the following is a primary protein database
   a) PIR b) PDB
   c) Genpept d) Refseq

66. Which of the following is a 3D structure database?
   a) Genpept b) NCBI
   c) PDB d) Swissprot

67. Which of the following database that classify proteins based on the structure in order to identify structural and phylogenetic relationship is
a) CATH b) SCOP
c) Both (a) and (b) d) None of the above

68. Which of the following is not a "nucleotide"
a) Genebank b) Unigene
c) SGD d) Genechip

69. Which is the retrieval system for searching several linked database for NCBI
a) Entrez b) Gene census
c) COG d) None of the above

70. Which of the following is related to gene expression?
a) Affymatrix b) Genechip
c) SAGE d) All of the above

71. Which of the following is a database for human?
a) Gene cards b) REGG
c) Both d) None

72. "nnPredict" is bioinformatics tool for
a) Protein secondary structure prediction
b) Protein tertiary structure prediction
c) Nuclic acid structure prediction
d) Both (a) and (b)

73. "Sequin" is a tool for?
a) Data submission tool b) ORF finder
c) An alignment vicuer d) All of these

74. A large and detailed monitoring of genome sequencing project produced by which of the following database
a) GOLD b) TIGR
c) EBI d) NCRI

75. Which of the following algorithm is used for global alignment?
a) Needle man- Wansch algorithm
b) Needle man algorithm
c) Smith-waterman algorithm
d) EMBOSS

76. Smith-waterman algorithm is used for
a) Global alignment b) Local alignment
c) Both d) None

77. Which of the following are progressive alignment programme
   a) Clustal W
   b) Clustal X
   c) Both (a) and (b)
   d) None of the above

78. Which of the following step is followed by clustal W?
   a) Perform pair wise alignment for all the sequence
   b) Use the alignment scores that gives a phylogenetic tree using neighbour joining method.
   c) The sequences are aligned using the phylogenetic relationship
   d) All of these

79. Match the following

A)	FASTA	i)	Compare a protein sequence to a DNA sequence
B)	TFASTA	ii)	Identify one or more region of similarity between two sequences
C)	LPASTA	iii)	Compares a protein sequence to an other protein sequence.
D)	PLFASTA	iv)	Presents a dot matrix plot of region of sequence similarity between two sequence

   a) A-(iii), B-(i), C-(ii), D-(iv)
   b) A-(iii), B-(iv), C-(i), D-(ii)
   c) A-(ii), B-(iii), C-(i), D-(iv)
   d) A- (iii), B-(ii), C-(iii), D-(iv)

80. Which of the following is a similarity search programme
   a) FASTA
   b) BLAST
   c) Both (a) and (b)
   d) None of the above

81. Which of the following technique is used for large scale identification of the proteome in a sample
   a) 2D-Gel electrophoresis
   b) SDS-PAGE
   c) 3D-Gel electrophoresis
   d) All of these

82. In 2D-Gel electrophoresis proteins are seprated on the basis of following
   a) pI and size
   b) Size and charge
   c) Charge and pI
   d) Size, charge and pI

83. In mass spectrometry proteins are separated according to their
   a) Mass to charge ratio
   b) Charge to mass ratio
   c) Charge to size ratio
   d) Mass to size ratio

84. Secondary and tertiary structure of proteins can be determined by
   a) Mass spectrometry
   b) X-ray crystallography
   c) Nuclear Magnetic resonance
   d) Both (b) and (c)

85. Which of the following is not a method of study of protein-protein interaction?
 a) Yeast two hybrid system b) Affinity chromatography
 c) DIPTM d) None of these

86. The resolution power of nacked eye is
 a) 0.2 mm b) 0.2 µm
 c) 0.2 nm d) 100 nm

87. The resolution power of light microscope is
 a) 0.2 mm b) 0.2 µm
 c) 0.2 nm d) 200 nm

88. The resolution power of electron microscope is
 a) 0.20 µm b) .2 nm
 c) 100 nm d) 200 µm

89. A homogenous protein of native molecular weight 100,000 kDa gave a single band of molecular weight 50,000 kDa on SDS-PAGE in presence of mercaptoethanol. N-terminal analysis gave two amino acids alanine and leucine in equal proportions. This:-
 a) Protein is homodimer
 b) Protein is contaminated with another protein
 c) Protein has two polypeptide linked by disulphide brigdes
 d) None of the above

90. A protein X was fused with GFP in a vector and expressed in E.coli. The lenth of protein X is 1000 amino acids and the molecular weight of GFP is 27 kDa. What is the total approximate weight of fusion protein in daltons?
 a) 137000 b) 138000
 c) 83000 d) 270000

91. A southern transfer of E.coli DNA after complete digestion with EcoR1 was probed with labeled cDNA probe of a gene which occurs only in the E-Coli genome. If the gene contains one EcoR1 cleavage site near its center, the number of radioactive bands you are most likely to find on autoradiography is/are.
 a) 0 b) 1
 c) 2 d) 3

92. Two restriction enzymes A and B have eight and four base pairs as their recognition site respectively. The ratio of the number of fragments they will generate on restriction digestion of a genomic DNA of E.coli is approximately
 a) 4 : 8 b) 8 : 4
 c) 1 : 64 d) 1 : 8

93. A Gene that does not contain intron has an EcoR1 site just down stream of translational termination codon in the 3' untranslated region. The size of the gene is 4kbp. The length of 3' UTR is 2kbp, the 5'UTR is 1kbp and the open reading frame is 1kbp. Upon probing a southern blot of an EcoR1 the digested genomic DNA with the radioactively labeled fragment containing only the open reading frame, the size of the band detected by hybridization would be
   a) 1kbp
   b) >2kbp
   c) 0.5 kbp
   d) 1.5 kbp

94. You are attempting to clone a gene. You cut a vector with the restriction enzyme, EcoRI. You mix your cleaved plasmid with an EcoRI fragment carrying the gene of interest to carry out a ligation reaction. Transform the ligation mix and plate the bacteria. When you examine the plasmid from individual colonies what do you primarily find?
   a) Plasmids that contain the EcoRI fragment
   b) Plasmid that contain concatamers of the EcoRI fragment carrying the gene
   c) Plasmid that do not contain EcoRI fragment carrying the gene
   d) Plasmid dimers held together by EcoR1 fragment carrying gene.

95. Bacterial artificial chromosomes (BACs) cosmids, phages, plasmids and yeast artificial chromosomes (YACs) are commonly used to clone vectors that differ in their cloning capacities with a range from approximately 100bp to 3000 kb. Which of the following is the proper order for these vectors in terms of increasing cloning capacity?
   a) BAC, cosmid, phage, plasmid, YAC
   b) YAC, BAC, cosmid, phage, plasmid
   c) Plasmid, phage, cosmid, BAC, YAC
   d) Plasmid, cosmid, phage, BAC, YAC

96. Which of the following statement gives a correct explanation for the use of vectors containing drug resistance genes in the cloning of recombinant DNA (cDNA) molecules?
   a) The products of drug resistance genes protect the cDNA from destruction by the host cells.
   b) The drug resistance genes provide additional base sequences that enable the vector to accommodate large inserts of cDNA.
   c) Entry of the vector containing the cDNA the drug resistance gene into the host cells renders the later indentifiable as it is now resitant to antibiotic drugs.
   d) The cloned cDNA imparts drug resistance upon any cellular system with which it is used.

97. What is the most logical sequence of steps for splicing foreign DNA into a plasmid and inserting plasmid into a bacterium?
    A) Transform bacteria with recombinant DNA molecules
    B) Cut the plasmid using restriction enzyme
    C) Extract plasmid DNA from bacterial cells
    D) Hydrogen-bond the plasmid DNA to nonplasmid DNA fragments
    E) Use ligase to seal the plasmid to non plasmid DNA
    a) A, B, C, D, E b) B, C, E, D, A
    c) C, B, D, E, A d) C, D, E, A, B

98. The annealing temperature at which the primers attach to template can be calculated by determining the melting temperature (Tm) of the primer template hybrid. What will be the Tm of the primer 5' TGACACAGAGTGTTCCC-3'
    a) 50°C b) 52°C
    c) 102°C d) 43°C

99. There are two different ways to determine the nucleotide sequence of a nucleic acid. The chemical sequencing method also known as Maxam- Gilbert method and enzymatic sequencing also known as Sanger method. The basic principle/advantage of the Sanger method is
    a) Different interaction of bases with particular dye.
    b) Extension of synthetic primer and reliable termination of DNA repair system.
    c) The correlation of restriction sites with the end label of the DNA
    d) The ability to sequence both strand of DNA duplex simultaneously

100. A certain purified DNA sample was cut with two restriction endonuclease E1 and E2. The following results were obtained from agarose gel electro-phoresis.
    Sample cut with E1 alone two bands of size 35kb and 15kb
    Sample cut with E2 alone two band of size 40kb and 10kb.
    Sample cut simultaneously with E1 and E2 hree bands of size 35, 10 and 5kb.
    From above mentioned data it can be inferred that the DNA has.
    a) Two sites for E1 and one site for E2
    b) One sites each for E1 and one site for E2
    c) One site for E1 and two site for E2
    d) Three sites for E1 and one sites for E2.

101. In order to identify the person who committed a crime forensic experts will need to extracts DNA from the tissue sample collected at the crime scene and conduct one of the following procedures for DNA finger-printing analysis
    a) Cut the DNA and hybridize with specific microsattelite probe.
    b) Cut the DNA and subclone the fragments

c) Determine the sequence of the subclomes
d) (b) followed by (c)

102. A mouse in which one particular gene has been replaced by its inactivated form is called
a) Transgenic mouse b) Knock out mouse
c) Nude mouse d) Mutant mouse

103. Which of the following method would give you the most precise and accurate information about where and when a given gene is expressed?
a) In situ hybridization b) DNA microarray
c) Protein microarray d) Reporter gene fusion including introns

104. Dideoxy DNA sequencing exclusively depends on one of the following
a) Termination b) ATP
c) Plasmid vector d) Vector primer

105. A plant genetic engineer wants to transfer and express a gene from sunflower into beans. Which of the following would be the vector choice?
a) Lambada phage b) PBR322 plasmid
c) Ti plasmid d) Maize streak virus.

106. Agrobacterium tumefaciens is an effective vector for use with?
a) Corn b) Rice
c) Wheat d) Soyabean

107. The essential component of Ti plasmid required for integration into plant genome is
a) Origin of replication b) Tumor inducing gene
c) Nopaline utilization gene d) All of the above

108. Beginning with 600 template DNA molecules, after 25 cycles of PCR how many amplicons will be produced?
a) 2×10^{10} b) 2×10^{12}
c) 25^{600} d) 600^{25}

109. An oligonucleotide is dissolved in 1.5ml of water. You diluted 50µl of the oligonucleotides into a total volume of 1000 ml and read the absorbance of diluted sample at 260nm. An A260 of 0.264 is obtained. How many O.D units are present on 1.5 ml of oligonucleotide stock?
a) 7.92 b) 79.2
c) .792 d) 792

110. A microorganism when viewed under a compound microscope with objective of 40X and eye piece of 10X magnification, measured 400µ in length. The same microorganism when viewed under a dissecting microscope with 10X lens would be

a) 100μ b) 10μ
c) 40μ d) 400μ

111. Histones have very high percentage of basic amino acids (15-30%). For this class of proteins which of the following reagents would be a suitable choice for generating peptides in determination of amino acid sequence of the protein.
a) Cyanogen bromide b) Chymotrypsin
c) Trypsin d) - Bromosuccinamide

112. If the 5'-termini of a linear DNA molecule with sticky ends are being modified in a way that the ends cannot be ligated with each other anymore (to form, a circular molecule) what enzyme was used to modify the molecule.
a) Methylase. b) Kinase
c) Phosphatase d) Dehydrogenase

113. An E. coli bacterial strain was mutated in lac permease gene and this bacterial strain was allowed to grow in glucose. What effect will be seen in this experiment:
a) Growth in glucose medium.
b) Growth in lactose medium.
c) No growth in lactose medium.
d) No growth in both glucose and lactose medium.

114. Restriction endonuclease which recognize and cut same recognition sequences are known as
(a) Isoschizomers (b) Isocaundromers
(c) Isoaccepting endonuclease (d) Isozymes

115. SmaI and Xma I are Isoschizomers. A circular DNA has two SmaI and one Xma I sites. How many fragments will be generated by digesion with XMaI?
(a) 1 (b) 2
(c) 3 (d) 4

116. P32 has half life of 14 days. After 3 month what should be the residual radioactivity of 1 milli curie of ATP labeled with P32.
(a) 62.5 μcurie (b) 6.25 μcurie
(c) 15.5 μcurie (d) 1.55 μcurie

117. What is the smallest distance between two closely spaced point which can be resolved by light microscope?
(a) 20nm (b) 200 nm
(c) 20 micron (d) 2 nm

118. Which of the following antigen-antibody reaction does not involve agglutination reaction
(a) RIA (b) Qucliterlony
(c) ELISA (d) Immunoelectrophoresis

119. Which technique is used to study de novo RNA syntheis?
(a) Southern blotting (b) Northern blotting
(c) Microarray (d) RT-PCR

120. An oligonucleotide DNA sequence tagged with fluorescent tag used to identify unknown gene by hybridization is termed as
(a) Probe (b) Reporter gene
(c) Ligand (d) cDNA

121. Principle of formation of image in phase contrast microscopy involves
(a) Interference of light waves
(b) Negative staining of object
(c) Use of flouroscent probes
(d) Enhancing contrast by differentiating the change in phase of light passed through specimen coming from ½ angle of cone of light entering through objective lens

122. In a poupation of 10 million individuals natality rate is 19 per thousand and mortality rate is 14 per 1000. Annual rise in population would be
(a) 50,000 (b) 5, 000
(c) 14,000 (d) 500,000

123. For constructing recombinant plasmid, plasmid and DNA to be inserted are digested with same restriction enzyme kept in the same reaction solution. To prevent self sealing of plasmid which of the following enzyme is utilized?
(a) Alkaline phosphatase (b) Polynucleotide kinase
(c) Terminal transferase (d) Ligase

124. An oligonucleotide is dissolved in 1.5ml of water. You dilute it 50ml and read the absorbance of diluted sample at 260nm. An absorbance at 260nm, 0.260 is obtained. How many O.D units are present in 1.5 ml of oligonucleotides stocks?
(a) 7.8 (b) 0.78
(c) 1 (d) 78.0

125. Molecules of DNA as large as 10 mb can be separated by
(a) Agarose gel electrophoresis
(b) Poly acrylamide gel electrophoresis
(c) Pulsed-field gel electrophoresis
(d) 2-D gel electrophoresis

126. A culture of an E. coli strain that is lysogenic for phage lambda is grown at 32^{0}C. Induction of the prophage from the host chromosome will occur when the culture is exposed to
a) 40^{0}C. b) ultra violet radiation
c) infra red radiation d) wild type *E. coli* culture.

[CSIR (NET/JRF) Exam. June 2011]

127. Which of the following methods of plant transformation can be used to introduce a gene into chloroplast genome?
a) Agrobacterium-mediated transformation
b) Particle delivery system
c) Permeabilization
d) Electroporation **[CSIR (NET/JRF) Exam. June 2011]**

128. Yeast artificial chromosome (YAC) vectors contain selectable markers. Loss of which marker at the cloning site distinguishes the religated YACs from the original vector marker?
a) TRP1 b) SUP4
c) URA3 d) CEN
[CSIR (NET/JRF) Exam. June 2011]

129. ELISA assay uses
a) an enzyme which can react with secondary antibody.
b) an enzyme which can react with the antigen.
c) a substrate which gets converted into a coloured product.
d) a radiolabelled secondary antibody.
[CSIR (NET/JRF) Exam. June 2011]

130. PCR based DNA amplification is an essential feature of which of the following combination of molecular markers?
a) RFLP, AFLP and SSR. b) AFLP, SSR and RAPD.
c) RFLP, RAPD and SSR. d) RAPD, RFLP and SSR.
[CSIR Model Paper 2011]

131. A biochemist purifies a new enzyme, generating the following purification table.

S. No.	Procedure	Total protein (mg)	Activity (units)
i.	Crude Extract	20,000	4,000,000
ii.	Salt precipitation	5,000	3,000,000
iii.	Ion-exchange chromatography	200	800,000
iv.	Affinity chromatography	50	750,000
v.	Size-exclusion chromatography	45	675,000

The most effective purification step is
a) iv. b) iii.
c) v. d) ii. **[CSIR Model Paper 2011]**

Part C

1. There were four experiments carried out for tissue transplantation.
   A) A tissue is transplanted between two different organism of two different species.
   B) A tissue is transplanted between two different organism of same species.
   C) A tissue is transplanted between monozygotic twins.
   D) Different areas of same individual.
   Where tissue graft acceptance will occur?
   a) A and C b) Only B
   c) B and D d) C and D

2. The average human genome has approximately 3×10^9 bp coding for various proteins. If an average protein contains 400 amino acids. What is the maximum number of protein that can be encoded by human genome .
   a) 2.5×10^6 b) 250 x 106
   c) 0.25 x 106 d) 25000

3. The polypeptides (A, B and C) whose masses are 55 KDa, 50 KDa and 75 KDa with pI of 6.5, 7.0 and 8.0, respectively, were subjected to standard reducing SDS-PAGE. The order of their separation from top to bottom would be .
   a) A, B and C b) B, A and C
   c) A, C and B d) C, A and B

4. Denaturation profiles of DNA are shown below.

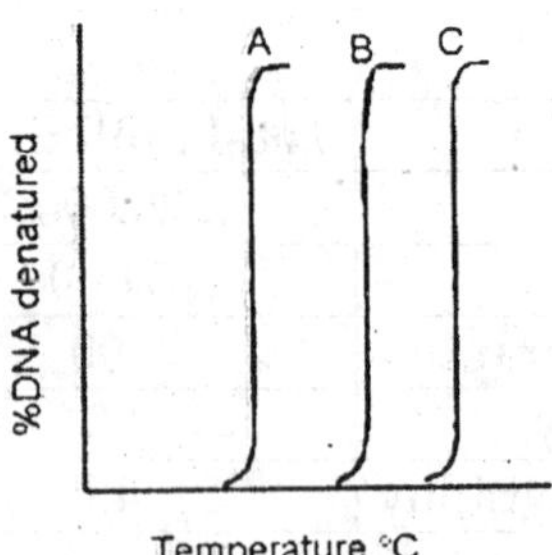

   The differences in the profiles arise because
   a) The DNA is single stranded but of different sizes.
   b) A + T content of A>B>C and the DNA are from complex genomes.
   c) G + C content of C>B>A in DNA of comparable sizes isolated from simple genomes.
   d) G + C content is identical but A + T content in A>B>C in DNA of comparable sizes isolated from simple genomes.

[CSIR (NET/JRF) Exam. Dec. 2011]

5. Cre/lox P system is used by phage PI to remove terminally redundant sequences that arise during packaging of the phage DNA. Cre-lox system can be used to create targeted deletions, insertions and inversion in genomes of transgenic animals and plants. Consider a series of genetic markers A to K. How should the Lox P sites be positioned in order that Cre recombinase can create an inversion in the EFG segment relative to ABCD and HIJK?

a) A B C D → E F G → H I J K
Lox P Lox P

b) A B C → D E F G → H I J K
Lox P Lox P

c) A B C D → E F G ← H I J K
Lox P Lox P

d) A B C D ← E F G ← H I J K
Lox P Lox P

[CSIR (NET-JRF) Exam. Dec. 2011]

6. Genomic DNA of transgenic plants (P1, P2 and P3) obtained by transforming with binary vector A whose map is depicted below, was digested with BamH I and Sal I and hybridized with a labelled fragment X

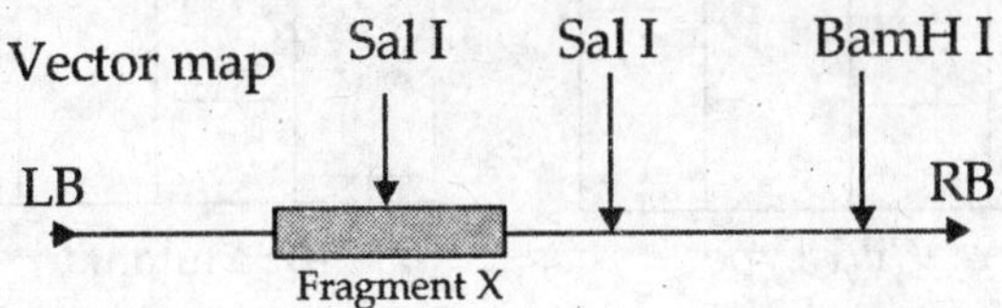

The pattern obtained in Southern hybridization is show below:

P1		P2		P3	
BamH I	Sal I	BamH I	Sal I	BamH I	Sal I
	—	—		—	—
—	—		—		
—	—		—		—

Based on the above, which of the following interpretations is correct:

a) All the plants (P1, P2 and P3) contain two copies of the transgene
b) P1, P3 contain one and P2 contains two copies of the transgene
c) P1 contains two, whereas P2 and P3 contain one copy of transgene each.
d) P1 and P2 contains two and P3 contains one copy of the transgene.

[CSIR (NET-JRF) Exam. Dec. 2011]

7. Figures A and B respectively represent the dideoxy sequencing gels obtained for partial sequences from 5'-ends of a bacterial gene and its mutant (with a point mutation).

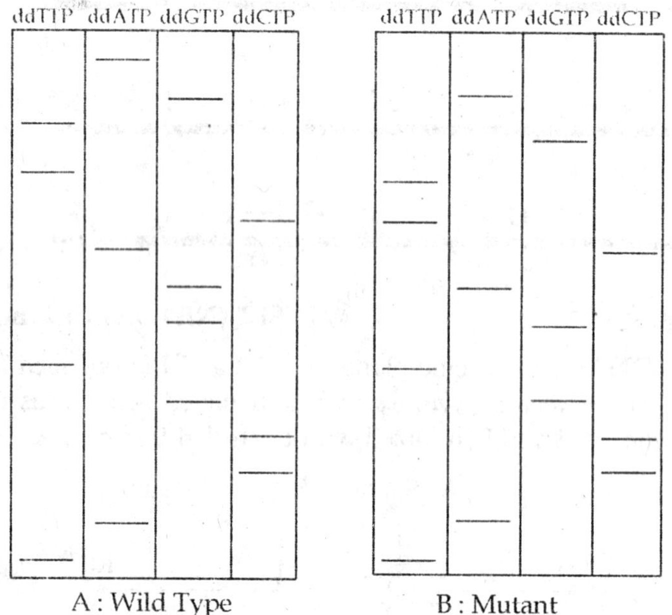

What type of mutation has occurred in the gene?

a) Nonsense
b) Missense
c) Frameshift
d) Transversion

[CSIR (NET-JRF) Exam. Dec. 2011]

8. A 1 meter tall object was placed 10 meter in front of a normal eye. The size of the image on the retina will be (consider distance between lens and retina = 1.7 cms)

a) 0.17 mm
b) 1.7 mm
c) 3.4 mm
d) 170 μm

[CSIR (NET-JRF) Exam. Dec. 2011]

9. A fixed smear of a bacterial culture is subjected to the following solutions in the order listed below and appeared red.
(A) Corbolfuchsin (heated)
(B) Acid-alcohol
(C) Methylene blue
Bacteria stained by this method can be identified as
a) Non-acid fast E.coli   b) Acid-fast Mycobacterium sp.
c) Gram-positive E.coli   d) Gram-negative Mycobacterium sp.
[CSIR (NET-JRF) Exam. Dec. 2011]

10. The following is a schematic representation of region (showing six bands) of the polytene chromosome of Drosophila, along with the extent of five deletions (Del1 to Del5):

1 2 3 4 5 6

Del 1
Del 2
Del 3
Del 4
Del 5

Recessive alleles a, b, c, d, e and f are known to correspond to each of the bands (1 to 6), but their order is not known. When the recessive alleles are placed against each of these deletions, the following results are obtained. The plus (+) in the table indicates wild type phenotype of the corresponding allele, while a minus (-) indicates the phenotype governed by the corresponding mutant allele.

	a	*b*	*c*	*d*	*e*	*f*
Del 1	+	-	-	-	+	+
Del 2	+	+	-	-	+	+
Del 3	-	+	-	-	+	+
Del 4	-	+	+	-	-	+
Del 5	-	+	+	+	-	-

Which one of the following indicates the correct location of the recessive alleles on the bands of the polytene chromosomes?
a) a-3; b-1; c-2; d-4; e-5; f-6   b) a-2; b-1; c-3; d-4; e-5; f-6
c) a-4; b-1; c-2; d-3; e-5; f-6   d) a-6; b-2; c-3; d-4; e-1; f-5
[CSIR (NET/JRF) Exam. Dec. 2011]

11. The following are statements about molecular markers in the context of plant breeding.
    A. Molecular markers can be used for elimination of undesirable traits.
    B. Molecular markers cannot be used for estimation of the genetic contribution of each individual parent in a segregating population.
    C. Molecular markers are used for mapping of QTLs, which is also possible by conventional techniques.
    D. Molecular markers can be used for selection of individuals from a population that are homozygous for the recurrent parent genotype at loci flanking the target locus.

    Which of the above statements are TRUE?

    a) A and B   b) A and C
    c) A and D   d B and C

    [CSIR (NET-JRF) Exam. Dec. 2011]

12. In 'TaqMan' assay for detection of base substitutions (DNA variant), probes (oligonucleotides) with fluorescent dyes at the 5'-end and a quencher at 3'-end are used. While the probe is intact, the proximity of the quencher reduces the fluorescence emitted by reporter dye. If the target sequences (wild type or the variant) are present, the probe anneals to the target sequence, down stream to one of the primers used for amplifying the DNA sequence flanking the position of the variants. For an assay two flanking PCR primers, two probes corresponding to the wild type and variant allele and labelled with two different reporter dyes and quencher were used. During extension the probe may be cleaved by the Taq-polymerase separating the reporter dye and the quencher. Three individuals were genotyped using this assay. Sample for individual I shows maximum fluorescence for the dye attached to the wild type probe, sample for individual II shows maximum fluorescence for the dye attached to variant probe and sample for individual III exhibits equal fluorescence for both the dyes. Which of the following statement is correct?

    a) Individual I is homozygous for the variant allele.
    b) Individual II is homozygous for variant allele.
    c) Individual II is homozygous for wild type allele.
    d) Individual III is homozygous for wild type allele.

    [CSIR (NET-JRF) Exam. Dec. 2011]

13. The most important property of any microscope is its power of resolution, which is numerically equivalent to D, the minimum distance between two distinguishable objects. D depends on three parameters namely, the angular aperture, , the refractive index, N, and wavelength, , of the incident light. Below are given few possible options to increase the resolution of the microscope.

A. Decrease the value of or increase either N or to improve resolution.
B. Moving the objective lens closer to the specimen will decrease sin and improve the resolution.
C. Using a medium with high refraction index between the specimen and the objective lens to improve the resolution.
D. Increase the wavelength of the incident light to improve the resolution.

Which of the following combination of above statement is correct?

a) A and C b) B and C
c) A and D d) C and D

[CSIR (NET-JRF) Exam. Dec. 2011]

14. Stem cell therapies are being used in regenerative medicine like forming new adult bone, which usually does not regrow to bridge wide gaps. Successful attempts have now been made in this area because the same paracrine and endocrine factors were found to be involved in both endochondral ossification and fracture repair. Few methods to achieve the above are given below:
A. Develop a collagen gel containing plasmids carrying the human parathyroid hormone gene and place in the gap between the ends of the broken leg.
B. Develop a gel matrix disc containing genetically modified stem cells to secrete BMP4 and VEGF-A and implant it at the site of the wound.
C. Make scaffolds of material that resemble normal extracellular matrix that could be molded to form the shape of a bone needed and seed them with bone marrow stem cell.
D. Develop a collagen gel containing plasmids carrying the human bone marrow cell. and place them between the ends of the bones.

Which of the above methods would you employ to develop a new functional bone in patients with severely fractured bones.

a) A and B b) A, B and C
c) A and C d) C and D

[CSIR (NET/JRF) Exam. Dec. 2011]

15. Match list I (Enzyme) with list II (charactersticks/activity) and select the correct answer using the codes given below the lists.

	List I (Enzymes)		List II (characterstics/ Activity)
A)	Terminal transferase	1.	Stable above 90^0C
B)	Polynucleotide kinase	2.	Cleave the end of linear DNA
C)	Taq DNA polymerase	3.	Adds PO_4^- to 5′OH end of DNA/RNA
D)	Exonuclease	4.	Adds numbers of Nucleotides to 3′ end of DNA/RNA
		5.	Regulated the supercoiling of DNA molecule.

a) A-5, B-4, C-3, D-2 b) A-4, B-3, C-1, D-2
c) A-1, B-4, C-5, D-2 d) A-2, B-3, C-4, D-1

16. Match the items in Group I with Group II

	Group I		Group II
A.	Circular dichroism	1.	Concentration
B.	X-Ray crystallography	2.	Sedimentation coeffecient
C.	Freeze drying	3.	Secondary structure determination
D.	Ultracentrifugation	4.	Tertiary structure determination

(a) A-4, B-1, C-2, D-3
(b) A-1, B-4, C-3, D-2
(c) A-2, B-3, C-4, D-1
(d) A-3, B-4, C-1, D-2

17. Protein protein interaction is studied by :-
A. DNA foot printing
B. Yeast two hybrid system
C. Ligase chain reaction
D. Mass spectrometry
Which of the following combination is correct?
(a) A and D
(b) A and C
(c) B and D
(d) Only B

18. Hypoxanthine aminopterin and thymidine is used for selecting the hybridomas based on following:-
I. Only hybridoma will grow since it inherited the HGPRT genes from B cells and can synthesize DNA from hypoxanthine
II. Myeloma cells will not grow is culture since de novo synthesis is blocked by aminopterin and due to the lack of HGPRT enzyme.
Which of the following is correct?
(a) Only I is true
(b) Only II is true
(c) Both I and II is true
(d) None of the above

19. A 200 µl of polymerase chain reaction has 100 template, DNA molecules and then reaction was performed for 10 cycles. How many molecules of amplicons will be generated and how many molecules of amplicons will be present is 0.1 µl of reaction.
(a) 1.024×10^4 amplicons and 102.4 molecules
(b) 1.024×10^5 amplicons and 102.4molecules
(c) 1.024×10^5 amplicons and 51.2 molecules
(d) 1.024×10^4 amplicons and 215 molecules

20. A new topoisomerase is discovered from an archaebacterium isolated from hot spring, which catalyses the ATP driven introduction of positive supercoiling into DNA. How might this enzyme be advantageous to the organism? Read the following statements
(A) It is a reverse gyrase type I DNA topoisomerase
(B) It functions as a DNA renaturase
(C) It functions as a DNA denaturase
(D) It has a biological function in sensing and eliminating unpaired regions in the genome.

Which of the following combination of the statement is true?
(a) A and D (b) B and D
(c) A, C and D (d) A, B and D

21. Centrifugation is a method by which we separate our preparations on the basis of sediment coefficient. Density gradient centrifugation method of separation separates DNA/RNA and other cellular components according to their density. If we want to separate a mixture of DNA containing linear double stranded DNA, nicked circular double stranded DNA and super coiled dsDNA by density dependent centrifugation method using ficoll then what would be the sequence from bottom to up after centrifugation?
(a) Linear ds DNA→ nicked circular ds DNA → super coiled ds DNA.
(b) Nicked circular ds DNA→ Linear ds DNA → super coiled ds DNA.
(c) Super coiled ds DNA→ nicked circular ds DNA→ linear ds DNA.
(d) Super coiled ds DNA→ linear ds DNA→ Nicked circular ds DNA.

22. The activity of the enzyme -galactosidase is easily monitored by including in the growth medium the chromogenic substance 5-bromo-4-chloro-3-Indolyl-β-D-galactoside (x gal). This compound is colourless but on cleavage releases a blue indolyl derivative; On solid medium colonies that are expressing active β-galactosidase are blue in colour while those without activity are white in colour. This is often referred to as blue/white screening.
The following statements are related with the mode of action of x gal.
(A) X gal is works as substrate and as well as a gratuitous inducer.
(B) X gal works as only substrate for -galactosidase.
(C) X gal works only as a gratuitous inducer for -galactosidase.
(D) complementation is generally based on this blue white selection principle.
Which one of the following is correct?
(a) A only (b) A and D
(c) B and D (d) C and D

23. Two E.coli culture A and B are taken. Culture A was earlier grown in the presence of optimum concentration of gratuitous inducer IPTG. Both the cultures are now used to inoculate fresh medium containing sub-optimal concentration of gratuitous inducer. It was observed that culture B was unable to utilize lactose, whereas culture A did so efficiently. The reason behind this is
a) pretreatment with IPTG has resulted in a mutation as a result of which lac operon is constitutively expressed.
b) IPTG has made the cell membrane more porous to small molecules and so lactose is taken up more efficiently by A as compared to B.
c) in culture A, lactose permease was induced to a high level, during pretreatment with IPTG, which allowed the preferential uptake of lactose.

d) in culture A, IPTG activated a receptor which bound lactose more efficiently, thereby triggering a signal.

[CSIR (NET/JRF) Exam. June 2011]

24. Molecular beacons (MB) and Taqman (TQ) are used as probes in Real time PCR experiments. Both these probes are based on the principle of FRET and employ a fluorophor (F) and a quencher (Q). However the mechanisms by which they function are different as illustrated below
At what stage of the PCR we would be able to detect fluorescence?
a) Annealing step for both.
b) Extension step for both.
c) Annealing for A and Extension for B.
d) Extension for A and Annealing for B.

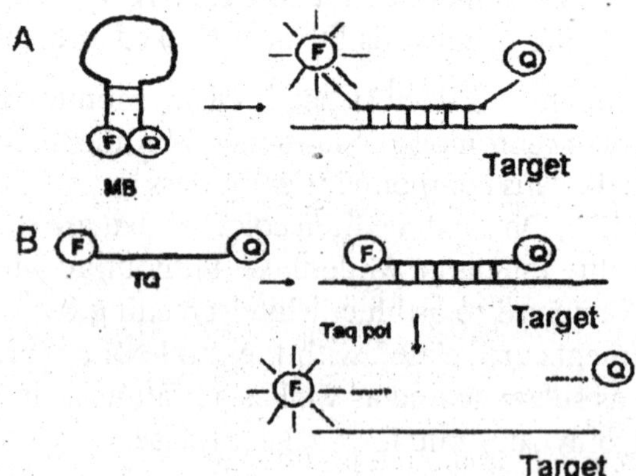

[CSIR (NET/JRF) Exam. June 2011]

25. Proteins in cells can be visualized by the following methods:
A. Express the gene (coding for the said protein) as a fusion with the green fluorescence protein (GFP) and directly visualize under a fluorescence microscope.
B. Express the gene (coding for the said protein) as a fusion with the -galactosidase gene (lac Z) and directly visualize under a phase contrast bright field microscope.
C. A fluorescence tagged antibody raised against the said protein could be used for visualization in a fluorescence microscope.
D. Overexpress the protein and directly visualize it under a scanning electron microscope.

Which of the following methods you would choose to visualize a protein in living cell?

a) A only
b) A and B only
c) A and C only
d) D only

[CSIR (NET/JRF) Exam. June 2011]

Answer Sheet

Part – B

1.	c	2.	d	3.	a	4.	d	5.	d	6.	a
7.	a	8.	c	9.	a	10.	a	11.	a	12.	d
13.	d	14.	d	15.	b	16.	c	17.	d	18.	c
19.	c	20.	d	21.	b	22.	d	23.	c	24.	d
25.	c	26.	c	27.	a	28.	b	29.	d	30.	d
31.	c	32.	a	33.	b	34.	a	35.	a	36.	c
37.	b	38.	a	39.	b	40.	c	41.	a	42.	b
43.	b	44.	d	45.	a	46.	a	47.	d	48.	b
49.	c	50.	d	51.	c	52.	b	53.	a	54.	c
55.	b	56.	b	57.	a	58.	c	59.	c	60.	b
61.	d	62.	b	63.	b	64.	c	65.	b	66.	c
67.	c	68.	d	69.	a	70.	d	71.	a	72.	a
73.	d	74.	a	75.	a	76.	b	77.	c	78.	d
79.	a	80.	b	81.	a	82.	a	83.	a	84.	d
85.	d	86.	a	87.	b	88.	b	89.	a	90.	a
91.	b	92.	d	93.	a	94.	c	95.	d	96.	c
97.	c	98.	b	99.	d	100.	b	101.	d	102.	b
103.	d	104.	a	105.	c	106.	d	107.	b	108.	a
109.	a	110.	b	111.	c	112.	c	113.	a	114.	a
115.	c	116.	c	117.	b	118.	d	119.	b	120.	a
121.	d	122.	a	123.	a	124.	a	125.	c	126.	b
127.	b	128.	b	129.	c	130.	b	131.	b		

Part – C

1.	d	2.	a	3.	d	4.	c	5.	c	6.	c
7.	c	8.	b	9.	b	10.	a	11.	c	12.	b
13.	a	14.	a	15.	b	16.	d	17.	d	18.	c
19.	c	20.	d	21.	c	22.	c	23.	c	24.	c
25.	c										